Merriam-Webster's
Medical Office
Handbook

Merriam-Webster's
Medical Office
Handbook

SECOND EDITION

Joseph Hamburg, MD, ScD, LHD
Consulting Editor

Merriam-Webster, Incorporated
Springfield, Massachusetts

A GENUINE MERRIAM-WEBSTER

The name *Webster* alone is no guarantee of excellence. It is used by a number of publishers and may serve mainly to mislead an unwary buyer.

Merriam-Webster™ is the name you should look for when you consider the purchase of dictionaries and other fine reference books. It carries the reputation of a company that has been publishing since 1831 and is your assurance of quality and authority.

Library of Congress Cataloging-in-Publication Data

Merriam-Webster's medical office handbook / Joseph Hamburg, consulting
    editor. — 2nd ed.
      p.   cm.
    —Title of 1st ed. Webster's medical office handbook.
    ISBN 0-87779-235-6 (hardcover)
    1. Medical offices—Management—Handbooks, manuals, etc.
2. Medical secretaries—Handbooks, manuals, etc. I. Hamburg,
Joseph. II. Title: Medical office handbook. III. Title: Webster's
medical office handbook.
R728.8.M47   1996
651.9′61—DC20   96-26851
                                                     CIP

Printed and bound in the United States of America
123456RRD010099989796

SECOND EDITION

Consulting Editor
Joseph Hamburg, MD, ScD, LHD
Dean Emeritus
College of Allied Health Professions
University of Kentucky at Lexington

General Editor
Jocelyn White Franklin
Merriam-Webster, Incorporated

Contributors

Joyce E. Beaulieu, PhD
Principal, JB Associates
Lexington, Kentucky

Robert D. Miller, JD
University of Wisconsin Hospitals & Clinics
Madison, Wisconsin

Samuel R. Bierstock, MD, BSEE
President, Computer Consultant
  for Professionals
Boca Raton, Florida

Physician Services of America
John E. Hill, MBA; Ruth Ann Ray, CMT;
  and Nancy Groves
Louisville, Kentucky

Gordon D. Brown, PhD
Director, Program in
  Health Services Management
University of Missouri at Columbia

Janet I. Pisaneschi, PhD
Dean, College of Health and Human Services
Western Michigan University
Kalamazoo, Michigan

Joan B. Conrad, CMA-A
Administrator, Towers Internal
  Medicine Associates
Grand Rapids, Michigan

Lou Ann Schraffenberger, MBA, RRA
Research Assistant Professor
Health Information Management
University of Illinois at Chicago

Kim Fox
President, Multi-Image Communications
San Jose, California

Charles R. Wold, CPA
President, HNF Consulting
Minneapolis, Minnesota

Patricia A. Ireland, CMT
Jacobson MSO Inc.
San Antonio, Texas

FIRST EDITION

Consulting Editor
John Rhodes Haverty, MD

General Editor
Anne H. Soukhanov

Contributors

Susan E. Abbe, RN, MS
Lorene Euler Berman, CMA-AC
Aileen J. Black, RRA
Keith D. Blayney, PhD
Helen G. Burzynski, RN, MA
Rita M. Finnegan, RRA, MA
J. F. Follmann, Jr.

Charles Willard Ford, PhD
Joseph M. Healey, JD
Melvin Morgenstein, EdD
Susan A. Orlowski, RN, CMA-C
Donald D. Scriven, PhD
Jolene D. Scriven, EdD

Contents

Preface   xi

1. Medical Ethics   1

Understanding Professional Responsibilities, 1 • Respect for
Persons and for Their Autonomy, 6 • Beneficence, 12 •
Justice, 14 • Additional Ethical Responsibilities, 17 •
Emerging Issues in Medical Ethics, 20

2. Health Law   23

Introduction, 23 • The Physician's Relationship with the
Patient, 24 • Regulation by Government, 29 • Certification and
Accreditation, 32 • The Relationship with Payers, 34 • Handling
Medical Information, 36 • Leases and Other Contracts, 38 •
Liability, 38 • Conclusion, 44

3. Quality of Care   45

The Importance of Quality in Medical Care, 45 • The Definition
of Quality, 47 • Measuring Quality—Historical Background, 48 •
Implementing TQM in the Medical Office, 53 • Integrating
TQM and QA Activities, 65 • Conclusion, 68

4. Managed Care   69

An Evolving System, 69 • HMO Models of Managed Care, 73 •
Other Models of Managed Care, 76 • Specialized Managed-
Care Models, 79 • Managing Utilization in HMOs, 82 •
Managing Health Benefits, 85 • Provider System
Models—Future Potential, 86 • Integrated Health Systems, 91 •
Managing the Health of Populations, 96

5. The Computer in the Medical Office   99

Introduction, 99 • General Principles and Operational
Techniques, 100 • Good Computer-Related Work
Habits, 107 • Computer Networks, 111 • Configuration of
Office Computer Systems, 112 • The Computer-Literate Asset
to the Practice, 119 • The Future, 120

6. Medical Office Components   124

Business Office Design, 124 • Clinical Office Design, 130 •
Medical Office Personnel, 141

7. Personnel Policies   150

Introduction, 150 • Personnel Policies Manual, 150 •
Recruitment of Medical Office Staff, 153 • The Hiring
Process, 156 • The Working Relationship, 161 • Terminating the
Working Relationship, 165 • Legal Requirements of a Working
Relationship, 169 • Benefits of a Working Relationship, 174 •
Death or Disability of a Physician, 176 • Conclusion, 177

8. Human Relations in the Medical Office   178

Introduction, 178 • Patient Service, 178 • The Telephone, 184 •
Human Relations among Staff Members and with Patients, 195 •
Conclusion, 200

9. Health Information Management   201

Components of Health Information Management, 201 •
Collecting Health Information—Appointments, 206 •
Patient Registration Information, 210 • Health Records
Information—Format, 212 • Health Records
Information—Content, 217 • Releasing Health
Information, 226 • Using Health Information for Insurance
Billing, 233 • Managing Health Information, 237 • Filing
Systems, 239 • Health Records Retention, 246 • Health Records
Disposition, 250 • Computer Use in Health Information
Management, 253

10. Financial Management   256

Introduction, 256 • Physician Fees, 257 • Billing and
Collection, 263 • Banking, 273 • Internal Financial
Controls, 277 • Budgeting, 279 • Taxes for Medical
Practices, 280 • Insurance for Medical Practices, 281 •
Retirement Plans, 284 • Conclusion, 286

11. Medical Transcription and Correspondence   287

The Transcriptionist in the Medical Office, 287 • Dictation/
Transcription Equipment and Reference Material, 290 •
Transcription in Practice, 29 • Medical Correspondence, 302 •
Proofreading and Editing, 305

12. A Guide to Punctuation and Style   325

Punctuation, 325 • Capitals and Italics, 359 • Plurals and
Possessives, 380 • Compounds, 388 • Abbreviations, 400 •
Numbers, 410 • References, 427

Appendix A. Career Development   431

You as the Job Applicant, 431 • Sources for Jobs, 436 •
Interviewing, 440 • On the Job, 444

Appendix B. Supplementary Information   446

Health Promotion and Disease Prevention, 446 • Schedules of
Controlled Substances, 449 • Glossary of Managed Care
Terms, 451 • National Practitioner Data Bank, 453 •
Immunization Schedule, 454 • Poison Control Centers, 454 •
Selected References, 461

Appendix C. Medical Abbreviations and Vocabulary   466

Abbreviations, 466 • Frequently Confused and Misused
Words, 486

Index   493

Preface

Today's medical office is part of the ever-changing health care environment. The roles of all medical office personnel are undergoing revision in response to the new requirements of health insurance and managed care plans, quality assurance demands, and the need for a more responsive patient-service medical office.

There are aspects of health care delivery that remain constant, such as medical ethics and the requirements for quality of care. The most important constant, usually overlooked, is that the bulk of health care is still provided in physicians' offices. Hundreds of thousands of these offices remain the major source of care in the United States. In the attempt to control costs, improve quality, and remain sensitive to the needs of the sick, the medical office continues to be the central focus of attention.

The first edition of this book was published in 1979. No one at that time could have predicted the tumultuous changes in health care that would occur in the next two decades. Aside from the ongoing scientific revolution, which has brought new approaches to the diagnosis and treatment of disease, the costs of treatment, the methods of delivery, and the modes of payment have changed enormously.

All the book's chapters have been completely revised with updated information, and five new chapters and appendixes have been added. The title of this new edition, *Merriam-Webster's Medical Office Handbook,* changed from its former title *Webster's Medical Secretaries Handbook,* reflects the broader intended audience for this book, which now includes all administrative employees in a medical office—from medical assistants to office managers and even to physicians. This essentially new book will be useful not only as an office resource but also as a supplementary text for allied health courses at community colleges.

The contributors to this edition are recognized authorities in their respective fields and come from a variety of backgrounds, some academic, some practice-oriented. In consultation with Joseph Hamburg, M.D., they have addressed the most important aspects of medical office administration. Included in this coverage are the following new topics:

- Quality of care and developing an in-office quality improvement program
- Managed care and the ongoing changes in health plans
- Computer uses in the medical practice

A new appendix of medical abbreviations and vocabulary includes a comprehensive list of the many terms useful in all medical settings. An appendix of supplementary information includes highlights of the government's *Healthy People 2000* project, a glossary of managed care terms, and a list of selected references to provide suggestions for further reading on the book's key topics.

In addition to the contributors who created the initial text for the various chapters, there are others who gave advice and information to some of those contributors, for which they acknowledge the following: the physicians and staff of Kalamazoo (Michigan) Internal Medicine and of Western Michigan University's Sindecuse Health Center; Linda Galbraith, CMT/ART, of D&T Medical Transcription in Parker, Colorado; Betsy Harlow, CMT, of the IMA Foundation in Tupelo, Mississippi; medical transcriptionists Deborah Herring in San Antonio, Texas, and Julie Naimi, CMT, in Seattle, Washington; and Alan Blitz of Blitz and Associates in Riverwoods, Illinois. The consulting editor for the book's first edition, John Rhodes Haverty, M.D., gave valuable advice at the outset of this project.

Editorial staff members at Merriam-Webster assisted in the preparation of this book in various ways: John M. Morse, executive editor, and Mark A. Stevens, senior editor, provided planning and conceptual advice; Stephen J. Perrault, senior editor, produced several computer-art figures; Maria A. Sansalone, associate editor, reviewed the chapter on health records; Joan I. Narmontas, associate editor, prepared the medical abbreviations section; and Florence A. Fowler keyboarded parts of the manuscript. Freelance editors Karen Singson and Robie Grant, respectively, proofread the text and prepared the index.

Merriam-Webster's
Medical Office
Handbook

Chapter 1

Medical Ethics

Understanding Professional Responsibilities   1
Respect for Persons and for Their Autonomy   6
Beneficence   12
Justice   14
Additional Ethical Responsibilities   17
Emerging Issues in Medical Ethics   20

Understanding Professional Responsibilities

Regardless of the medical practice setting, a critical factor for effective patient care is the quality of the relationship between the patient and the health care provider. The nature and integrity of that relationship are of such importance that they are defined and safeguarded by law and by formal professional codes of ethics. In addition, the special field of medical ethics or bioethics has developed over the past three decades to explore this relationship. It is essential that all who participate in the delivery of health care understand and reflect on the ramifications of the relationship with their patients.

Because of the complexity of the delivery of care, two additional interactions are essential for effective patient care—the relationship of the health care provider to other professionals and staff members of the health care team, and to society.

There are a number of responsibilities entailed in these three professional relationships. In many instances, the principal obligations fall to the physician or other caregiver. In others, the obligations are shared by all members of the health care team.

In contemporary medicine, most care is not provided by a single physician but by a team of various health care professionals, each contributing a special knowledge and expertise. The patient must also be a member of the team. The complexity of modern medicine has necessitated this team approach in order to achieve effective care. Being a member of the health team does not diminish the moral responsibility of each member of the team.

Just as the health care team or staff must know and agree to the way in which the members will provide care, they must discuss and agree on the ethical dimensions of their practice. In all cases, each person who participates in the art and science of healing must be aware of the full spectrum of professional responsibilities and of each person's specific role in meeting these responsibilities.

Limitations of the Law

Understanding the stipulations of the law with regard to professional relationships is important for every member of the medical office staff. Adherence to the law alone, however, will not insure that all of the commonly accepted responsibilities have been met, because many of these are ethical in nature.

Ethical or moral responsibilities toward patients are not always identical with the legal obligations. So too, the ethical rights of patients are not always identical to their legal rights. There are some patient rights which may be legal but which an individual patient would not consider as ethical; for example, the legal right of a woman to an abortion. There are some rights that an individual patient may hold to be ethical or moral even though they may not be legal, such as the right of a terminally ill patient to end his or her life. To understand the responsibilities of health care providers and medical office staff members, therefore, it is important to know more than just the law; you must know something about ethics and morality.

Importance of Professional Codes

As a guide to identifying and meeting ethical responsibilities, medicine and other health professions have formulated and promulgated statements of ethics for their members. The history and tradition of these professional codes of ethics probably began even before the appearance in the fourth century B.C.E. of what is known as the Hippocratic oath. Hippocrates was the founder of a Greek school of medicine, and some of his students and followers are credited with writing commentaries on the practice of medicine from which the Hippocratic oath was drawn. (A modern version of the oath is shown in Figure 1.1.)

Fig. 1.1 Modern Version of the Hippocratic Oath

At the time of being admitted as a Member of the Medical Profession
I solemnly pledge myself to consecrate my life to the service of humanity;
I will give to my teachers the respect and gratitude which is their due;
I will practice my profession with conscience and dignity;
The health of my patient will be my first consideration;
I will respect the secrets which are confided in me;
I will maintain by all the means in my power, the honor and the noble traditions
  of the medical profession;
My colleagues will be my Family;
I will not permit consideration of religion, nationality, race, party politics or
  social standing to intervene between my duty and my patient;
I will maintain the utmost respect for human life; even under threat, I will not
  use my medical knowledge contrary to the laws of humanity.
I make these promises solemnly, freely and upon my honor.

Fig. 1.2 Principles of Medical Ethics of the American Medical Association

The medical profession has long subscribed to a body of ethical statements developed primarily for the benefit of the patient. As a member of this profession, a physician must recognize responsibility not only to patients, but also to society, to other health professionals, and to self. The following Principles adopted by the American Medical Association are not laws, but standards of conduct which define the essentials of honorable behavior for the physician.

I. A physician shall be dedicated to providing competent medical service with compassion and respect for human dignity.

II. A physician shall deal honestly with patients and colleagues, and strive to expose those physicians deficient in character or competence, or who engage in fraud or deception.

III. A physician shall respect the law and also recognize a responsibility to seek changes in those requirements which are contrary to the best interests of the patient.

IV. A physician shall respect the rights of patients, of colleagues, and of other health professionals, and shall safeguard patient confidences within the constraints of the law.

V. A physician shall continue to study, apply and advance scientific knowledge, make relevant information available to patients, colleagues and the public, obtain consultation, and use the talents of other health professionals when indicated.

VI. A physician shall, in the provision of appropriate patient care except in emergencies, be free to choose whom to serve, with whom to associate, and the environment in which to provide medical services.

VII. A physician shall recognize a responsibility to participate in activities contributing to an improved community.

(Reprinted by permission of the American Medical Association)

Following in the tradition of the Hippocratic oath, the American Medical Association (AMA) periodically revises its Principles of Medical Ethics, first issued in 1847. These principles describe the physician's basic responsibilities not only to patients but also to other health professionals, to society, and to self (see Figure 1.2 for a copy of the principles). The Council on Ethical and Judicial Affairs of the AMA is responsible for interpreting these principles. When needed, the Council issues recommendations concerning new practice or social policy issues for approval by the AMA delegates. In 1994, for example, the Council's report on ethical issues in managed care was adopted by the AMA membership.

The bylaws of the American Association of Medical Assistants (AAMA) include both a code of ethics and a creed for its members (see Figure 1.3). The American Nurses' Association (ANA) has published a code for nurses since 1950, and the latest restatement was revised in 1985 (see Figure 1.4).

Although all these formulations of ethical responsibility are similar in

Fig. 1.3   Code of Ethics of the American Association of Medical Assistants

The Code of Ethics of AAMA shall set forth principles of ethical and moral conduct as they relate to the medical profession and the particular practice of medical assisting. Members of AAMA dedicated to the conscientious pursuit of their profession, and thus desiring to merit the high regard of the entire medical profession and the respect of the general public which they serve, do pledge themselves to strive always to:

1. render service with full respect for the dignity of humanity;
2. respect confidential information obtained through employment unless legally authorized or required by responsible performance of duty to divulge such information;
3. uphold the honor and high principles of the profession and accept its disciplines;
4. seek to continually improve the knowledge and skills of medical assistants for the benefit of patients and professional colleagues;
5. participate in additional service activities aimed toward improving the health and well-being of the community.

Creed
I believe in the principles and purposes of the profession of medical assisting.
I endeavor to be more effective.
I aspire to render greater service.
I protect the confidence entrusted to me.
I am dedicated to the care and well-being of all patients.
I am loyal to my physician-employer.
I am true to the ethics of my profession.
I am strengthened by compassion, courage and faith.

(Reprinted by permission of the American Association of Medical Assistants)

purpose, they are not identical in content. There are, however, a number of significant common obligations or values that they share. These include the following:

- Professional competency
- Respect and compassion for the patient
- Avoidance of harm to the patient
- Patient confidentiality
- Respect for and loyalty to the profession

The three contemporary codes—those of the AMA, AAMA, and ANA—share two additional professional duties: (1) the obligation to study continually to improve a member's professional knowledge and skills, and (2) the responsibility to improve the health of the community or of society. The AMA and the ANA principles counsel members to respect and work together with other health professionals, while the AAMA creed speaks of being loyal to the physician-employer.

Fig. 1.4   Code for Nurses of the American Nurses' Association

1. The nurse provides services with respect for human dignity and the uniqueness of the client, unrestricted by considerations of social or economic status, personal attributes, or the nature of health problems.
2. The nurse safeguards the client's right to privacy by judiciously protecting information of a confidential nature.
3. The nurse acts to safeguard the client and the public when health care and safety are affected by incompetent, unethical, or illegal practice by any person.
4. The nurse assumes responsibilities and accountability for individual nursing judgments and actions.
5. The nurse maintains competence in nursing.
6. The nurse exercises informed judgment and uses individual competency and qualifications as criteria in seeking consultation, accepting responsibilities, and delegating nursing activities.
7. The nurse participates in activities that contribute to the ongoing development of the profession's body of knowledge.
8. The nurse participates in the profession's efforts to implement and improve standards of nursing.
9. The nurse participates in the profession's efforts to establish and maintain conditions of employment conducive to high-quality nursing care.
10. The nurse participates in the profession's efforts to protect the public from misinformation and misrepresentation and to maintain the integrity of nursing.
11. The nurse collaborates with members of the health professions and other citizens in promoting community and national efforts to meet the health needs of the public.

(Reprinted by permission of the American Nurses' Association)

The Need for Medical Ethics

Although the professional codes provide a useful list of responsibilities, they alone are not sufficient to assist the health care provider in daily practice. Professional codes are only basic guidelines; they do not and cannot include every ethical issue that will occur in clinical practice. In addition, professional codes cannot tell how to judge specific clinical situations in which two obligations may conflict, such as confidentiality and protection of the community.

In spite of the limitations of professional codes, they are valuable guidelines in the effort to provide quality care. The codes are also public declarations of common standards of conduct, announcing to all what should be expected of health care professionals. Knowledge of the codes, however, must be supplemented by the study and understanding of medical or health care ethics.

The Meaning of Ethics

The word *ethics* commonly refers to what philosophers term "general normative ethics"—the study and establishment of principles and values that should be used in deciding what people ought to do or how they ought to behave.

Medical ethics is the formal study of the nature and application of general normative principles specifically to medicine and health care. The professional codes are an attempt to apply normative ethical principles and values to professional practice. Individual members of the health care team must also understand and apply these principles to their own practices.

Ethical decision making usually concerns two sorts of questions: (1) What is the morally right action for me to take in this situation? (2) What is motivating my action? or What sort of person am I being when I take this action? The first question relates to the ethical nature of the act and the obligation to do what is right, for example, to divulge or not to divulge confidential information. The second question relates to the ethical character of the professional taking the action and the responsibility to practice what may be called professional "virtues," for example, compassion or loyalty. Medical ethics attempts to identify the basic principles and values that should guide ethical decisions about both sorts of responsibilities.

The Application of Ethical Principles to Medical Practice

The ethical principles most frequently cited as the major guides for consistent decision making in medical practice are:

1. Respect for persons and for their autonomy or self-determination
2. Beneficence and its complement, nonmaleficence
3. Justice

These major ethical principles can be viewed as either responsibilities for the health care provider or as rights of the patient. The American Hospital Association (AHA) has emphasized the rights of the patient and created "A Patient's Bill of Rights." However, this chapter focuses on the basic ethical principles in terms of the responsibilities of health professionals rather than in terms of patient rights. In any case, whichever perspective is used—as health provider's responsibilities or as patient's rights—the same ethical obligations pertain.

These principles do not exhaust all the ethical values needed in a medical practice, but they do cover a majority of issues that you will encounter in the medical office. It is important to note that sometimes more than one of the principles may apply in specific cases, and sometimes two of the principles may even be in conflict. Situations in which two ethical principles are in conflict are usually called ethical or moral *dilemmas*. These are the most difficult ethical problems that you will face, and they require the greatest amount of reflection and discernment. Each of these principles and their applications in the medical practice is examined in the following pages.

Respect for Persons and for Their Autonomy

Respect for the patient as a person is perhaps the pivotal ethical principle in the patient-physician relationship, and it includes the greatest number of responsibilities. This principle means that insofar as the patient is a person, he or she should not be involuntarily used or exploited to meet someone else's purposes. There are two critical facets of this principle for the health care provider: the first concerns the general regard for the patient as a person; the second deals with the person's fundamental characteristic of being an independent decision maker.

Respect

From the patient's first phone call to the medical office, the relationship between the patient and the health care staff begins and so too does the responsibility for respect. The relationship between the patient and the health care provider places the patient in a position of dependence on the knowledge, skill, time, and cooperation of the health care provider. There is an imbalance of power within the relationship which should not be exploited by the provider. In this relationship, respect requires more than politeness; it requires the recognition of the dignity, worth, individuality, beliefs, and values of the person.

Opportunities for showing such concern are present in the manner in which you address patients—for example, using the surname until invited to use the given name—or in the way you discuss potentially sensitive issues regarding anything from billing issues to intimate health-related practices. Respect for the patient as a person also requires that any differences in socio-economic status, race, gender, generation, culture, or ethnicity do not diminish the obligation to show respect or to provide care.

This facet of the principle of respect for the patient as a person may be challenging for the health care professional. The patient is after all a *patient* and therefore someone who may not be at their best. The patient may be in pain, confused, frightened, even angry. Maintaining respect can be especially difficult when a patient has lost all self-esteem and is overbearing, verbally abusive, or does not respect you as a person. However, this obligation of respect for the patient as a person calls upon you to be tolerant, patient, understanding, and sensitive.

Autonomy

The second critical aspect of the principle of respect for persons relates to the essential element of personhood, that is, independent decision making. To be a person means to have the ability and power to make independent decisions and to be self-determining. Some persons, however, may lack or may lose the mental capacity to make independent decisions. Infants and children are in the process of achieving this capacity. For those without the capacity for self-determination, parents or legally appointed guardians or surrogates assume the responsibility of decision making.

The health care worker must respect the independent decision-making authority or autonomy of the patient. However, there is an inevitable dependency of the patient on the physician and other staff members. Specifically, the patient asks for and is dependent on their knowledge, skill, and expertise. Respect for the autonomy of the patient in such a relationship is a complex obligation.

Providing information   To enable the patient to make a sound, autonomous decision, the health professional must provide the competent, adult patient with all of the pertinent information that is needed. In some instances, the health professional must even educate the patient about his or her basic right to autonomy in medical decision making. Providing the patient with all the necessary information to make an informed, autonomous decision means that the health care provider must be

- knowledgeable and skillful in the medical matter in question;
- aware of the patient's medical history and relevant personal history and beliefs;
- truthful and open in sharing the pertinent medical information with the patient, exaggerating neither the risks nor the possible beneficial outcomes;
- skillful and clear in communicating the necessary information;
- perceptive about the patient's level of ability to understand the information provided;
- able to determine when a patient does not have the capacity to make an informed decision or when this capacity is questionable;
- sensitive to and able to assuage a patient's unreasonable and obstructive fears; and
- facilitative but not controlling of the collaborative decision-making process.

Advocating for autonomy   Sometimes the physician or other health care provider must protect and advocate for the patient's right to autonomy. This may apply not only to the individual patient but also to a physician's entire patient practice if a managed care organization is involved. In this latter context, the physician may need to insist that patients be informed of the full range of treatment options available and appropriate for their use, including those that may be disallowed as too costly by the managed care organization.

Protecting elderly patients   The need for advocacy for the individual patient often occurs in the case of the frail elderly who may have some increased dependence on others but who still retain the mental capacity for decision making. For example, spouses, adult children, or even other service providers such as home health workers may urge the primary physician to initiate a change in an elderly patient's medication or other treatment regimen. The reasons for their request may be in what they consider to be the patient's best interest. The physician, however, is obligated to make certain that the change requested is indeed what the patient wants and needs.

Determining capacity for autonomy   Sometimes a patient's capacity for making autonomous decisions may become questionable or uncertain. In such situations, it is important to seek the help of appropriate family members or, in some instances, friends, to help determine if the capacity of the patient has been diminished. A patient's family or friends can often provide the physician with a better understanding of the patient's values and desires about the quality of life.

The health professional must continue to be an advocate for any patient with diminished decision-making capacity, even after a legal guardian or surrogate for the patient has been appointed. Cases do occur when guardians or surrogates abuse their position by neglecting their responsibilities or by demanding medical interventions that the physician judges to be contraindicated. Sometimes a health professional who cannot prevent harm to a patient by irresponsible surrogates may be forced to seek legal intervention.

Protecting children and adolescent patients   Ethical dilemmas regarding informed consent may also arise in the case of pediatric and adolescent patients. This is the case even though, as noted earlier, autonomy and informed consent are usually defined in terms of the competent, adult patient. Few would dispute the rights and responsibilities of parents or guardians with respect to decision making for their children. So too, few would dispute that children also have rights—both legal and ethical. The health professional must understand these rights and sometimes both protect and advocate for them on behalf of the pediatric patient. The healing relationship in pediatrics must include the child or adolescent as well as the parent or guardian.

The rights of the parent of the adolescent or young adult patient in matters of informed consent and confidentiality are sometimes problematic for the health professional. Part of the problem is the difficulty in determining when a child or adolescent is intellectually and psychologically competent. Achieving competency may well occur before the legal age of majority. In such cases, it may become very difficult for the health professional to mediate between the wishes of a parent or guardian and the ethical rights of the adolescent or young adult.

The health professional is obliged when appropriate to advocate for the minor as the patient and to protect the minor's right to be informed of and to understand the status of his or her health and care plan. Examples of some of the difficulties that may arise include cases in which the parent requests drug testing for the minor without the adolescent's knowledge or consent, or in which the parent demands the continuation of therapy (such as kidney dialysis) which the adolescent is refusing.

To be an advocate in such instances will require the health professional to form a trusting relationship not only with the child or adolescent but also with the parents or guardian. The health professional will also need to respect and not violate the legitimate and trusting relationship between the parent and the child. However, the health professional must intervene if the decisions of the parent or guardian are detrimental to the well-being of the minor.

There is even legal precedence for such intervention in cases where parents have refused on the basis of religious convictions to allow their children to receive life-saving therapies, such as blood transfusions.

Collaborative relationship   Informed decision making in health care is essentially a collaborative process between the provider and the patient. Although the final decision rests with the fully competent adult patient or a duly authorized surrogate, the role of the health professional is essential. The better the collaborative relationship between patient and professional, the smoother will be the decision-making process. The catalyst in any good relationship is trust. The health professional must trust the honesty and candor of the patient; the patient must trust the competence and loyalty of the health professional. Both must show that they are worthy of trust.

Privacy and Confidentiality

The obligation of all health professionals to protect the privacy and confidentiality of patients is often linked to the principle of respect for persons. A patient's body, personal life and history, as well as physical and emotional health, are part of who a patient is as a person. The patient, alone, owns and is the custodian of his or her body and life story.

Privacy of the body   Part of the obligation to protect the privacy of the patient includes the responsibility to be sensitive to and protect a patient's need for modesty with regard to his or her body. Regardless of what may be perceived as contemporary society's inhibitions regarding nudity, the health care professional must assume that patients wish to be treated with careful regard for their physical modesty. Where patients are placed and how they are asked to disrobe, who is present during an examination in addition to those who are directly providing care—all affect the privacy of the patients. For example, a patient's permission should be sought if other health professionals, such as medical students, are to observe a procedure.

Confidentiality   Although the obligation to maintain the confidentiality of patients is perhaps one of the most widely recognized obligations in health care, it continues to be problematic. One of the reasons is that an ever-growing number of health professionals may legitimately have access to a patient's confidential information. With the computerization of patient records, there are new possibilities for breaching confidentiality, requiring new safeguards to protect patient information.

Threats to confidentiality   The safeguards to patient information are, of course, only as trustworthy as the persons who legitimately collect and access the information in the first place. The age-old and common threats to confidentiality continue to challenge health care; they include (1) gossiping or sharing patient information with persons, including other health professionals, who have no right to the information; (2) legitimately discussing patient issues in inappropriate places (such as elevators or reception desks) where the conversation can be overheard; (3) careless handling of patient records, either written or computerized; and (4) inappropriately responding to inquiries from a patient's family or friends.

Third-party requests for information   Dealing with a third party who requests or in other ways seeks information about a patient can be difficult. How should a health professional respond to inquiries about the condition of a competent adult patient made by the patient's spouse or children? What about the spouse who insists on remaining with the patient throughout the examination and conference? In all such cases, patient confidentiality must be protected unless specifically waived by the patient. Handling anxious, worried, or even meddlesome relatives in a respectful manner requires patience, compassion, and tact by all medical office staff.

Waiving the right to confidentiality   Patients are routinely asked to waive their right to confidentiality. This is the case when patients are asked to authorize the release of their information for insurance or other claims for reimbursement or for the purposes of medical research. These situations always require, even by law, that the patient or legal guardian or surrogate duly authorize both the release of information and the kinds of information to be released. The health professional must be sure that the patient not only signs the authorization forms appropriately but also fully understands what is being signed.

As with the principle of autonomy, confidentiality regarding both adult patients whose competency is uncertain and pediatric or adolescent patients presents additional challenges. With adult patients whose competency is questionable or diminished, the physician is obliged to make the family or legal surrogates of the patient aware of the medical condition. The family or surrogate then can assist in the decision-making process in behalf of the patient.

Confidentiality for adolescents   With adolescent patients, the responsibility of the health professional to share information with parents or guardians is not always clear. There are a number of medical conditions or concerns that are critical to the well-being of adolescent patients but which they may be unwilling to discuss with their parents. Issues of contraception, pregnancy, sexually transmitted diseases, and drug addiction are concerns that adolescents most often do not want shared with parents. Health professionals when asked (often begged) by adolescents to withhold such information from parents face a difficult choice among several ethical values: the trust of the adolescent patient, the compliance of the adolescent patient, the trust of the parent, the integrity of the relationship between the parent and child, and, most essentially, the health and well-being of the adolescent. Each such dilemma must be judged individually, weighing the ethical values and principles involved and making that choice which ensures the well-being of the adolescent.

Breaching confidentiality   There are circumstances in which breaching confidentiality is morally, and often legally, required. Situations in which confidences may be broken usually involve a conflict between the patient's right to privacy and some other right of greater importance. This more important right may be one that pertains to the patient, to some other person, or to society. Some of the instances in which confidentiality is sometimes breached include cases of known or suspected child abuse, criminal activity, potential suicide, and certain infectious diseases.

As noted earlier, revealing the confidences of patients can be viewed as a violation of the person, robbing patients of what is their own property. It can also be viewed in some circumstances as the potential destruction of their reputation. The possibility of their medical history being divulged to others can sometimes keep patients from seeking the medical assistance needed, resulting possibly in greater illness or death; this can be seen in instances of unwanted pregnancies, illegal abortions, and in the late diagnosis of AIDS. The consequences of violating the confidentiality of patients must be taken seriously. The obligation to maintain confidences, although sometimes confusing and challenging, must be met by health care professionals.

In safeguarding confidentiality and privacy, the health care provider once again contributes to the development of a trusting and productive relationship with the patient. To maintain this trust, the health care team must create an environment that the patient experiences as safe, trustworthy, respectful, and competent.

Beneficence

The ethical principle of beneficence and the corollary of nonmaleficence are underscored in the writings of Hippocrates and his followers. In an early version of the Hippocratic oath, physicians are told to practice medicine "for the benefit of the sick." Elsewhere in Hippocratic writings, physicians are admonished: "As to disease, make a habit of two things—to help or at least to do no harm." There are continuing debates about what "to help" includes and what "to do no harm" forbids.

To Benefit the Patient
One aspect of the obligation to benefit the patient is rather clear. The care provided should enable patients to achieve their goals of health or well-being. Health care is not to be provided solely to promote the self-interest—whether financial, emotional, or scientific—of the health professional. For example, to prescribe harmless but marginally useful, or even useless, drugs or other sorts of therapies that might financially profit the provider violates the provider's obligation to benefit the patient. The interest of the patient is primary.

Limitations   There are, however, medical and social limits to what individual patients may expect in order to achieve their health care goals and, concomitantly, to what the health professional is obliged to do to benefit the patient. The individual patient is never totally independent and autonomous. Each patient is a member of various collectives—a medical practice, a health care delivery plan or organization, a community or society. As a member of these groups, the patient's individual rights and expectations will be limited by those of other members and by the available medical resources. What the individual patient can expect as "beneficial" will usually in some way be limited. More will be said about the limitations on health care services in the section on the principle of justice.

Paternalism   From another perspective, it is possible for a health professional to have an exaggerated sense of beneficence, which could rob a patient of his or her autonomy. The health professional, committed to curing the patient, may not be able to convince the patient to accept a medical intervention that the professional believes will be beneficial or even essential to the patient's health. An overzealous health professional might forcibly (or by some ruse) medically intervene, overriding the patient's wishes and justifying action by claiming the necessity of beneficence. Most health professionals would not condone this extreme paternalistic behavior, because it so blatantly violates the patient's autonomy.

Some health professionals and ethicists believe, however, that the health professional cannot practice beneficence without being to some degree "paternal," that is, being simultaneously a protector, a goad, an adviser, and one who cares. Indeed, determining where empathetic caring for and protecting the well-being of a patient ends and where unwarranted paternalistic intrusion on the patient's autonomy begins is not always easy. Here, as with other patient care dilemmas, ethical principles clash for precedence, and resolving the conflict requires careful reflection, appropriate consultation, and prudent judgment.

To Do No Harm to the Patient

The corollary ethical principle stated in the Hippocratic oath, "to do no harm" (expressed by the phrase *primum non nocere*), includes the obligation both to refrain from injuring a patient and to prevent potential injury where possible. There are a number of obvious applications of this principle in everyday practice. Examples of violations of this principle include culpable errors in diagnosis or in prescribing harmful drugs or other therapeutic regimens; negligence in the performance of potentially dangerous procedures; sexual, psychological, or physical abuse of patients; and failure to report any type of malpractice, fraud, or negligence. Health professionals can also allow harm to occur by not effecting adequate follow-up for a patient or by not educating patients about relevant disease-prevention strategies, such as stopping smoking or the practice of safe sex.

Dilemmas   Some health professionals use the principle of nonmaleficence to support their opposition to either discontinuing or not initiating life-support

systems (respirator, parenteral nutrition, etc.) or other life-prolonging therapies (kidney dialysis, chemotherapy, etc.). The argument used is that to allow
a patient to die is to do harm; discontinuing (or not initiating) life support
or life-sustaining procedures could result in death; so to discontinue or not
initiate such procedures is to do harm. For this argument to be valid, of
course, the basic premise equating death with harm must be valid. Many
would not accept this equation of death with harm without qualifications.

The decision to discontinue or not initiate life support or life-sustaining
therapies must involve a number of considerations, such as the ethical and
religious values and desires of the patient; relevant legal considerations, including the patient's durable power of attorney or living will; medical or
scientific data, such as the nature of the patient's condition and prognosis;
and other related factors, such as the availability and cost of the medical
resources needed.

A related and even more problematic dilemma involving the principle
of beneficence is that of "doctor-assisted" suicide of the terminally ill patient.
The clash in this case between the obligation to do what is of benefit to
the patient and the obligation to do no harm is perplexing for most health
professionals. Even at the level of law, the dilemma of assisted suicide, regardless of who provides that assistance, has not been consistently adjudicated.

In all, the obligation to beneficence—to do what is of benefit and to do
no harm for patients—provides challenges that range from the simple to the
complex. Beneficence requires that health professionals be caring, compas-
sionate, loyal, and attentive as well as competent, prudent, accountable, and
reliable.

Justice

A variety of definitions and theories of justice have been proposed by philosophers over time. Most often justice is defined in terms of fairness or of giving
to others what they deserve. There are, however, a variety of ways in which
someone may be deserving, for example, because of a formal promise or
contract or because one is a human being. Medical ethics is concerned with
justice as it applies to the individual and to society.

Justice to the Individual Patient

In the context of the relationship between the individual and the health care
provider, justice is central. The principle of justice is different in one sense
from the other ethical principles so far reviewed. If you were to define all of
the ethical principles in terms of "rights" of a person, the principle of justice
would be the ground for all other principles. Although there is overlap among
the principles, there are some issues in medical practice that are more obviously issues of justice.

Professional standards   The relationship between the health care provider and the patient is usually viewed as a form of tacit contract or promise—whether there is monetary remuneration for the services provided or not. This contract morally requires that the health professional fulfill a specific role as a health care provider.

The health professional must *be* and *do* exactly what he or she professes to be and do. For example, if the health professional is a nurse, he or she must be a prepared and capable nurse, having all the knowledge and skills that a nurse is professionally expected to have. The nurse also must provide a level of care that will benefit and not harm the patient and that will meet the acknowledged standards of nursing care. The commitment of the health professional to be and to do what is professionally required also entails an obligation to accountability—to assessing and assuring that the knowledge and skills and the care provided meet acknowledged professional standards.

Appropriate remuneration   In exchange for the quality services provided, the health professional has a right to financial remuneration from the patient. In most cases the cost of patient care is provided indirectly by the patient through insurance, managed care arrangements, or the like.

Justice for the patient would require that all financial charges be fair, relative to the amount and kind of service provided and to some acknowledged community standard. Justice would also require that all of the policies and procedures established by the health professional regarding financial arrangements (such as the method of collection) be fair. The health professional must guard against pricing levels or policies that are abusive or exploitative of the patient, taking unfair advantage of the patient's need for medical services.

Undue advantage   Health professionals must avoid other related practices that may take undue advantage of patients, such as inappropriate or unnecessary prescription of drugs or referral for diagnostic or therapeutic services in order to gain financial incentives. On the other hand, the opposite practice, in which health care providers gain financial incentives by cutting back the services provided to individual patients, can be unjust if it results in inadequate or ineffective care for the patient.

Patients' obligations   The patient, as partner in this contract, also has obligations related to justice. For example, patients owe the health professional the following:
- Honesty in providing relevant medical information
- Openness to and compliance with medical advice
- Willingness to assume the responsibilities of personal decision making
- Clarity in the directives provided to the physician
- Respect for health professionals' integrity by not asking them to perform actions that would diminish that integrity (such as altering insurance claims)
- Payment for services

In addition, patients have the responsibility to understand the limits of what they might expect in health care and to temper their demands, in light of the competing demands for service, the scarcity of some resources, and the costliness of care.

Termination of the relationship   Under special circumstances, the health professional may find it necessary and justifiable to terminate the professional relationship with a patient. These circumstances often involve the patient's repeated purposeful failure to meet one or more of the obligations delineated above. To prevent possible harm to the patient when justifiably terminating the professional relationship, the health professional must provide the patient with referrals for continuing care. Similar assistance should be provided to patients when a health professional is forced to reduce or close the medical practice because of illness or disability.

Justice in the Context of Society

It is impossible to speak of what is owed to the individual patient without recognizing the limits that are necessarily placed on what the patient can claim as fair. Medical resources (such as health personnel, equipment, or drugs) are not limitless. All the other members of a practice, a health system, a community, or a society have competing claims for access to these finite resources. Various theories of distributive justice (that is, how the goods of a society should be equitably or fairly dispersed) are used to address the issue of the allocation of medical resources. However, there is so far no consensus on any one of these theories or on the issue of whether all persons have a fundamental right to health care. There is not even agreement among those who believe that people do have a right to health care as to what that right ought to include.

Guidelines   Even though there is no societal consensus, health professionals know that guidelines are needed to adjudicate the competing patient claims for care, including claims for scarce resources such as transplant organs, and to control the ever-growing cost of care.

Federal and state governments have attempted to provide some regulation of the cost and availability of health care services in our society, through Medicaid, Medicare, and other programs. However, systemic health care reform by government has not succeeded. Therefore, an increasing number of health care delivery organizations are emerging in an attempt to address these issues through a variety of managed care systems.

Managed care   In considering the medical ethics of justice to the individual and to society, concerns have been raised by health professionals about the cost-saving and cost-cutting approaches taken by some managed care organizations. Some of these common concerns include the following:

- Individual patients may be prevented from obtaining the care they need
- Many uninsured patients will continue to go uninsured and uncared for

- Individual physicians will be forced to make cost-related decisions that in fairness ought to be made by society
- Patients may not be informed of those treatment options that may be medically indicated but which are costly
- Patients will lose the freedom to choose physicians or to retain those with whom they have established strong relationships

Whatever accommodations are made by managed care organizations to address these concerns, they must achieve the following goals: (1) maintain the quality of patient care, (2) protect the rights of patients, (3) maintain the integrity of the relationship between health professional and patient, and (4) recognize and address the serious problems of social justice in terms of access to medical and health care resources. (For details on managed care, see Chapter 4, "Managed Care.")

Therefore, the principle of justice requires health professionals, to be and to do precisely what they promise and to be accountable and fair to their own patients while being prudent and unwasteful in the use of society's limited health care resources.

Ensuring Ethical Practice

All of these ethical principles can serve as guides for initiating and maintaining sound and productive professional relationships with patients. Although a number of applications of these principles have been described, there are many more examples that you were probably able to draw from your own experience.

To ensure that medical office staff members do not lose sight of these principles and of the ethical dimension of your practice in the hectic pace of daily work, the following strategies may be helpful.

- Incorporate into office policies and procedures manuals reminders of the major ethical responsibilities specifically related to your medical office.
- Develop and publish procedures that enable staff members to report with impunity any unethical activities or conduct which they might discover.
- Encourage staff members to identify and circulate articles on ethical issues related to your practice.
- Create an atmosphere in which it is acceptable to talk about the philosophy and ethics of the medical practice.
- Schedule periodic opportunities for the staff to review and reflect together on the moral dimensions of their service and the quality of the caring relationships that they have formed with patients in the practice.

Additional Ethical Responsibilities

The professional codes cited earlier in this chapter point out several ethical obligations that health professionals have to one another and to society.

Obligations to Other Health Professionals

For the most part, the ethical obligations that health professionals have to one another derive from the obligations they have to their patients. Working collaboratively, often with health professionals from a variety of disciplines, has become necessary in contemporary health care in order to meet the complex needs of the patient. There are a variety of collaborative working groups or teams that can be found in health care, for example, the surgical team, the rehabilitation team, the home care team, as well as the health care personnel who staff a medical practice.

Responsibilities of team members   The leadership of these different teams will vary, usually depending on the basic function of the team. Even though the leadership may vary, the ethical responsibility for the care provided is always shared by each member of the team. To fulfill the team's obligations to the patient, the team members must be able to count on one another. This requires that all team members understand and perform their responsibilities relative to the overall task that must be accomplished. Members of the team must understand and mutually agree to the way in which the team will work together and to the values that they will collectively strive to maintain.

Common values   In some medical practices, it is critically important that this understanding of values be established before the individual health professional agrees to join the team. An example of such a setting would be that of the obstetrics-gynecology practice where the issue of abortion might be raised. Potential conflicts between a health care professional's personal ethical or religious values with those of the patient or the health care team should be anticipated and resolved to avoid the disruption of quality patient care.

Health care team members owe each other competence, reliability, integrity, cooperation, support, and loyalty. These are all necessary insofar as they enable the team to serve the patient ethically, effectively, and efficiently. If loyalty to other members of the team would in some way jeopardize the responsibility to the patient, however, loyalty to the patient must prevail. The patient's legitimate needs and well-being have priority.

If the relationship among members of the health care team is characterized by animosity, arrogance, competitiveness, miscommunication, divisiveness, or discord, the patient may lose trust in one or all of the team members, the patient's care may be jeopardized, and the patient may be harmed. The quality of the relationship among the team of professionals providing care to patients, therefore, is important since it can impact both the quality of care provided to patients and the level of satisfaction patients may have for that care.

Obligation to the employer   In this discussion of obligations to one another, you cannot ignore the obligations to the employer. The quality of the employer-employee relationship can also impact the overall quality of the care provided to patients. For the most part, if responsibilities to patients and colleagues are fulfilled, then the obligations to the employers are also fulfilled. In one sense, the patients are the employers. There are, however, several responsibilities to the formal employers that should be singled out.

The health care worker, according to the principle of justice, owes the employer the time, knowledge, and skills negotiated in the employment agreement. You also owe the employer professional respect and compliance with organizational policies and procedures, as well as respect for property or resources of the employer. This latter obligation precludes misusing, mismanaging, or misappropriating monies or other resources such as sample drugs. As in the relationship with your health care colleagues, for these obligations to your employers to be binding, they must be consistent with the legal and ethical obligations to the patients.

Obligation to the employee   The health care employer has reciprocal ethical and legal obligations to the health care staff. The employer must meet all of the employment promises and provide an environment in which the employee is professionally respected and is able to practice competently, legally, and ethically. Employers cannot ethically ask or require health care employees to provide services that exceed their professionally recognized scope of practice or to engage in any illegal or unethical activities such as falsifying insurance claims or accreditation reports.

Obligations to Society

In living one's life, the individual person is inextricably linked to other persons and to communities of other persons. The health and well-being of the individual person is similarly linked to others in a community or society. The health and well-being of the individual patient are affected by many factors, including genetic inheritance; environmental conditions such as soil, water, and air quality; an adequate food and water supply; infectious diseases such as measles or HIV; poverty; the availability of and access to suitable medical resources; chance destructive occurrences such as automobile accidents or even hurricanes; violent crimes; and war.

Broader responsibilities   The health professional in caring for a patient cannot ignore the significance of these broader social, economic, environmental, and political factors. If individual patients are to be protected from harm and effectively cared for, these issues must also be addressed by someone. Many believe that because of their special knowledge, skills, and responsibilities, health professionals, individually and collectively, have an obligation to provide leadership in addressing these public or societal issues. The AMA, AAMA, and ANA professional codes underscore the public obligation of health professionals to improve and safeguard the health of the community.

To effectively fulfill these social or public responsibilities, individual health professionals and the professional associations could enter into collaborative efforts with others in the community to solve the health problems these broad societal factors have created. Both individual health professionals and professional associations have shown their willingness to assume these public responsibilities by advocating for such things as health care reform or legislative bans on smoking. More must be done, however, both to educate health professionals about their responsibilities to the public and to address the pressing social issues that affect the health and well-being of all patients.

To create and maintain a strong professional relationship with patients, therefore, is only part of the overall challenge of the health care professional. The trusting relationship between professional and patient, nurtured by a mutual commitment to respect, beneficence, and justice, must be extended to embrace professional colleagues and the community.

Emerging Issues in Medical Ethics

Concerns and debates about the ethical practice of medicine are certainly not new. Interest in and the formal study of medical ethics have intensified, however, over the past three decades. This growth has paralleled the growth in the understanding and application of the science and technology of medicine, whether in terms of the importance of sanitation in the prevention of disease or of the utility of laser physics. With each new revolutionary discovery in medicine and medical technology, health professionals are challenged to sort out its impact on the relationship with patients or with society and on the ethical principles that support and guide these relationships.

Human Genome Project

One such recent intriguing project of science that has stimulated debate as to both its ethical and social implications is the Human Genome Project. The primary purpose of this international scientific project is to develop genetic and physical maps of the human genome. These maps will provide extensive information about the genetic basis of the human body's functions and disease. James D. Watson, the first director of the National Institutes of Health Office of Human Genome Research, predicted in the April 6, 1990, edition of *Science:*

> Although the final monies required to determine the human DNA sequence of some 3 billion base pairs (bp) will be an order of magnitude smaller than the monies needed to let men explore the moon, the implications of the Human Genome Project for human life are likely to be far greater. A more important set of instruction books will never be found by human beings. When finally interpreted, the genetic messages encoded with our DNA molecules will provide the ultimate answers to the chemical underpinnings of human existence. They will not only help us understand how we function as healthy human beings, but will also explain, at the chemical level, the role of genetic factors in a multitude of diseases, such as cancer, Alzheimer's disease, and schizophrenia, that diminish the individual lives of so many millions of people.

The strategy envisioned is that once the genes related to specific human diseases or disabilities are located and analyzed, tests can be developed either to make or confirm a diagnosis or to screen for the presence of potentially deleterious genes. The next step is to develop various therapeutic techniques to obstruct, redirect, supplant, or in some way suppress the impact of the gene. A number of advances have been made in genetic mapping and in the development of diagnostic tests and gene therapies.

Concerns about the social and ethical consequences of the Human Genome Project were expressed early in the push to obtain legislation in the United States to fund it. Monies were set aside by the two principal agencies funding genome research to support studies exploring the ethical, legal, and social implications of the research. This special program has been identified by the acronym ELSI. With each renewed request for funding, United States legislators have insisted on the establishment of guidelines to prevent the misuse of the information that has and will result from the Project.

Although the ethical, legal, and social implications of the Project may not be radically new or unique, they are nonetheless challenging. One fundamental question that is raised by some is whether it is morally right for the mapping of the genome to be done at all in light of the potential power it provides to shape the human race, for better or for worse. Such fears are not new to science or to medicine. Most see the progression of the genome research to be inevitable, however, and focus their concern on the ethical use or application of the information that will result from it.

Some of the many ethical questions that we must face regarding the impact of genome research include the following:

- If we have the ability to screen everyone for genetic predispositions to disease, should such screening ever be mandatory?
- Should persons suspected of being at risk for serious genetically related diseases be forced to be screened in order to undergo therapy, if such is available, to avoid costly therapies later?
- Should screening be required for parents at risk of producing offspring with serious genetically related disease conditions or disabilities?
- Should prenatal screening be allowed to enable parents to manipulate the phenotype of their child, such as blue eyes or curly hair?
- What is the potential for a person's genetic information being used to discriminate against him or her, such as by employers or by insurance companies fearful of future claims?
- Under what circumstances would it be morally acceptable to divulge such information without the person's consent?
- Who should have access to genetic screening and the related therapies, and who should pay for these procedures?

Although the context of these questions, that is, the analysis and manipulation of the human genome, may be novel and awesome to us, the ethical questions themselves are not. Similar questions have been raised with regard to the use of HIV/AIDS testing, for example. To respond to these questions, health professionals must rely on the same guidelines or principles that apply to the ethical challenges that arise in the daily clinical practice.

Conclusion

To practice or to participate in the practice of healing and caring is a special privilege and carries with it serious responsibilities. These responsibilities grow out of the special human relationships that are essential to the health care practice. A report on health education by the Pew Health Professions Commission describes health care as an activity that involves many people in a mixture of personal, professional, and community relationships. It is not a "grand machine," but is instead "an essentially human activity, undertaken and given meaning by people in relationships with one another and their communities, both public and professional."

Chapter 2

Health Law

Introduction   23
The Physician's Relationship with the Patient   24
Regulation by Government   29
Certification and Accreditation   32
The Relationship with Payers   34
Handling Medical Information   36
Leases and Other Contracts   38
Liability   38
Conclusion   44

Introduction

There are many aspects of law that have an impact on medical practices and the operation of medical offices. Some of these aspects include the following:

- The relationship with the patient
- Regulation by government
- Certification and accreditation
- The relationship with payers
- Handling medical information
- Leases and other nonemployment contracts
- Liability

Legal issues are becoming more important for all those involved in providing medical care. Public concern with the access to care, the way care is provided, the cost of care, and adverse outcomes have resulted in increasing use of the law to channel the way care is provided and to impose sanctions on physicians and other providers for a widening range of behavior.

All branches of government are involved in these efforts. Congress and state legislatures are passing laws that have a direct impact on practices in medical offices. The federal and state executive branches are adopting regulations, targeting enforcement of laws on physicians and other health care providers, and using the contracting and spending power to obtain arrangements that affect the way medical care is delivered. The judicial branch is also having a direct influence on the way medical care is provided through imposition of liability in malpractice and other civil suits and through judicial interpretation of the laws.

Laws that address medical practice often vary from state to state and may even vary within a state due to county, city, or other local laws. Thus, it is important to consult with an attorney who is familiar with local law before adopting procedures that minimize legal liability.

Through medical malpractice and other civil-law suits, courts and juries become involved in deciding what behavior is not permitted and imposing liability for violations. The rate of medical malpractice suits and the average cost of the suits varies, but they remain significant. It is prudent to structure medical office activities to avoid claims and to maximize the ability to defend claims.

Malpractice should not be the only legal concern in the medical office. In addition to statutes and regulations, physicians need to be concerned about the contracts they enter. Increasingly, contracts are an important tool for structuring medical care delivery. Although it is still rare, criminal law is also used to punish the behavior of physicians and other health care providers. Therefore, it is important to know what behavior is being targeted for criminal sanctions.

The Physician's Relationship with the Patient

How the Relationship Is Started

In a physician-patient relationship, the physician has legal duties to the patient. The physician has a responsibility to care for such patients until the relationship is ended. Most physicians depend significantly on their office staff to assist them in fulfilling these duties. The relationship can start in several ways.

Individuals The first, and usually the most common, way is for the physician to agree to accept an individual patient. Without a special agreement as described below, physicians have broad latitude to decide whether to accept an individual patient, as long as they do not base their decisions on discriminatory reasons.

There have been legislative proposals to require physicians to accept certain patients. For example, in 1994 Tennessee considered a rule to require physicians who were accepting any new patients to accept patients in the state Medicaid program; however, the proposal was withdrawn before it became a rule.

Groups The second way to begin the physician-patient relationship is for the physician to agree to care for a group of patients. When one of the patients covered by the agreement seeks care from the physician, the physician assumes the duties of the relationship even though the physician has never seen the individual patient before. Examples of this second type of relationship are (1) agreements to provide on-call coverage to a hospital emergency room; (2) contracts to care for a panel of patients for an HMO or other managed care organization; and (3) agreements with companies, jails, prisons, nursing homes, schools, athletic teams, or others to provide certain kinds of coverage.

Office staff responsibilities   When a physician begins caring for a patient, the law will often assume that the physician has agreed to accept the responsibilities of a physician-patient relationship. In some states, listening to the patient's symptoms on the telephone or commenting on the patient's case may be sufficient to create a relationship. Thus, it is important for office staff members to be instructed about the correct responses to telephone and other inquiries, and to follow those instructions. This will help to assure that patients receive the care they need, and that duties are not inadvertently created which the physician is not able or willing to fulfill.

There are many ways that physician assistants, nurses, and others in medical offices are properly used to provide more efficient care. They assist the physician in fulfilling the duties of the physician-patient relationship, with the physician retaining the ultimate responsibility. Professional and technical staff need to understand, to fulfill, and to stay within the scope of their assigned duties, assuring that the physician becomes directly involved when needed.

Office staff members should follow the policies and practices established by the physician in responding to persons seeking appointments or consultation, so that needed care is given to those who are entitled to such care. When busy schedules cause delays in available appointments, careful attention should be paid to priorities to assure that emergency and emergent conditions are diagnosed and treated in a timely fashion.

Responsibility to attend patient   Physicians should not assume the responsibility of admitting a patient to a hospital unless the physician can attend the patient. A Florida physician admitted a patient to a hospital as a favor when the physician was at home recovering from an illness. The physician never saw the patient and attempted to limit his duty so that it would not include treatment after admission. The patient's brain abscess was not diagnosed before the patient died in the hospital a few days later. A Florida court ruled that the physician-patient relationship required that the physician see the patient; therefore, the physician could be sued for malpractice.

How the Relationship Is Ended

Once a physician-patient relationship is established, the physician has a duty to the patient. The physician must continue to provide timely medical care until the relationship is properly ended. A physician who fails to care for a patient with whom there is an ongoing relationship can be liable for "abandonment'' of the patient. The physician-patient relationship can end for any of the following reasons:

- Medical care is no longer required
- The patient ends the relationship
- Another physician accepts the transfer of the care of the patient
- The physician terminates the relationship with a proper notice of withdrawal that gives the patient enough time to find another physician

Contracts with HMOs, managed care groups, and other organizations may require specific procedures to be followed before the physician can withdraw from the relationship with patients covered by the contract, so such contracts should be reviewed before terminating the relationship with a covered patient. In addition, the physician can be temporarily excused from the duties to patients when unable to provide care, due to serious illness or the more pressing needs of another patient, but to the extent possible the physician should seek to arrange for alternative coverage.

Consent and Refusal

One important aspect of the physician's responsibility to the patient is the duty to obtain informed consent for certain procedures. The patient has the legal and moral right to decide which of the available treatments to accept and whether to have any treatment. The physician has a duty to provide the information necessary to make this decision an intelligent one.

Implied consent   Consent is implied for most minor procedures in physician offices. When a competent patient submits to a standard procedure with apparent knowledge of what is involved in the procedure, consent is implied. Thus, patients who hold out their arms for an injection give implied consent to the physical injection. This is why a signed informed consent is not obtained for many procedures.

However, when the patient will be anesthetized, when there are risks associated with the procedure that are not known to most patients, or when there are accepted alternatives some patients might choose, express consent should be obtained and documented when possible.

Informed consent   Obtaining informed consent is more than just the formal step of getting a signature on a consent form. For the consent to be informed, the patient must be given information concerning the procedure and the alternatives.

Physicians can delegate the explaining and the obtaining of the signature to others in the office. Staff members who are given this responsibility should inform the physician of questions that they cannot answer so that the physician can have further discussions with the patient before any consent form is signed. Patients should not be pressured to sign forms while they still have unanswered questions and concerns.

Refusal of treatment   Competent adult patients have a broad right to refuse treatment. While physicians and their staff may encourage acceptance of needed, appropriate treatment, the patient's ultimate decision should be respected, except in the rare cases where the state steps in to compel treatment, such as in child abuse cases or in commitment for mental illness.

Some patients cannot make their own decisions due to age, injury, or disability. In that case, someone else must make decisions for them.

Consent for minors   A parent or legal guardian can make most medical decisions for a minor child, as long as the decision is not considered child abuse. In situations where parental rights have been taken away or restricted or where custody has been adjudicated by a court in a divorce proceeding, local law must be examined to determine who may make medical decisions.

When a mature minor disagrees with a parental decision and consensus cannot be reached between the parents and child, local law must be examined to determine whether the parental consent is sufficient. In most states, the outcome will vary depending on the patient's condition and the nature of the procedure. For example, a parent may need the minor's concurrence to refuse life-sustaining treatment or to authorize cancer chemotherapy with a low rate of success, while a minor probably cannot refuse low-risk treatment that is likely to prevent or cure a condition that threatens death or significant harm.

Many states have special rules concerning consent for treatment of minors for sexually transmitted diseases, substance abuse, reproductive matters, and other conditions. These special rules often permit minors to consent without parental involvement and may prohibit informing parents of the treatment. Special arrangements should be made for payment for care that is subject to such confidentiality, because a bill sent to the parents' health insurer could violate the confidentiality requirement.

Incapacitated patients   When an adult is unable to make medical decisions, a surrogate previously designated by the patient or a legal guardian can make most medical decisions.

In most states, the law is less clear on when spouses or others can make decisions for incapacitated adult patients; they clearly have no authority to decide when the patient has the capacity to decide. Generally, when the wishes of the patient are not known and decisions concerning treatment can be deferred until the patient regains capacity, major decisions concerning treatment should wait until the patient can again decide. However, when the decisions cannot be deferred, many physicians accept the decisions of the spouse, next of kin, or other adults who have assumed responsibility for the patient.

In most states, this practice is usually acceptable. Before accepting such decisions concerning major procedures, local law should be checked. When there is more than one possible decision maker available and they disagree, legal consultation is advisable to determine if one decision maker has priority or there is a need for a court to resolve the disagreement. It is clear that family members cannot make decisions that are contrary to the known directions or preferences of the patient.

Referrals

No physician can know all of medicine, so every physician will encounter patients that need to be referred to other physicians or facilities. Physicians have a duty to recognize their limits and to make such referrals.

Managed care networks Managed care organizations (MCOs) increasingly have an influence on referrals in several ways. Many MCO networks are structured so that primary care physicians assume the responsibility for a wider range of conditions, thereby reducing referrals and costs. This places additional responsibility on primary care physicians to assure that they develop and maintain the knowledge to perform at this level. However, there remains a duty to refer when the patient's condition requires expertise that is outside the primary care physician's expertise.

Failure to make necessary referrals may be attacked not only as malpractice but also as discrimination. Recently a federal court ruled that a primary care physician in a managed care organization could be sued under the Americans with Disabilities Act for allegedly failing to treat or refer an HIV-positive patient.

On the other hand, patients cannot use nondiscrimination laws to force unnecessary referrals. In 1993, when an HIV-positive patient sued seeking to require more appointments with an HMO physician, the court ruled that nine appointments in ten months, plus three referrals to specialists, demonstrated that there was no discrimination.

Inside the MCO network Many MCO networks are structured to keep referrals within the network. In some cases this is in the contract between the physician and the network. Even where it is not in the physician's contract, the physician should be attentive to network panels when making referrals, because patients frequently will not have any coverage or will have reduced coverage for out-of-network services.

Although patients should assume the responsibility for keeping track of their own networks, many fail to do so and become angry when they receive a bill after being referred to a specialist who is not part of the network. Thus, the medical office staff can help the physician to keep track of the various, changing networks.

Outside the MCO network There will be situations where physicians may feel it necessary to refer patients to specialists outside the network. The physician should inform the patient that the referral is out-of-network and may cost the patient more in medical bills, and give the reasons for recommending an out-of-network referral, so the patient can have an opportunity to decide whether to accept the referral or seek an alternative.

Nondiscrimination

Physicians and their office staff cannot discriminate against persons on the grounds of race, color, national origin, or disability in deciding which patients to accept or how services are provided. In some localities other grounds for discrimination may also be prohibited.

Title VI of the Civil Rights Act of 1964 forbids discrimination on the basis of race, color, or national origin by anyone who receives federal financial assistance, which includes Medicare or Medicaid payments.

The Americans with Disabilities Act (ADA) forbids discrimination based on disability in privately owned places of public accommodation, which is defined to include the professional offices of health care providers. In 1994 a federal court decided that a dentist could be sued under the ADA for refusing to treat HIV-positive patients in his office.

The Rehabilitation Act of 1973 also prohibits discrimination against the disabled. This is the law that initially required offices to be made accessible to wheelchairs. In 1995 a federal court ruled that a deaf patient could sue a physician under the Rehabilitation Act for refusing to provide an interpreter in the office.

Under state law, a dentist in New York was accused of discrimination for taking extra precautions while treating an HIV-positive patient. A state administrative agency found that this was humiliating to the patient, but a court overruled the agency, finding that the precautions were not discriminatory. There is still sensitivity concerning steps taken to avoid transmission of HIV. Care should be used to assure that any precautions can be scientifically justified.

Discrimination on the basis of other characteristics, such as sexual orientation, is forbidden by some state or local laws.

Regulation by Government

Individual Licenses

Physicians, nurses, physician assistants, and many other professional and technical persons must have individual licenses or other permits from state and/or local governments.

Medical offices need to keep copies of the licenses and permits for the physicians and all other staff members who are required to have a license or a permit. The office also needs a tickler system to assure that each license and permit is renewed as needed. Although not required, many licensing agencies voluntarily send reminders for renewals, but the medical office should also have a system for tracking required renewals for its staff.

Continuing education   Many states require health care professionals to participate in a specified amount of continuing education to be eligible for license renewal. Since it can be disruptive to office scheduling for the licensees to fulfill the entire requirement just before the deadline, offices need a system to keep track of continuing education hours completed and to remind those involved not to postpone compliance. Many hospitals and other organizations have programs that count toward these requirements, and participating in these programs can make compliance easier.

Scope of practice   The law specifies what scope of practice is permitted for persons with each license or permit. The law also addresses what functions may be delegated by licensed persons. The scope of practice of the profession and the scope of permitted delegation varies from state to state.

Increasingly, more sophisticated functions are being performed by persons with less comprehensive medical training. This generally has occurred more rapidly in practice than has been permitted by the actual legal requirements. Occasionally physicians, nurses, and others have been criminally prosecuted or have been sued for malpractice for violating scope-of-practice restrictions. Thus, the fact that a particular practice pattern is occurring in other medical offices in a locality is not an assurance that the practice is permitted. Scope-of-practice issues include the following distinctions:

- Who may order procedures and medications
- Who may accept such orders
- Who may perform procedures or administer medications
- Whether procedures or medication administration must be performed under supervision
- What degree of supervision is required
- Who may interpret results or diagnose conditions
- Who may modify ordered procedures and medications

In addition to professional and technical licenses which are usually issued by the state, many localities require a local business license. Local business licenses usually do not have an impact on scope of practice; they are usually just procedures to register businesses and collect taxes.

Organizational Licenses

Hospitals, ambulatory surgery centers, and a variety of other health care organizations require organizational licenses. Medical offices usually do not require such licenses unless the offices expand to where they constitute an ambulatory surgery center or they provide other services that require an organizational license.

Building Permits

Medical offices like other buildings must comply with local land-use and zoning restrictions and must obtain required building permits and certificates of occupancy before they can be used.

X-Ray and Other Equipment Permits

All states have special licensure or permit requirements for radiology equipment. Medical offices that have radiology equipment must comply with the applicable regulations and maintain the required licenses or permits.

Some states require licenses or permits for other equipment, so local requirements should be investigated.

In some states that still have certificate-of-need requirements, physicians may have to obtain a state certificate of need before acquiring some expensive equipment.

Narcotic and Drug Regulation

Narcotic and other drug possession, prescription, and use is heavily regulated by both the federal and state governments. A practitioner must have a certificate from the Drug Enforcement Agency (DEA) to possess or prescribe controlled substances, or must fall within the list of persons exempt from registration, which includes resident physicians acting under a hospital DEA registration and some agents of practitioners.

Controlled substances   Controlled substances are divided into five groups, called schedules. Each schedule has a different level of control, with Schedule I having the most controls. Schedules I through IV require an order of a practitioner before they can be dispensed. The order must be in the form of a prescription that includes all of the information required by federal law. There is an exception that permits a chart order to be used for patients who are hospital inpatients. (For details of each schedule, see Appendix B.)

When a practitioner signs a blank controlled-substance prescription and someone else later fills the prescription in, both the practitioner and the person who fills in the blanks commit federal crimes. Thus, office personnel should avoid this practice.

When controlled substances are stored in the office, there must be adequate precautions and procedures to protect against theft and diversion. An accurate record of all drug utilization must be maintained. Medical office staff can assist the physician in avoiding violations in the following ways:

- Keep careful, required records
- Control access to prescription pads
- Lock places where drugs are stored
- Assure that drugs are stored under appropriate conditions
- Dispose of drugs properly when expiration dates are reached or when a portion of a drug remains after the ordered amount is administered to a patient

Investigational drugs   Drugs and devices must be approved by the U.S. Food and Drug Administration (FDA) before they can be used outside of investigational contexts. Before such approval, an investigational new drug (IND) or a device that is subject to an investigation device exemption (IDE) can be used only in the context of approved research or certain other limited clinical uses.

There are extensive record-keeping requirements with which physicians using these investigational drugs and devices must comply. Falsifying these records has led to criminal prosecution of physicians. Medicare, Medicaid, and most third-party payers refuse to pay for some or all use of INDs and IDEs. Thus, when billing for services to patients that involve INDs and IDEs, applicable restrictions need to be checked to assure that a prohibited bill is not submitted.

State laws   Some states impose additional requirements for uses of drugs and devices, so local law should also be checked. For example, some states limit the circumstances in which drugs can be dispensed from physician offices without a special permit under the state pharmacy law. The definitions of the terms in these laws need to be read carefully. Restrictions on dispensing generally apply only to giving drugs to patients to take home for use outside the office. Administration of drugs within the office is generally not considered to be dispensing.

Office Laboratories

The federal Clinical Laboratory Improvement Act (CLIA) regulates nearly all laboratories, including laboratories in physician offices, unless only a very narrow list of tests are performed which are exempt from the Act. The Act requires all nonexempt laboratories to comply with detailed regulations; for example, the persons performing the testing must meet certain standards, the accuracy of the testing periodically must be checked with a reference laboratory, and extensive records must be kept. Some medical offices stopped performing laboratory testing when the Act took effect, but many others complied and continue testing.

Other Rules

There are other governmental rules that apply to physician offices. For example, biohazardous wastes must be disposed of in accordance with law. Occupational Safety and Health Act (OSHA) rules mandate steps to protect health care employees from blood-borne diseases.

Certification and Accreditation

In addition to government regulation, there are many kinds of private certification and accreditation. Physicians and their offices are not required by government to comply with the requirements of these certification and accreditation agencies, but as a practical matter approval by these agencies may be essential to practices in many settings. When in those settings, these private requirements must be taken seriously.

Hospital Medical Staff

Most physicians need to be authorized to admit patients to a hospital in order to practice. The major exception is some physicians who have an entirely office-based practice. However, physicians with office-based practices need medical-staff membership in a hospital to be eligible for some managed care contracts.

A physician must be a member of a hospital medical staff to admit patients to the hospital. The physician is then authorized to treat the patient within the scope of the clinical privileges granted by the hospital.

Requirements   Physicians do not have a right to be admitted to the medical staff of any hospital; they must first prove that they meet the requirements. Then they must continue to meet the requirements or they can be removed from the staff. Most hospitals mandate physicians to adhere to the following requirements:

1. To provide continuous care for admitted patients, promptly responding to calls from hospital staff
2. To complete medical records promptly
3. To attend meetings
4. To demonstrate a level of activity at the hospital
5. To participate in scheduled emergency room on-call status
6. To inform the hospital promptly of events such as licensure complaints and malpractice cases

Medical office staff can assist physicians in keeping track of and meeting their hospital obligations.

Managed Care Organizations (MCOs)

Increasingly, managed care organizations (MCOs) are requiring that all their providers meet certain standards. As MCOs control where their patients go for care, it is essential in many settings to meet their standards and to contract with them in order to maintain a practice.

One of the accrediting bodies for managed care organizations, the National Committee for Quality Assurance (NCQA), requires that the MCOs conduct a site visit of physician offices, so that the physical facilities, organization, and record keeping in the office can be checked. Medical office staff should become familiar with NCQA requirements. (For a description of NCQA standards, see Chapter 3, "Quality of Care.")

Some physicians and their office staff have expressed concern about the legality of allowing site reviewers to have access to medical records for the review. Each office should check its state law on this issue, but in most states the review can be conducted either on (1) records of patients of the MCO (who will have signed releases as part of the enrollment process) or (2) blinded records of other patients. Blinded records are copies of the records with all identifiers deleted (such as names, addresses, phone numbers, patient numbers). Usually a copy of the original record is made and then, on the copy, the deleted material is covered with opaque tape, marker, or fluid. This deletion process is usually performed by office staff, so that patient identities are not disclosed outside the office without patient consent.

Board Certification

There are many private organizations that certify that their members meet the standards of the organization. The number of certifying bodies has expanded rapidly, so they have varying degrees of acceptance and recognition. The core medical, dental, osteopathic and podiatric boards have achieved considerable recognition. The American Board of Medical Specialties (ABMS) recognizes 23 medical specialty boards, but there are over 100 other medical boards that the ABMS does not recognize.

Certification usually requires the following: (1) successfully completing an approved training program, (2) performing a specified number of procedures under supervision, and (3) passing an examination.

Certification is generally voluntary; few if any states require it for licensure. However, many physicians seek certification because of its importance to their practices. Many hospitals and MCOs prefer board-certified physicians, and it is often easier to obtain specialty clinical privileges in hospitals when board-certified.

Some hospitals require board certification, but this violates the Medicare prohibition on requiring board certification, so most hospitals provide an exceptions process by which physicians can demonstrate their training and experience in a specialty in other ways. It can be difficult to make a sufficient demonstration, so physicians desiring to practice in a specialty generally prefer to obtain board certification.

Some boards require physicians to complete continuing education in their specialty or other requirements in order to periodically renew certification. It is important for office staff members to keep track of these requirements in the same way that licensure requirements are tracked.

The Relationship with Payers

Contracts

Physician practices are increasingly dependent on maintaining contracts with hospitals and third-party payers—such as health maintenance organizations (HMOs), preferred provider organizations (PPOs), and managed care organizations (MCOs)—or with organizations that contract with third-party payers on behalf of the physician and others, including independent practice associations (IPAs), physician-hospital organizations (PHOs), and other integrated delivery systems.

Each medical office should have a procedure for administering these contracts, to assure compliance with their varied requirements by both the physician and the other party to the contract. This tracking of contracts is also necessary so that opportunities for renewal or termination are not overlooked.

Contract requirements can include, for example, mandatory reports, prior approvals, billing restrictions, and copayment and deductible conditions that must be met by the patient. Thus, it is important to identify which contract governs each patient. Since patients or their employers often change plans, office staff members should always inquire of each patient whether there has been a change in plan.

The other party to the contract has also made promises; these may include assigning a certain number of patients, making certain payments at certain times, and other steps. Compliance should be monitored by the medical office. Violations may simply be oversights that can be corrected if called to the attention of the other party. However, violations may also signal that the other party is having problems, either financial or administrative. Many providers have lost substantial amounts of money when third-party payers have failed. Early detection of problems may permit steps to correct the problems or to minimize the adverse impact on the physician's practice.

Prior Approvals

Many third-party payers require prior approval for many procedures. In some HMO situations, this may mean local approval by the primary care gatekeeper. In many situations, prior approval must be obtained from an external approver, generally by a telephone call to a distant and often unavailable approver. This is one of the more frustrating aspects of operating a medical office today. Unfortunately there is no shortcut; the only solution that has yet been found is persistence and patience.

Such approvals are essential. Only in very rare emergency situations can third-party payers be compelled to pay when the required prior approvals were not obtained.

When approvals are obtained, they should be well-documented. However, third-party payers can sometimes avoid paying for procedures even after giving approval, if they later determine that the person was not covered by the plan or that false or inaccurate information concerning the patient's condition was supplied when obtaining the approval. Thus, it can be helpful to document what information was given concerning the patient's condition. It is also important that the records of the approved care document all of the aspects of the patient's condition that were reported to the third-party payer in obtaining the approval.

Capitation

Capitation describes a plan whereby a provider or network of providers contracts to provide all the necessary care for a group of persons at the rate of a fixed amount per person per month. Sometimes single-specialty physician networks contract to provide all the care in a specialty on this basis. The network assumes the risk that the demand will exceed its ability to provide services; the network benefits when demand can be kept within projected bounds. Careful analysis is required to determine whether the network has the resources to prudently assume the risk.

Capitated specialty groups usually require approval from primary care gatekeepers in order to keep demand within the costs covered by the capitation payment. Other procedures are needed within the network to assure that there are appropriate controls over procedures and that needed procedures are not being denied to patients. (For details on capitation and managed care, see Chapter 4, "Managed Care.")

Coding, Billing, and Collections

Under most payment systems, records of services must be generated, coded, and converted into a bill. Proper coding is important. Inaccurate coding either can result in less payment than the physician is entitled to or can be considered a false claim that exposes the physician and those doing the coding to criminal and other penalties.

Unless an outside billing and collection service is used, the physician's office staff will have the primary responsibility to generate an accurate bill and pursue initial collection steps. There are state and federal restrictions on the steps that can be taken to collect consumer debts, including the federal Fair Debt Collection Practices Act and the Fair Credit Reporting Act. These laws are designed to protect consumers from harassment and from misrepresentations. Billing and collection procedures and practices should be designed to comply with these restrictions. (For details on billing and collection, see Chapter 10, "Financial Management.")

Two special rules should be kept in mind in billing. First, when a patient files for bankruptcy, the office must stop all efforts to collect directly from the patient and may need to make a claim in the bankruptcy proceeding before the deadline. It is a violation of federal law to continue billing the patient directly. Second, when a patient dies, there is usually only one way to collect from the patient's estate and that is by making a claim in the estate proceeding. Most states have deadlines for making such claims.

Handling Medical Information

Record Keeping

Physicians are required by law to maintain adequate records to document the services that they have provided. This is required both for individual licensing and for payment.

Accurate record keeping is also necessary to provide proper care and to prove that proper care has been given. Thus, accurate and proper records are important to avoid malpractice and to defend malpractice claims. The integrity of the contemporaneous record must also be maintained. Alteration of a record can cast doubt on the entire record.

The medical office should have a procedure for assuring that records are completed and filed so that they are readily available for subsequent care. Records needed to be flagged to assure that needed follow-up contacts are made. (For details on medical records, see Chapter 9, "Health Information Management.")

Confidentiality

Patients disclose sensitive information to their physicians in order to assure proper diagnosis and care. It is the physician's duty to maintain the confidentiality of this information and only to release the information when permitted by the patient.

The entire office staff must be carefully trained and disciplined to maintain confidentiality. There should be clear policies on what disclosures are permitted and when patient consent to disclosures should be obtained. Whenever office staff members have any doubt whether a disclosure is permitted, they should check with the physician.

Confidentiality applies to any discussion about patients and their health around the office or elsewhere where others may hear.

Confidentiality also includes not permitting unauthorized persons to have access to files and computer databases. In one instance, a secretary in a Florida clinic permitted her daughter to use her computer terminal. The daughter copied down patient names and phone numbers and called the patients, telling them falsely that they were HIV-positive. The daughter was indicted and the mother lost her job.

Most states have special rules concerning disclosure of information concerning HIV status. There are federal and state rules restricting disclosure of information concerning substance abuse treatment. These and other special confidentiality rules should be considered in structuring disclosure policies in offices.

Required Reports and Disclosures

State and local laws require that some events and conditions be reported, including births and deaths, many contagious diseases, child abuse, and elder abuse. Some states and localities require reporting of domestic violence, gunshot wounds, other wounds of violence, industrial accidents, and radiation incidents. State and local law should be reviewed to determine what reports are required, so that procedures can be established to assure that required reports are generated and submitted to the proper authorities.

Leases and Other Contracts

Office and Equipment Leases

Many physicians lease their offices and some of the equipment in the offices. Office staff members should keep track of the leases, so that the physician can do what is required to comply with the lease, take steps to assure that the other party is fulfilling its duties, and prepare for the termination of the lease, by arranging for an extension or arranging for alternate space or equipment.

Many leases are one-sided in favor of the landlord or equipment owner. When the lease is first entered or when the other party wants an extension, it is often possible to negotiate changes in some of the more one-sided provisions.

Some states have laws that give tenants and landlords rights that are not spelled out in the lease. Thus, in disputes concerning leases, a review of state and local law is often helpful. Landlords frequently have legal procedures to expeditiously remove tenants who do not pay the rent that is due, even if there is a dispute over the amount. Therefore, it is important to involve an attorney before withholding rent.

Employment Contracts

Contracts between physicians and medical practices vary according to the type of practice. Office staff members usually do not have contracts but letters of agreement; these also vary according to the type of practice. (For details, see Chapter 7, "Personnel Policies.")

Liability

Medical Malpractice Liability

Patients who have injuries caused by the failure to fulfill medical duties can sue for medical malpractice. They generally must prove four things to establish liability:

1. Duty
2. Breach of duty
3. Injury
4. Causation

The patient is usually the plaintiff (the person bringing the suit), but in some circumstances it is possible for others to sue on behalf of the patient or for their own related injuries.

Duty   There are two aspects to duty that must be proven. First, it must be shown that a duty was owed to the person harmed. Second, it must be shown what that duty was. This scope of the duty is often called the *standard of care.*

Proving that there is a physician-patient relationship proves the first aspect, although this becomes more complicated if there is a question whether a relationship has started or if someone with no direct relationship with the physician claims a duty. For example, sometimes persons who are injured in automobile accidents with patients who are on medications or have epileptic seizures sue the patient's physician, claiming the physician owed them a duty to warn the patient not to drive. Sometimes family members or others who contract contagious diseases from patients sue a physician, claiming the physician owed them a duty to prevent the spread of the disease. Courts vary on when they find duties to others in these and other circumstances.

In proving the second aspect (what the duty was), the patient must prove what the provider should have done differently under the circumstances. This is usually proven by having another physician testify. Sometimes written standards can be used to prove the standard of care.

Many medical organizations are developing practice parameters and other guidelines for how various conditions should be handled by physicians. Following these guidelines will establish that the physician met the standard of care.

A few states have passed laws giving certain guidelines extra weight in determining the standard of care. Physicians should become familiar with the guidelines that apply to their type of practice, in order to take advantage of these protections and to avoid the possibility of increased liability from not following the practice guidelines.

Breach of duty   The plaintiff must then prove some act or omission that deviated from the standard of care. This can be proven by showing that there was some action performed that should not have been performed or by proving that there was some action that should have been performed which was not.

Injury   The plaintiff must prove some legally recognized physical, financial, or emotional injury. In most malpractice cases, it is not difficult to prove some injury, so that the dispute focuses on the dollar amount to assign to that injury.

Causation   The plaintiff must prove that the injury was caused by the deviation from the standard of care. This is often the most difficult part of the case for the plaintiff. Plaintiffs can usually prove that something was not done correctly and that there was a bad outcome, but this is not enough for liability without showing that there was a substantial likelihood that the incorrect action caused the bad outcome. There are often many other more likely causes for the bad outcome.

Responding to Complaints and Incidents

Many patients who could file lawsuits decide not to do so. The way that the physician and the office staff treat patients and the way that they respond to complaints and incidents can help to avoid suits. Establishing and maintaining a good relationship with the patient can create an atmosphere for dealing with incidents within the relationship. When complaints and incidents occur, the physician should be promptly informed, so that they can be responded to and so necessary reports can be made to insurers and lawyers.

Records related to patients involved in such incidents should be protected and should not be altered.

By promptly and constructively addressing any adverse situation, further problems can often be minimized.

Responding to Suits

When suits are filed (or letters of intent to sue are received), it is important to promptly turn them over to an attorney for defense. When the physician is insured, the insurer should be informed and will usually designate the attorney to use for defense.

In the unusual case where office staff members are named as defendants in the suit, then a determination will be made whether the insurer is covering their liability and whether the physician's attorney will defend them or if they need their own attorney.

The case should not be discussed with anyone and records should not released to anyone, except as directed by the defense attorney. Many states have complicated procedures that must be followed in the stages before malpractice suits and after the suit is filed. Failure to follow these steps can jeopardize the defense of the suit, so it is important to cooperate with the defense attorney. Records should not be altered or misplaced.

Depositions At some stage of the suit, it is likely that office staff members who witnessed the events will have their depositions taken. This is an official question-and-answer period with the plaintiff's attorney, during which the questions and answers are recorded by a court reporter. It is important to prepare well for depositions. If a different answer is given at the trial, the deposition can be used at the trial to demonstrate that the story has been changed, casting doubt on the truth of the witness or the ability of the witness to remember the events.

A deposition is usually not the time to try to tell your side of the story or to blame others. Answers should be focused on the questions asked. Listen carefully to the questions, and when questions are not understood, ask for clarification before answering.

Insurance

Most physicians maintain liability insurance for malpractice and for other liability that can arise out of operation of an office. It is important to make sure that the insurance policies are kept up to date and that premiums are paid on time. (For details on insurance, see Chapter 10, "Financial Management.")

In some areas, malpractice insurance is so expensive for certain specialities that physicians do not obtain malpractice insurance. Some states have special requirements that uninsured physicians must meet.

Liability and the Office Staff

When there is a malpractice suit due to actions of the office staff that cause injury to patients, usually the employing physician is sued. It is unusual for medical office staff members to be sued in malpractice cases, since employers are liable for the negligent acts of their employees under the doctrine of *respondeat superior,* "let the master answer."

However, it is possible for the office staff member to also be sued. Anyone who performs a function has a duty to perform that function properly. When that duty is breached, causing injury to someone, there is the possibility of liability. Thus, you and other office staff members should find out whether you are covered by the physician's professional liability (malpractice) insurance policy. Such coverage is advantageous to both you and the physician because it assures that there is a common defense. When physicians are uninsured, you should determine what arrangements have been made for responding to lawsuits.

Lawful orders Office staff members need to carry out the reasonable and lawful orders of the physician. It is important to be familiar with the licensing laws and rules in your state to know the limits of what the physician can order you and other office staff to do.

Some duties can be performed only by physicians or other licensed personnel. An illegal order to a person without the necessary license to perform one of these duties cannot be followed. Some functions can be performed only under supervision. You and other office staff performing the function should determine that the required level of supervision is available before undertaking such functions.

Office staff members need to stay within the boundaries established by the physician. A physician does not have to delegate any function to the office staff. The physician can limit the scope of activities of even licensed persons in the office.

Whenever you or other staff members are uncomfortable with or do not understand an order, you have a responsibility to seek clarification before carrying out the order. Sometimes orders may appear to be erroneous; you should check such orders with the physician to avoid mistakes. Each person should be aware of his or her own level of competence and not venture outside that level. Level of competence can change with training and experience, but there needs to be appropriate training and closely supervised experience to assure that patients receive appropriate care during the process.

Written task list It is helpful for the physician to give assistants who are assigned clinical tasks a written list of the clinical tasks that the assistant is expected and permitted to perform. The list should indicate the degree of supervision required and when direct orders from the physician are required. The licensing laws of the state, the skills of the assistant, and the practice pattern of the physician will determine the content of the list.

Patient outcomes   Never promise a patient a good outcome. Office staff members need to be careful whenever reassuring patients that they do not inadvertently promise a specific outcome. It is possible to create a contract, so that there can be liability for failing to achieve the outcome without any errors in the treatment. Some states require "contracts to cure" to be in writing to be enforceable, which provides some protection against inadvertently creating a contract in those states. However, in all states it is best to avoid appearing to promise too much, because unrealistic expectations increase the risk of ultimate patient dissatisfaction.

Prior care   Office staff should not evaluate or criticize care the patient has received prior to coming to your medical practice. If you are given the job of questioning the patient about prior medications, record the answers, but do not comment on whether the medications were good or bad. Only the physician should make judgments about the appropriateness of medications. Moreover, neither you nor the physician knows what the patient's condition was when the prescription was made, so it is inappropriate to criticize. It is better for the physician to make needed adjustments in the medications and discuss prior medications only to the extent that they have a bearing on the future condition and care of the patient.

It is not the job of office staff members to diagnose the complaint or to prescribe medications, except for staff who are licensed and authorized to diagnose and prescribe. In some states, physician assistants, nurse practitioners, and registered nurses can make some diagnostic decisions and can write selected prescriptions. Other staff members should not assume these roles.

Potential liability   Office staff can help to avoid other areas of potential liability by taking the following steps:

1. Avoid slippery floors. Be alert to spills and have them cleaned up promptly. When floors are washed or waxed, be sure that staff and patients are alerted to slippery spots and are kept off them to the extent possible.
2. Help patients who require assistance with walking, dressing, getting on examination tables, and other preparations for examinations.
3. Do not leave patients who need assistance unattended in examining rooms and toilet areas. Very ill, infirm, infant, and very young patients frequently require special attention.
4. Keep equipment in a clean, safe, operating condition.
5. Follow appropriate precautions to avoid the spread of transmissible disease.

Other Civil Liability

There is a possibility of civil liability on grounds other than medical malpractice. There are what are called *intentional torts,* which include assault and battery, defamation (libel and slander), false imprisonment, invasion of privacy, and intentional infliction of emotional distress.

Assault and battery You commit an *assault* when you put another person in fear of being touched in a way that is offensive, insulting, provoking, or physically injurious, unless you have legal authority of consent. When such touching actually occurs, you have committed a *battery*. Assault or battery can occur when medical treatment is given without consent or other legal authority. They can also occur when trying to restrain patients when the law does not permit such restraint.

Defamation You commit defamation when you wrongfully injure another person's reputation. When defamation is written it is called *libel;* when spoken, it is called *slander*. When you release inaccurate medical information or you make untruthful statements about other persons you can commit defamation. It is best to avoid all gossip about others.

False imprisonment When you restrict another person's freedom without legal authority you commit false imprisonment. Patients who are detained in a hospital or office or are committed to mental institutions sometimes claim that it is false imprisonment. This is an unusual occurrence in most medical offices. If the physician's practice involves such detention, it is important to be familiar with state law concerning when detaining the patient is permitted and what procedures need to be followed.

Invasion of privacy Unauthorized release of patient information can result in claims of invasion of privacy. This is another reason to follow office policies as to the release of information and not to discuss patients outside the office or in the office in places where patients and others can hear the conversation.

Intentional infliction of emotional distress When emotional trauma is caused by outrageous conduct, there is the risk of liability for the intentional infliction of emotional distress. In one instance, an Ohio physician was found liable for this tort when he had his office staff send repeated reminders to a deceased patient's family to have her come in for a checkup. The family had sued the physician for her death. The court noted that while the first reminder could have been an error, the office should have had a procedure to update its records when a patient died. However, after the family informed the office of the first reminder, there was no excuse for the subsequent reminders.

Criminal Liability

Physicians and medical office staff need to be aware of the increasing use of the criminal law to address activities that affect physician offices. Three such areas have already been discussed:

1. Bills for services that were not provided, were not billable, were improperly coded, or were otherwise in violation of law can result in criminal prosecutions for false claims, mail fraud, and other criminal violations.

2. Violations of the laws concerning prescribing and handling controlled substances can result in criminal prosecutions.

3. Violations of licensing laws can result in criminal liability for the illegal practice of medicine or for the violation of licensing laws concerning other professions and services.

Conclusion

The law will continue to have an impact on how medical care is provided as long as the public continues to place a high value on appropriate medical care. All interaction with the law cannot be avoided, but some precautions can maximize compliance and minimize negative encounters with the legal system.

This chapter has been designed to help you spot some of the areas where precautions may be helpful. A short chapter like this cannot provide definitive answers, but it should give you some of the steps and help you to know when to ask questions about other important issues.

Chapter 3

Quality of Care

The Importance of Quality in Medical Care   45
The Definition of Quality   47
Measuring Quality—Historical Background   48
Implementing TQM in the Medical Office   53
Integrating TQM and QA Activities   65
Conclusion   68

The Importance of Quality in Medical Care

All providers of health services, regardless of their size or specialty, want to believe they provide high quality of care for their patients. In recent years, however, the groups that pay for medical care have focused attention on the need for improved quality, given the increasing amount of money being spent on health care. This concern over quality in health care stems from several sources.

Current Concerns

Regional variations One source is research that consistently shows variations among physician practices in different parts of the United States as to the number of surgeries and the types of medical procedures used to diagnose or treat the same illness. These variations in treatment are accompanied by variations in outcomes (such as infant mortality) among different popula-tions. For instance, if physicians in one region of the country perform twice the number of cesarean sections, without a measurable improvement in the health of mothers and infants, then are cesarean sections being performed too often in that region?

Uniform agreement Another source of concern is the lack of uniform agree-ment about the best diagnosis or treatment for a condition, which often results in physicians performing different tests and treatments for the same condition, again without measurable improvement in the patient's health. Which diagnosis or treatment should be followed? To provide physicians with information about the best practices or methods, expert panels of physicians in some specialties study the evidence supporting care that results in better outcomes. The information is then disseminated to practicing physicians to help them choose the best course for their patients. Whenever available, this information on the best practices should be used by medical offices to assure quality of care.

Reimbursement   A third source of concern about quality of care originates from reimbursement entities—such as insurance companies, Medicare, Medicaid, employers, and other third-party payers—as well as from patients and their families. Questions focus on such issues as whether early detection and prevention should be a covered benefit, whether experimental treatments should be covered, under what circumstances certain tests or treatments should be administered, or whether co-payments and deductibles should be required to discourage unnecessary use of medical services. Reimbursement decisions have a profound effect on a patient's quality of care because they also affect the access to care.

Access to care   This last concern—an individual's access to quality health care—is based on the important physician-patient relationship. If a physician performs the right procedure for the right condition in a textbook fashion but does not also address the patient's needs or questions, the patient may not return for follow-up care, may refuse to comply with the treatment, or may lose confidence and trust in the physician. The patient-physician relationship is a vital factor in the quality of care, contributing to a patient's satisfaction with the physician and the medical office staff.

Medical Offices

Medical offices must also be concerned with the quality of their services. In the current health care environment, they must respond to the demand for quality from a wide range of interested parties: government regulators (notably the Health Care Financing Administration, which runs Medicaid and Medicare, and state licensing and payment agencies); private payers (indemnity insurers and health maintenance organizations); and medical providers with which a physician or medical group engages in contracts for services (managed care companies, hospitals, nursing homes, and others). Each group wants some assurance that the services it regulates, pays for, or contracts for meet its quality criteria and standards.

In this chapter, staff members and managers in the medical office will learn how to measure quality of care in order to meet the demands for information from these various groups. In addition, staff members will learn methods of continuous monitoring and improving quality of care, as set forth in the principles of Total Quality Management (TQM). TQM permits the medical office to continuously improve its services, to become more efficient and effective, and to involve physicians, nurses, clerical staff, and other medical office workers in a quality improvement team.

The Definition of Quality

While it is true that quality is an elusive concept and definitions of quality may vary, a medical office must have a set of objective criteria and standards against which it can measure its services.

Simply stated, *quality* is the degree of excellence of medical care. As defined by the Institute of Medicine, "Quality of care is the degree to which health services for individuals and populations increase the likelihood of desired health outcomes and are consistent with current professional knowledge."

Outcomes of Care

Note an important element of this definition: it focuses on *outcomes* of care. Despite whatever services a physician has rendered, if the care given does not increase the likelihood that the patient will have a positive outcome, the care is not of the highest quality. To focus on health outcomes means also that quality is not assured merely by the physician's education, credentials, and technical performance. While these factors may improve the likelihood of quality, quality itself is proven by the health outcomes resulting from the services provided by the physician.

This definition of quality also requires that the outcomes are *desired.* The process of care has included the patient's wishes, desires, and needs. The physician and the patient have decided together on the course of care and the expected outcome. The patient and/or the patient's family have been given options, understand the consequences of different approaches to diagnosis and treatment, and are full partners with the physician in the patient's care.

Current Professional Knowledge

In addition, the definition of quality states that the health services *are consistent with current professional knowledge.* Quality is time-bound because professional knowledge changes rapidly. Outcomes achieved by certain methods today may be improved tomorrow by knowledge gained in future research. For instance, in the 1960s patients with ulcers often received a treatment involving freezing of ulcerated tissue, with mixed results; today new drugs make treatment for ulcers safe and effective. In the 1970s cataract surgery required surgical procedures to be performed under general anesthesia; today new surgical techniques provide many patients with outpatient treatment. A treatment which is commonplace today will probably be replaced by a more effective treatment in the future.

But current professional knowledge is not defined merely as the practice currently in use by most physicians. Many current medical practices come into common use before they are thoroughly tested for their effectiveness. The federal government has taken a lead role in assessing the effectiveness, safety, and utility of new drugs and devices, but many new procedures or medical technologies are adopted for widespread use by physicans without the necessary tests to determine the types of patients and health conditions for which they are most effective. Some new procedures are adopted merely because they are new, before their effectiveness can be determined. Only through amassing the necessary research about a procedure, surgery, treatment, or diagnostic test can physicians know the most effective treatment in terms of health benefits. Therefore, physicians and medical office staff members are responsible for keeping abreast of the results of research inquiries and incorporating them into their practice.

Measuring Quality—Historical Background

One of the first treatises on quality was the Hippocratic oath, which outlined an ethical code in which the physician, at the least, promised to do no harm. It did not, however, outline how to do the patient good.

In the 20th century, as medical care became more effective, issues of access to services and their cost and efficiency began to arise. In the 1930s a national committee was charged with studying the medical care system and recommending ways to make it more accessible. A set of fundamentals of good medical care was the result, which emphasized the following:

1. Scientifically based care
2. Importance of prevention
3. Informed patient input into decisions
4. Treatment of the whole patient and not merely the disease
5. Continuity in the physician-patient relationship
6. Coordination with social work services and other medical services
7. Comprehensiveness of care

In the 1940s and 1950s various individual researchers tried to measure the quality of medical practices, but the real impetus for a more systematic method to assess quality of care came after the passage of Medicare and Medicaid legislation in the mid-1960s.

Structure, Process, and Outcomes

One of the first to shape the quality movement was the physician and U.S. university professor Avedis Donabedian. Beginning in the 1960s, his use of the terms *structure, process,* and *outcome* defined the efforts to measure the quality of care.

Structure The *structure of care* refers mainly to the physical facilities, the medical staff, and the administrative organization. Examples of structural measures of quality include the following:

- Qualifications of physicians and other staff members
- Existence of written policies and procedures for performance of care
- Adequate staff-to-patient ratios
- Access to appropriate equipment for the diagnosis and treatment of patients
- Safe and clean waiting, exam, and treatment facilities
- Adequate patient charts and medical information systems

Donabedian states that structural measures of quality are based on two assumptions: (1) that qualified physicians, better physical plants, or good organization increase the likelihood that care will be better; and (2) that we know what better structural aspects of care look like. The structure of care can only set the stage for quality.

Structural aspects are easy to measure and have been popular with health care accreditation and licensure entities. Many such groups also require process and outcomes measures as well.

Process   Another measurable aspect of quality, the *process of care* includes diagnosis, treatment, and follow-up services provided directly by health care professionals. Process includes the technical application of knowledge and the interpersonal skills to listen and respond to the patient's need for information and reassurance.

The quality of the process is best assessed by comparing the process to accepted norms or standards for diagnosis and treatment of given health conditions. The amount, type, and frequency of services, as well as the professional's adeptness in performing services, contribute to the overall quality of care. For instance, a physician may diagnose and treat a patient's high blood pressure, but also may stress the importance of the patient's complying with medication; this results in a better process than if the patient were not counseled in medication compliance.

In addition, many studies of the process of care have shown that the best care is given by physicians who perform at least a minimal number of procedures. For instance, better heart surgeries are performed by physicians who have done a certain number of heart surgeries over a minimum time period. In other words, the technical quality of the process of care usually improves with the physician's experience.

However, the *process* of care is harder to measure than the *structure* of care. Measuring process requires access to medical records, direct observation of services or the patient-physician interaction, laboratory results, health insurance claims, or direct evidence of care, and comparing these measures against a standard. It also assumes that the most appropriate process of care for each health condition is understood and that it results in the best health outcome. This may not be true, given the changing nature of medical knowledge, the lack of systematic evaluation of many processes for diagnosis and treatment, and the tendency of physicians to follow the norms of practice in their community, despite a practice's lack of proven effectiveness.

Outcomes   Since the ultimate goal of medical care is improvement in a patient's health, the *outcomes of care* become important, when added to the other two aspects of care.

Outcomes include death, disability, surgical survival, surgical complications, physical functioning of the patient, physiological measures, emotional health, well-being, symptoms, and the satisfaction of both the patient and the provider. Using outcomes of care to measure quality assumes that other influences on health status (such as patient compliance, nutrition, or genetics) are small, or that they can be accounted for.

A paradox of only using outcomes to measure quality is that some patients' health may improve despite bad care or no care at all, and that bad outcomes may occur despite care considered to meet all the currently known standards.

Interrelated aspects   The structure, process, outcome model conceived by Donabedian assumes a relationship among the three aspects of care (see Figure 3.1). Good structure should provide a basis for good process, which should result ultimately in good outcomes. Some believe that measuring only one aspect of care is not enough. Many of the quality assurance mechanisms in place in the 1970s measured two aspects: structure and process. Current quality improvement methods require measurement of any or all three aspects of care, but they focus more on measuring outcomes.

Fig. 3.1   The Three Aspects of Quality

Structure ⇨	Process ⇨	Outcome
Facilities	*Technical Aspects:* Prevention	*Health Status:* Mortality
Equipment		Morbidity
Materials	Diagnosis	
Organization of resources	Treatment	Symptoms
Administrative structure	Patient education	Physical functioning
Financial resources	*Interpersonal Aspects:* Communication between patient and medical staff	Mental functioning
Medical staff		Well-being
Nonmedical staff	Joint decision making for desired outcome	*Satisfaction:* Patient satisfaction
		Staff satisfaction

(Adapted from Donabedian 1969, 1980)

Programs to Measure Quality

Government programs With the unexpected rise in medical costs shortly after the implementation of Medicare and Medicaid, many questioned the necessity and quality of services under these public programs. At the same time, insurance companies began to use the same quality methods for contracting with hospitals and physicians for services. The Joint Commission on Accreditation of Hospitals (JCAH) was formed in 1951 to accredit hospitals for participation in insurance reimbursement. Most of the JCAH criteria measured the structure of care: the physical plant of the hospital, its organizational structure, and its professional staff qualifications. Other aspects of assuring quality of health care were handled at the state level through licensure standards for health care professionals and for health facilities.

In 1972 Congress passed a law requiring services provided under Medicare to undergo *peer review*, whereby professionals judge other professionals' quality of work. The law set up Professional Standards Review Organizations (PSROs), composed of physicians and other medical professionals, to review the admission and continuing stay of Medicare patients in hospitals. The process used by the PSRO to review hospital length of stay became known as *utilization review*. Some large Blue Cross organizations and other insurance companies also used similar utilization review systems in the 1960s and 1970s. (For details on utilization review, see Chapter 4, "Managed Care.")

Private programs In the 1980s most insurance companies and HMOs used this system of hospital admission and continued-stay authorization for payment. In the early 1980s the PSRO system was replaced by the PRO (Peer Review Organization) system; and the new Medicare DRG (diagnosis-related group) system of payment—based on the average length of stay for a particular diagnosis—made review of claims for length of stay redundant.

Accreditation standards for hospital, and later for ambulatory care facilities and HMOs, required them to institute a quality assessment and assurance program as an ongoing process of monitoring and implementing system changes to improve the quality of services. Most hospitals created departments of quality assessment—to perform data collection and length-of-stay review—and formed quality assurance committees—to carry out medical audits and chart reviews.

TQM

By the mid-1980s, however, other systems of quality improvement began to cross over from industry, where they had gained momentum in response to competition from Japan and other countries for quality and efficiency in production. After World War II, several Japanese industries had asked the American quality-control experts W. Edwards Deming and Joseph Juran to teach Japanese workers the system of quality improvement known as Total Quality Management (TQM) or Continuous Quality Improvement (CQI).

These methods were then adopted by the Joint Commission on Accreditation of Healthcare Organizations (JCAHO, the former JCAH) and incorporated formally into accreditation standards in their Agenda for Change.

The philosophy of TQM/CQI includes the following features:

1. Systems and processes, not people, are the causes of defects
2. Workers actually involved in a process, not managers, are the best sources of ideas for process improvement
3. Empowerment of workers to improve processes enables teamwork and results in improved satisfaction for all internal and external customers of a process
4. Improvement in a process results in improvement of the quality of the final product

The term *process* used by TQM means any activity in the health care setting, not just the process of care.

TQM and QA compared   TQM differs in several respects from quality assurance (QA). First, QA seeks out the *people* who are not performing up to standard and sanctions them to perform better; while TQM seeks out the *processes* that do not perform well, tries to find causes and solutions, and then implements solutions.

Second, QA is based on a review of events after they have taken place, while TQM provides a means for preventing adverse events in the first place, through improving processes continually.

Third, QA seeks to meet a set of predetermined standards, based on the norms of practice; while TQM seeks to improve the overall performance, and is not bound by current standards.

Fourth, the actors differ in the two systems. QA efforts are defined, measured, monitored, and focused on clinical areas and topics, led by medical professionals and managers. TQM involves all medical office employees—from receptionists to medical department heads—in a team effort to improve all of the following: office functions, patient flow, patient information, communication among workers, laboratory testing and information, patient scheduling and telephone response, patient diagnosis and treatment processes, and any other activities of the office.

Criteria   TQM and CQI are now required in many accreditation criteria for medical organizations by such accrediting bodies as the National Committee for Quality Assurance (NCQA), JCAHO, the Accreditation Association for Ambulatory Health Care (AAAHC), and others.

While the science and art of quality measurement and assurance are changing rapidly, the medical office can be certain about the continuing need to measure itself and improve all its activities, in order to compete for patients, for reimbursement, and for good physicians, nurses, and other staff. The next section describes the methods of TQM as they apply to the medical office. The implementation of quality improvement techniques is very complex, and medical office staff members charged with these duties should obtain further information and training before attempting to direct a quality improvement effort.

Implementing TQM in the Medical Office

As mentioned earlier, TQM describes a philosophy of medical office management as well as a method of tracking, measuring, and implementing change to improve the quality of care. All activities or processes of the office rely on each other, and problems in one process lead to problems in other processes. The output of a process might be a patient, information, materials, or ideas; that output then becomes the input into another process.

Interrelationships

The output from a process benefits not only the patients but also the staff members of the medical office. (In business, these beneficiaries are "customers.") Within the medical office, everyone affects and relies on each other's work: physicians receive patients and patient information; patient scheduling requires good telephone communications systems; billing and claims clerks receive information from other staff members. These tasks involve the "internal customers" of a process.

The patients served by the medical office, the health plans that pay for medical-office services, and the other health care organizations that provide medical services (such as hospitals, labs, medical supply companies, and pharmacies) are the "external customers" of a process. In addition, customers of one process are also suppliers for another process. Therefore, quality improvement in the medical office leads to improved customer satisfaction with all its services.

Using a single process   An example from a large multispecialty group practice illustrates the importance of using a single process for different situations. Two letters were received from two different patients. The first letter, from the dissatisfied family of a patient diagnosed with pancreatic cancer, reported that the physician did not adequately listen to their concerns or address the patient's problem with chronic pain. The second letter, from a satisfied patient, reported that the physician listened carefully to a problem with recurrent abdominal pain; the patient was very happy with the attention received from the physician.

These two opposite letters involved the same physician. The patients' different reactions to their treatments lay in the scheduling of their visits. The first patient was seen in a 20-minute slot for urgent visits, by the physician on call for the day. When the physician realized the complexity of the patient's pancreatic cancer but could not obtain all the necessary information within the time allotted, an appointment was made with the patient's primary care physician for the next day. The on-call physician was not satisfied with the short visit and knew that the patient was also dissatisfied.

The second patient was seen during a longer, 40-minute visit. The physician obtained a full history of the patient's problem, and presented the theory that the gastrointestinal pain might be caused by lead-based paint the patient used as an artist. The physician had ample time to listen to the patient's concerns and to order appropriate tests. The patient's visit fell within the allotted time frame, and both the physician and the patient were satisfied after the visit.

In both instances, peer review of the cases showed that the physician performed the correct procedures for each patient, given the allotted time. But the office scheduling procedure did not allow the more complicated patient to be allotted a longer appointment time. Had office procedures allowed a review of the patient's complexity and subsequently a more appropriate scheduling, both the patient and the physician would have had better experiences, and the reputation of the physician and the clinic would not have suffered.

Benefiting from the process   In this illustration the process—the appointment system—affects or benefits the internal customers (medical office staff), which include the clerks, appointment managers, physicians, and the staff member who received the letter. A problem in a process can affect patient satisfaction, use of resources, and physician efficiency and satisfaction.

CQI   In TQM the goal is to make processes exceed customer expectations through incremental improvements, thus the term "continuous quality improvement" (CQI). After initial problems are identified, solutions may be attempted and monitored for their effects, then changed again.

As shown in Figure 3.2, this cycle of TQM is sometimes described by its component steps:
- Plan
- Do
- Check
- Act

The *plan* phase involves identifying problems in processes, measuring current performance to find the causes of problems, putting together teams involved in the process, and developing a detailed plan of action for process improvement. The *do* phase is the implementation of the improvement plan. The *check* phase measures the action's effects on the process. The *act* phase involves standardizing the actions that work. The cycle then begins again. Specific methods for use in each phase of TQM are described in the following pages.

Plan

In the planning phase, techniques are used to identify problems in the medical office in any activity, to measure their current performance, to analyze

Fig. 3.2   The TQM Cycle

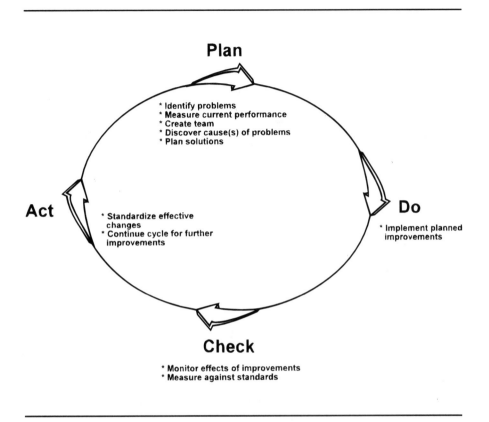

the process and its problems, and to choose actions to improve the process. At the end of the planning phase, a statement for improving the process is produced, including a time frame for action and standards of measurement to determine if the actions have effectively solved the problems. Each of the steps in the *plan* phase is described below.

Identify problems   Problems in the functioning of the medical office arise daily. Administrative and medical staff are all aware of problems that are chronic in nature or that interfere with office procedures such as effective patient care, scheduling, billing, communication, or the efficient use of staff members. A good candidate for a quality improvement project is a process that has one or more of the following characteristics:

- It causes serious downtime for staff.
- It affects many other office processes, even though in itself it seems to be small.
- It is expensive for the office to operate, and may not seem worth the time, effort, or money it uses.

- It is the source of many complaints from either patients, physicians, nurses, office staff, or nonpatient customers such as hospitals, labs, or suppliers.

Measure current performance   Sources of improvement projects come from office and medical staff, from patients or other outside groups, and from reports of medical offices that have performed a similar improvement project. At some point in the process of project identification, the group steering the quality improvement process (often called the *quality council*), will want more documentation on the extent and seriousness of the problem.

For instance, if the problem is that lab results are taking too long to be returned to the patient's chart, the quality council may query another medical office served by the same lab. Is the turnaround time for that office's lab reports similar? If it is, the council reexamines its office's own processes to further define the problem. A quick survey of medical-records staff then reveals that the incoming lab reports are the last items to be filed every day. The problem is then identified as the filing process used by the records staff.

Another example of problem identification could be patient complaints with phone access to physicians. A survey of physicians at the weekly staff meeting reveals that they would be glad to return phone calls during the day between appointments, but the phone messages are not available in their mailboxes or the messages are often unclear. The staff might then keep a log of complaints from patients and staff about phone messages to determine the volume and type of problems with the phone system. Or a phone survey of the patients calling the office during a week might ask if their messages were received. Or the physicians might simply jot down problems as they occur.

TQM tools for problem identification and performance measurement   Specific tools for data collection, problem identification, and performance measurement have been borrowed from business management and are widely used in TQM.

One of these tools is the *flowchart*, a visual diagram of the major points of activity in a process. A flowchart can help identify all the activities and decision points in a process and indicate the flow of patients, materials, information, or other work along the process. Wasteful movements or errors along the process will become clearer. A flowchart of a lab report, from patient sample to lab and finally to filing in the patient chart, is shown in Figure 3.3. After the current flowchart of a process has been drawn, another chart can be drawn to show the process in its ideal state, using it to work on solutions.

Another tool for problem identification is the *cause-and-effect diagram*. In a team meeting, or through information gathered from the staff involved in a process, the causes of a problem can be listed. A cause-and-effect diagram of the problem of lab results being filed late in patient charts is shown in Figure 3.4. A cause-and-effect diagram can show the multiple theories about the cause of a problem. Different team members will often have different perspectives about a problem and, therefore, different theories of its cause. Identifying all potential causes will help pinpoint the real problem in a process.

Fig. 3.3   Flowchart

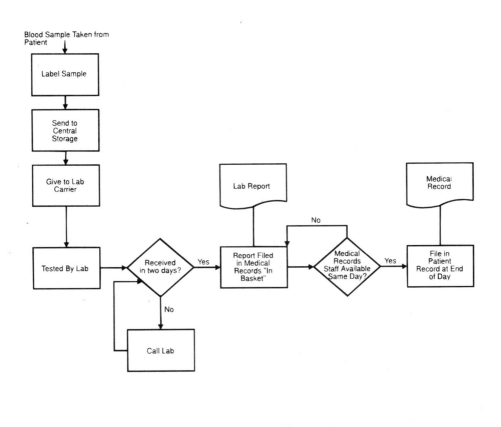

A tool used for data collection is a *data sheet*. Figure 3.5 shows one used to collect data on patient complaints with the phone system. Data sheets can be developed by a medical office to meet the specific data collection needs of the project.

Assemble the team   Either before or after measuring the current system's performance, a team of staff members is assembled, including a physician who works closely with the process under review. The team's task is to collect data on the problem and its causes, to develop workable innovations and plan their implementation, then to measure the innovations' effectiveness and to make changes in policies and procedures that standardize the improvements.

Fig. 3.4   Cause-and Effect Diagram

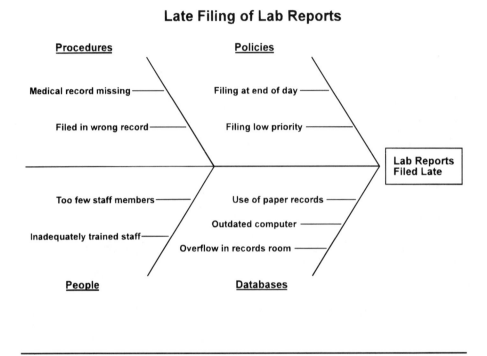

Late Filing of Lab Reports

Team development is an important feature of TQM. Assembling effective teams in medical care can be difficult because of barriers to involving physicians, the small staff of some medical offices, and the difficulty of scheduling time away from patient care. One solution is to ask an outside consultant or a quality expert from a local hospital to aid the team in its formation and with its data collection and analysis tasks. However, the key to a workable quality improvement program is that it remain the responsibility of the medical office staff and not be run solely by managers or an outside consultant. Without the involvement of the medical office staff, improvements will be harder to implement and may not work because of a lack of understanding or a perception that changes are being thrust upon them from above.

TQM tools for use by teams   Management tools exist to help teams identify problems, work on solutions, and plan implementation. Among these tools is the use of *brainstorming,* the process of getting team members to suggest as many ideas as possible, without criticism or editorial comment on an idea's

Fig. 3.5   Data Collection Sheet

Phone Complaints Log

Week	Line Busy	Placed on Hold	Tardy Callback	Incorrect Message	Other	Total
5/6	I		I	III		5
5/13		I	III	II		6
5/20			IIII	I		5
5/27	I	I	III	III		8
6/3	I		ЖΗΛ I	II		9
6/10		I	IIII	II	I	8
Total	3	3	21	13	I	41

usefulness. Brainstorming can be carried out in several ways: one is to ask each person of the team to suggest an idea, going around the table until all ideas have been heard; another way is for all team members to submit their ideas in writing. This second method is useful when staff members may be intimidated in a meeting with more authoritative or assertive people.

Another TQM tool for team members is *nominal group technique,* whereby a team comes to consensus about a problem or a solution. A list of the issues, problems, or solutions to be considered is distributed to each member of the team, who then ranks the items by priority. For instance, if five solutions to the problem of lab-report filing have been listed, each team member ranks them from best to worst. All the votes are tallied, and the solution with the highest overall ranking is the consensus of the group. (An alternative to this method is to delete the lowest-ranking items after the first vote, and to continue voting on the remaining items until a clear "winner" emerges.)

Nominal group technique has the advantage of being able to sort through multiple items on an agenda, allowing all team members to have input. Because it uses anonymous voting, it is especially useful for voting on controversial issues.

Develop and plan solutions   At this stage of TQM, the team will consider and choose among various solutions to the problems identified, and plan to implement the changes they believe will result in the desired outcomes. The plan for improvement should state (1) what is to be changed, (2) how the change will be accomplished, (3) what the deadlines will be for implementing the change, and (4) what outcomes will be expected in a specific time frame.

For example, with the problem of delayed phone messages from patients, assume that the team has decided to institute a change in the phone system, so that physicians will now receive a direct voice-mail message from the patient. This system will allow the physicians to answer up-to-date messages during a lull in office activity, and patients will feel that they have greater access to the physician. A date is set for the new system of voice mail to be instituted by the phone company, which agrees to train all office staff and physicians on the new system.

TQM tools for developing plans for improvement   These tools are similar to the tools used in earlier phases of the planning process. Brainstorming, nominal group technique, cause-and-effect diagrams, and flowcharting can all be useful for deciding the courses of action to solve a problem. Other planning methods, such as Gantt charts, help outline the objectives and timetables for the actions, define responsibility of staff for the actions, and provide clear statements of what measurements will be taken during implementation. The planning stage for a TQM improvement may become incorporated in the strategic planning for the overall organization.

Do

In the second or *do* stage of TQM, the improvements decided on in the planning stage are implemented. The team follows the agreed time frames, keeps the staff on task, assures that the implementation of improvements is as effective as possible, and gathers data on the entire process.

In the example of implementing a new voice-mail system, the telephone company is kept to its dates for training, and those staff who are trained then train others who missed the original session. Physicians are given instructions in a medical staff meeting. At first there may be resistance to learning a new telephone system, but the physician representative on the TQM team explains all the reasons for the new system and that phone messages will be easier to handle and more accurate. A few glitches on the first days of implementation are followed up immediately by the phone manager of the clinic.

Check

In the third or *check* stage, the TQM team monitors the progress of implementation on a continuing basis. At the end of the planned implementation, the team meets to review information about the improvements and to decide whether the goals have been met.

Monitoring the process   Several different charting methods can be used to check on implementation, such as a bar chart, Pareto chart, or run chart. These methods may also be used to diagnose a problem, before implementing a change.

Bar chart   A *bar chart* is a summary of data collected over time, presented in the form of a graph. A bar chart of data collected for patient complaints

Fig. 3.6 Bar Chart

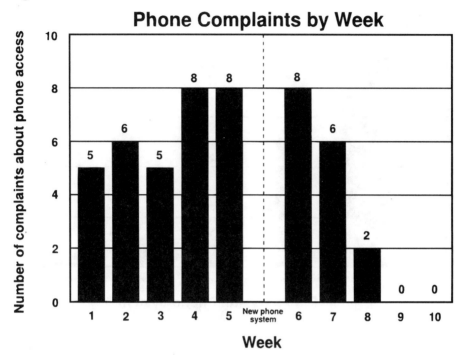

about the telephone system is shown in Figure 3.6. The bar chart shows the relative frequency of the number of complaints from patients tracked by week, both before and after use of the new telephone system. The decline of complaints after the new telephone system can be seen easily.

Pareto chart A *Pareto chart* presents a summary of data much like a bar chart but shows causes of problems by order of frequency, and therefore focuses the analysis on the worst problems in a process. A Pareto chart is based on the principle that a small number of causes ("the vital few") are usually the main source of overall system problems. These vital few problems can then be targeted for solutions. Figure 3.7 charts the information from the data collection sheet for telephone complaints. It is easy to see that most complaints are about lag time in returned calls, and inaccurate messages.

Using a Pareto chart helps the team focus on the problems that have the greatest potential for improvement and is therefore useful in the problem identification stage. The Pareto chart can also be used to track changes in problems after an innovation has been implemented. For the phone-system example, the TQM team would analyze another Pareto chart of the number and type of patient complaints after implementing the voice-mail phone sys-

Fig. 3.7 Pareto Chart

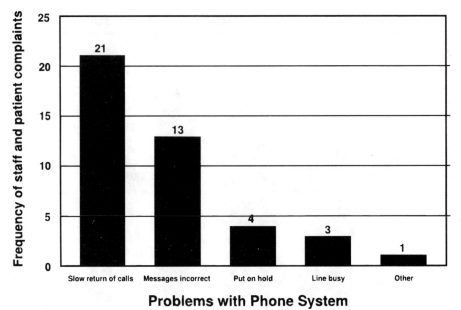

Problems with Phone System

tem. The team would expect fewer total complaints and a lower distribution of complaints.

Run chart Similar to a bar chart, a *run chart* allows a team to track performance over time, looking for trends and patterns. It can help detect changes in a process due to planned or unplanned innovation, and can help predict future trends in a process. In the phone-system example, the number of complaints was tracked over time (see Figure 3.8). The first change noted was due to the implementation of the new voice-mail phone system. The second change was caused when a receptionist was unavoidably absent and a replacement had to be trained.

Act

In the fourth or *act* phase of TQM, the information gathered during the implementation is reviewed by the team. If the change has had the planned effect, the team may recommend that the change become permanent. In the example of the new voice-mail system, a quick survey several weeks after its installation shows that staff members are happy with the new system, after they have become used to it. Data show that it reduces phone complaints from patients and physicians. The team recommends that all staff have voice mail throughout the office.

In some cases, the data may show a need for further improvement. If, for instance, there are fewer complaints about incorrect messages but continuing

Fig. 3.8   Run Chart

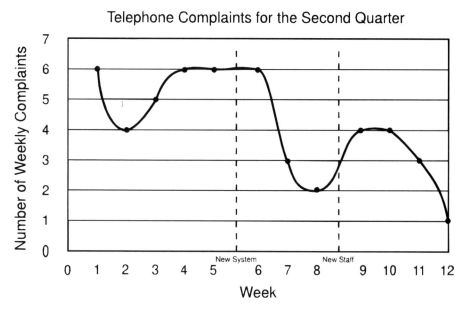

complaints about lag time in physicians returning phone calls, another team-driven TQM process would start again, beginning with brainstorming about ways to correct that problem.

The final part of the *act* stage involves writing new policies and procedures to institute the new changes.

Using TQM

The scenario below follows a hypothetical problem through the four phases of TQM—planning, doing, checking, and acting.

> **Plan**   A medical office has begun to have cash-flow problems, as noted by the physician-owner, Dr. Smith, and the office manager, Ms. Barnes. Because both are very busy with daily office management, they decide to involve other staff members in solving the cash-flow problem. An initial meeting is called with the billing clerk; Dr. Smith states that it is his goal to have all accounts receivable resolved within 90 days of the medical service given to a patient. With this standard in mind, the billing clerk and the office manager begin a TQM process with the office's accounts receivable.
>
> *Identify the problem*   There are many accounts from which the office receives reimbursement, including Medicare, Medicaid, private insurance, workers' compensation, and managed care contracts. Since the office has recently begun to see a larger volume of Medicaid patients, both the clerk and Ms. Barnes suspect a problem with Medicaid claims.

Assemble the team   They assemble a team to resolve the problem, adding a clerical staff member who does both medical records and business office tasks and a clerk from the business office. The first meeting of the team is spent brainstorming all the potential problems that might be causing delays in Medicaid payments. They build a cause-and-effect diagram showing the following causes: office billing and coding errors; Medicaid check-writing delays; Medicaid eligibility errors; medical records delays; and delays in depositing Medicaid checks. One member of the team is assigned to gather more information on each cause and to report at the next meeting.

In the second meeting, team members report on their investigations of the various causes of delayed Medicaid payments. There are no eligibility problems of note—Medicaid check-writing has not changed from the usual 40–60 days during the last year; and there has been no delay in depositing checks. However, since the office has nearly doubled the number of Medicaid patients, a few small errors in claims have caused delays in receiving large Medicaid payments. The billing clerk reports a claim error rate of 5 percent, the same as in the previous year but causing double the number of denied claims, which had to be resubmitted.

For the next meeting, the team brings every claim that was resubmitted during the past year for study. They tally the different types of claim errors on a data sheet, noting whether the claim was returned for the wrong diagnostic code, the wrong service code, the wrong doctor or patient identifier, and other problems. When all the claims have been tallied, the largest number of errors is found to occur in diagnostic coding.

Plan the solution   With this information in hand, the team reports to the executive staff of the medical office, and obtains approval for special training by the Medicaid claims office. It is planned that all clerical staff and medical records staff will receive training by Medicaid on the diagnostic coding system that they use. The training is arranged for a date of implementation, and the plan includes having the trained staff train any new office staff for the next three months.

Do   The plan is implemented, and the office manager assures that all the appropriate staff members receive training and that the Medicaid trainer certifies they are capable of effectively coding claims using the Medicaid system. During the next three months, no new staff members are hired. The office manager observes the number of Medicaid claims and notes when any claim is returned for any error. Claim errors are marked on a data sheet.

Check   At the end of the three months, the team meets again and goes over the data, which have been graphed in a line graph for easy interpretation. The number of claim errors has dramatically dropped to only 0.5 percent during the entire three months, and has stayed at this low level. The team concludes that the training has been effective.

Act   In order to assure that claims errors remain low, the team prepares a one-page report to the executive staff stating the effectiveness of training and requesting that the personnel policies be changed to include Medicaid claims training for newly hired clerical staff. The new change is approved and written into the personnel policies. The office manager monitors Medicaid claims carefully for the next year, and checks to assure that two new staff are given appropriate training.

Multiple TQM Projects

The TQM process may involve more than one project at a time, for resolution of different problems by different teams of staff members. However, the medical office staff should not attempt too many TQM projects simultaneously. First, data collection for multiple projects may become burdensome and time-consuming. Second, simultaneous changes in more than one process may become confusing and the effects difficult to distinguish. This is especially true in cases where the processes being changed are closely related.

Integrating TQM and QA Activities

Many medical offices are already dealing with the needs of managed care organizations (MCOs), and accrediting and licensure bodies for data about their performance. Performance data gathered for these purposes can easily serve as the basis for TQM activities to improve patient satisfaction, patient care outcomes, and relations with other providers. Some specific areas of performance in the medical office are being scrutinized by MCOs as precondition to a contract with an MCO. These areas of performance should be part of any TQM process, to aid the medical office in its ability to respond to MCOs and to compete for patients.

NCQA Standards

The National Committee for Quality Assurance (NCQA) requires that MCOs conduct site visits to all primary-care physician offices and to the offices of specialists with a high volume of the MCO's patients. The following are scrutinized in the site visits:

- Physical accessibility of the office: ability of the patient to enter and exit the office easily, despite any disability
- Physical appearance of the office: cleanliness and safety; attractiveness and comfort
- Adequacy of waiting and examining room space: size and comfort of waiting areas; ratio of exam rooms to number of patients treated
- Adequacy of medical records: filing; maintenance of confidentiality
- Adequacy of medical record-keeping system

In the site visit, the MCO credentialing staff may perform a review of a sample of records. NCQA standards require that medical records be maintained "in a manner that is current, detailed, organized, and permits effective patient care and quality review." Records must reflect all aspects of patient care, including ancillary services, and must be available to health care practitioners at each encounter. The medical office may be asked by the MCO to conduct periodic audits of medical records for their accuracy, completeness, and legibility; or the MCO itself may perform such audits, according to their contract with the medical office. (For more on medical records, see Chapter 9, "Health Information Management.")

Practice Guidelines

Another aspect of quality monitoring builds on the problems and prospects of past quality systems. One current effort is to establish valid and reliable measures of the outcomes of health care by implementing standard practice guidelines developed by national medical experts in various specialties.

Measuring outcomes   The effort to reliably measure the outcomes of care is based on (1) the rising costs of care; (2) competition for services, partly due to the growth of managed care and the reduction in hospital beds; and (3) a variation among physicians in their use of technology, surgery, hospital care, and other services, with little or no difference shown by their patients' outcomes.

Federal studies   The federal Agency for Health Care Policy and Research (AHCPR) has funded the Medical Treatment Effectiveness Program, with the special-project Patient Outcomes Research Teams (PORTs), to analyze the effectiveness of the diagnosis and treatment of discrete diagnoses. The studies focus on patient-centered health outcomes, including patient functioning, emotional health, and satisfaction with care.

Using research findings and the expert opinion of panels of professionals (consensus panels), practice guidelines are produced by the AHCPR, by physician specialty groups, and by other health care organizations. *Practice guidelines* are statements to help the practitioner and the patient decide about appropriate care for specific clinical conditions, based on review of available scientific evidence. According to the AHCPR, practice guidelines "specify processes of care that are known or believed to be associated with good outcomes." Practice guidelines may be used in the future by reimbursement entities to define reimbursable care for patients with specific diagnoses.

Critical Paths

Closely related to practice guidelines in their goal to improve the process and outcomes of care are critical paths or patient care protocols. Borrowed from business TQM terms, a *critical path* is described as an optimal timing of interventions by physicians, nurses, and other staff for a particular diagnosis or procedure, designed to minimize delays and resource utilization and to maximize the quality of care.

Critical paths (or pathways) deal with interactions among providers of all services, showing specific timelines for the occurrence of interventions. Patients are managed by a case manager who assures that the interventions and their timing keep on schedule. Critical paths have been developed by teams of health professionals (such as physicians, nurse specialists, nutritionists, therapists, and others) for high-risk, high-cost treatments.

Most critical paths have been developed to cover a hospital stay, an entire episode of care from doctor's office to posthospitalization, or a specialized management of chronic illness. The use of critical paths aims to standardize the patient care plan, to improve the efficiency of care and communication among the team of providers, and to reduce errors and waiting time for medical orders.

Report Cards

Another effort to improve quality care is the use of the *report card*, a term used for a standardized mix of structure, process, and outcome measurements to assess the performance of a single physician, group of physicians, or other health providers such as MCOs, hospitals, and health plans. As managed care becomes more widespread, payers of care want the best physicians and providers for the least cost. Also, there is an increasing quest by patients and their families for comparative information about the quality of their health providers.

There currently is no consensus about the information that should be required in a report card. It may encompass the following:

1. Structural standards—such as the adequacy of the medical office's parking space, hours of operation, number of staff and their qualifications; and the physician's education, board certification, malpractice history, and admitting privileges
2. Process standards—such as the use of practice guidelines or critical paths, standards for the treatment of particular chronic diseases, preventive services and education of patients (for example, the percentage of women age 45 and older receiving appropriate breast cancer screening), or hospitalization patterns
3. Outcome standards—such as preventable deaths or surgical complications; the percentage of children immunized; and patient satisfaction with the office, its staff, and the care received

Report-card data are now required by some state agencies for licensure, by MCOs, by employer groups wishing to contract with physicians for their employees, and by insurance companies and others. The type of performance data required in the future may resemble that being piloted by the NCQA using HEDIS (Health Plan Employer Data and Information Set). HEDIS was developed nationally by employer groups and managed care organizations to provide data for employers to use when comparing competing health plans. The NCQA report-card pilot project includes data on the following:

- Member satisfaction
- Quality and access—rates of immunization of children, cholesterol screen-

ing, mammograms, Pap smears, prenatal care, diabetes retinal screening, illness care, asthma hospital admissions, and low birth weight
- Physician network—rate of physician turnover, and board certification
- Utilization—rates of coronary bypass surgery, angioplasty, cardiac catheterization, cholecystectomy, hysterectomy, prostatectomy, laminectomy, cesarean sections, readmissions for certain diagnoses, OB hospital stays, and total hospital days
- Membership and finance—various measures of insurance performance, including membership disenrollment

This is only one example of report-card performance data being considered for use on a nationwide scale. Medical offices should keep informed about developments in their own states, as well as developments on the national level.

Conclusion

Quality measurement, monitoring, and management are extremely important to the ultimate goal of improved patient health. In addition, medical offices must increasingly respond to internal and external sources to provide data about the quality of their patient care, especially patient outcomes. Prepared medical offices will be able to respond to the need for quality measurements, and to compete successfully for patients, reimbursement, and managed-care contracts.

This chapter can serve as the initial springboard for discussions among medical office staff members on their quality activities. Staff given the responsibility for quality assurance and improvement should do further reading, as noted in the list of references (see Appendix B). Quality assurance and improvement requires good data collection and analysis skills in an efficient search for better patient care, and many methods are available for specific use in these activities. Medical office staff should be aware of and able to use these tools.

New quality requirements should be constantly monitored by medical office staff. A good way to maintain access to the latest information is to become involved in a local or state chapter of quality assurance personnel.

With proper training and updated information, any medical office can implement and effectively maintain a quality improvement program. The well-prepared medical office should be able to provide the best quality patient care with the use of these tools and information.

Chapter 4

Managed Care

An Evolving System   69
HMO Models of Managed Care   73
Other Models of Managed Care   76
Specialized Managed-Care Models   79
Managing Utilization in HMOs   82
Managing Health Benefits   85
Provider System Models—Future Potential   86
Integrated Health Systems   91
Managing the Health of Populations   96

An Evolving System

Definition and Concept

Managed care is a concept for which there is no single definition or accepted set of principles. It describes particular types of organizational relationships within a health financing and health delivery system that is itself undergoing fundamental change. Thus, the concept of managed care is evolving.

Managed care is a term used historically to define a new type of health financing system—namely, a capitated system as opposed to a fee-for-service system—and the controls introduced to manage the new set of risk relationships. At the most general level, the term has been used to describe the relationship between the financing system (such as a health plan) and a delivery system (such as a medical practice). At a more specific level, managed care is used to describe controls introduced over medical costs by "managing" unit costs, the utilization of services, and the benefit package.

Managed care has been viewed by most providers in its relation to a health plan, the health plan being the managed care entity. It is frequently seen in terms of *them* and *us*, and frequently them *versus* us. This describes the nature of the traditional relationship between providers and a financing entity, in that managed care has consisted of a reformed financing system overlaid on a traditional health delivery system. However, because the capitated financing system received its payments based on a per-member–per-month fee for an enrolled population, it became at risk financially for the health services provided to that population; thus it had to introduce controls over the cost of providing care in order to manage that risk. The financing system therefore imposed external incentives and regulations on the delivery system and created an adversarial relationship.

The controls imposed by managed care on physicians and other delivery institutions were designed to change the behavior of providers who were accustomed to the incentives for increasing utilization and costs under the fee-for-service health systems. To a large degree, however, these externally imposed controls are being replaced by a process of shifting risk to the delivery system itself, which results in the development of internal structures for managing and controlling costs and assuring quality. These structures are only now emerging in the health system and are appropriately considered part of the managed care concept; in fact, they will increasingly serve as the basis for defining the concept of managed care.

In summary, managed care is a concept that describes (1) a type of financing mechanism where an organization becomes financially accountable for providing "needed health services" to a defined population, and (2) a related set of controls for managing costs and quality in the delivery system. These controls can be externally imposed on the delivery system, or the system itself can assume the financial risk and develop internal controls for managing care. These control structures are varied and complex, and need to be understood in terms of what they are intended to produce, what they actually produce, and how they affect various parts of the organization.

Reform of the Financing System

Historically, the health care system has been described as an "illness system" driven by the demand for medical care. When a person became ill, contact with the medical system was initiated with considerable freedom of choice by the patient. An assessment was made by a health professional, usually a physician, and services were provided. Payment was made through a fee-for-service structure, where physicians, hospitals, and other providers were paid for services rendered. As technology increased, the cost of services, particularly specialized services, became too high for individual patients and their families to pay.

Private plans　Private health insurance plans evolved out of the need to distribute to a broader population group the individual risk of incurring a major financial loss due to an expensive medical procedure. Blue Cross is credited with establishing the first sustained private health insurance plan in the early 1920s, by enrolling a group of teachers in a plan developed by Baylor University Hospital. The teachers paid an annual fee or premium and were provided coverage for 21 days of hospital care. Due to the large number of individuals enrolled in the plan, all were willing to pay a small amount to cover the risk of illness resulting in hospital care. These insurance plans, called *indemnity plans*, were established on the principle of retrospective reimbursement, provided on a cost-plus basis and designed to cover high-cost and high-tech hospital services. It is not surprising that these plans rewarded the utilization of inpatient hospital care, particularly high-tech care.

Capitation payments   Capitation payment systems totally altered the basis for payment and the incentives for utilizing health services. *Capitation* is a form of financing where a health organization accepts a predetermined amount of money per individual in a defined population—that is, on a capitated basis—expressed in terms of a per-member–per-month fee. It reverses the incentives of an organization from providing more health services to (1) keeping the enrolled population healthy and (2) reducing the utilization of expensive medical services, thus reducing the costs of health care. The incentives to "maintain" health gave rise to the term *health maintenance organization*, used initially as a general phrase to describe a feature of capitated health plans, and later as a label to identify them.

Capitation and health maintenance organizations (HMOs) became synonymous with managed care. While these terms include important aspects of managed care, they do not in themselves represent the full range of managed care concepts. However, they have served to define managed care over the last 25 years, and to a large degree they still do today.

Historical Background

The historical context of managed care can be best understood through two related organizational developments: the creation of medical group practices, and the development of capitated health plans. The structure of the clinical process rests on the relationship between a doctor and a patient, each having the freedom to participate in defining the course of treatment. This freedom of choice assured protection from rules, policies, or other interference by organizations.

Independence   The independent decisions of a doctor and patient, free from organizational control, provide the basic structure of health organizations and of the health system. As a result, physicians have practiced in independent private practices, accepting monetary or in-kind payment for services rendered. Physicians working for organizations or physicians receiving salaries were considered by the profession as an unacceptable form of organizational control. The relationship between physicians and hospitals was characterized by the same independence; the medical staff was separate from the hospital and granted privileges to practice based on its own recommendations.

This independent relationship was the basic building block of organizational structure that was, and still is, characteristic of the health system in the United States. Health maintenance organizations have developed within this fundamental structure of the health system. They have introduced new incentives that have changed clinical behavior and altered the structure of institutions, but they have not fundamentally altered the structure of the clinical process or the basis of clinical decision making.

The formation of early medical group practices was brought about, in part, by the need to create an organization that could receive prepaid capitation fees and assume risk for providing health care to a population. Even though early capitation agreements were rudimentary by today's standards, they were a major force in bringing physicians into group practices.

These fledgling plans were small and widely scattered, and went relatively unnoticed as a social development. They did create a furor in county and state medical associations where they occurred, because they threatened the autonomy of the doctor-patient relationship. The organization, with its policies and incentives, was in a position to alter the clinical function. This change was more threat than reality initially, but it did introduce the organization as an important factor in the clinical decision-making process.

Development of Managed Care Plans

One of the earliest private group practices was formed in the 1880s, when William and Charles Mayo joined with their father to build a large general practice with an emphasis on surgery. This practice was not formed for the purpose of receiving capitation payments but as a means of structuring medical practice among a group of physicians. The Mayo brothers wanted to specialize in surgery, so they recruited additional physicians as diagnosticians, allowing the brothers to concentrate on surgery. Initially, the clinic was a proprietary enterprise controlled by the Mayos, with profits distributed to all of the practicing physicians. It was later converted into a nonprofit organization, with all physicians becoming salaried staff. The practice became a prototype for the development of other prepaid group medical practices throughout the country.

Early cooperatives   During this period, early prepaid capitated plans began to emerge as alternatives to traditional practice and indemnity insurance. In fact, some HMOs often trace their history to several large cooperatives established between 1920 and 1950. These cooperatives, many of which are still in existence today, provided some of the best demonstrations of coordinated prepaid systems.

Unlike their successors, early cooperatives were not primarily motivated by cost containment. Many were driven to make specific health care reforms that met immediate needs of employee groups and families within their respective communities.

Prepaid prototype   Perhaps the best known of the early prepaid prototypes was the Kaiser Permanente Medical Care Program, established in 1938 to provide medical care to Kaiser construction employees and their families working on the Grand Coulee Dam. Similar programs to provide comprehensive services were developed for Kaiser shipyard and steel-mill workers in three different areas. Through its own complete facilities, which offered hospitals and clinics to its members, Kaiser Permanente was able to produce even greater efficiencies than other models. Following several expansions, which included opening up the membership to the public, Kaiser Permanente is today the nation's largest nongovernmental prepaid program for hospital and medical care.

HMO Models of Managed Care

Early Models

Models of managed care organizations have been designed historically around capitation and its relationship with physician groups. In fact, early models were developed by physicians and frequently became the basis for organizing physicians in a group practice. Managed care organizations were later formed by insurance companies, concerned that the indemnity insurance market could be eventually converted to capitated health plans. These health plans, or HMOs, needed to develop organizational linkages with physicians in order to control risk. Initially, the HMOs employed the physicians and later formed linkages with medical groups or created independent practice associations (IPAs). (For a glossary of terms used in managed care, see Appendix B.)

Medical group practice and other structures of medical practice were an essential part of managed care organizations, because health plans needed mechanisms to control unit costs and the utilization of health services, as a means of managing risk. By linking with and controlling the behavior of physicians, hospital utilization could also be controlled. Thus, the structure of managed care organizations became defined as the relationship between the HMO, or the financing function, and the organization of physicians, or the delivery function.

The relationship between HMOs and hospitals has evolved over the years from indifference or hostility by the hospitals to one of dependence. In the early years, when the percentage of the population enrolled in HMOs was small and hospitals still had a high level of utilization, the bargaining position of HMOs for reduced prices was limited. Later, as the percentage of patients in HMOs increased and the level of hospital utilization decreased, managed care organizations were able to negotiate considerable discounts for hospital services.

Three types of HMOs developed as the organizations became more prevalent: the staff model, the group model, and the network model.

Staff Models

In staff-model HMOs, the medical staff who serve the beneficiaries of the health plan are salaried employees of the plan. They are generally not allowed to serve fee-for-service patients. Staff-model HMOs tend to be large and to retain on staff a full range of medical specialists as well as primary care physicians. If needed medical services are not available inside the HMO, they are obtained through contracts with other physicians in the community.

Popularity with physicians The development of HMOs was initially based heavily on the staff model, although it represented the most extreme form of organizational control over physicians, in terms of the patient's freedom to select them. The popularity of staff models was partly due to the appeal they had for group physicians who believed in this form of organization of health services and who were not interested in forming independent practices. In addition, these physicians would endure less criticism about capitated health plans from their colleagues if they were within group practices than if they were practicing in community settings. Also, staff models were facilitated by the HMO Act of 1973, which provided capital resources for developing staff-model HMOs.

Staff-model HMOs were considered by many to be inherently superior models, because they eliminated financial incentives for physicians to increase utilization through repeat consultations, referrals, or hospitalization. These HMOs did achieve significant reductions in utilization over the traditional fee-for-service insurance plans with which they initially competed. However, as these HMOs came into competition with other HMO models, the superiority of the staff model to control utilization was less clear. Staff-model HMOs have also been criticized as being less productive, due to the removal of the financial incentive for physicians to increase productivity.

Advantages and disadvantages There are pros and cons when the staff-model HMO tries to strategically position itself in new areas. When it moves into a new market, it must secure a clinic, equipment, and staff to start operations. The clinic has to absorb the start-up costs until it becomes profitable, requiring significant capital outlays. This condition was compounded when the HMO Act of 1973 eliminated its grant-and-loan program. However, staff models have the advantage of being able to replicate their management and clinic systems, corporate culture, name recognition, and good will.

Staff-model HMOs have greater restrictions on the freedom of patients to select a physician, due to the self-contained nature of the HMO and its medical staff. This restrictive nature goes against the traditional culture of patients who feel that they have the right select their own physician and to go to the hospital of their choice.

Although staff-model HMOs have been described as having the greatest control over the clinical practice of the physician, this is true only in relative terms. The physician is restricted as to the panel of patients seen and is provided incentives for changing utilization behavior; however, the HMO does not fundamentally alter the clinical decision-making process, and physicians function in large part as independent professionals in the organization. Though physicians are employees of the HMO, clinical behavior is changed by introducing incentives and controls outside the clinical decision-making process, not by restructuring the clinical process itself.

Group Models
Group-model HMOs contract with multispecialty group practices that agree to provide services for the beneficiaries of the health plan. Physicians are

members of the group practice and not the health plan and are paid either on a salaried basis or through some other income distribution formula. The group model is considered a *closed panel*, because physicians have to be members of the group in order to participate in the plan. The group selects, evaluates, and rewards its members. The group might contract to assume all risk for the subscribers of the health plan, or it might contract to provide services on a predetermined cost basis.

Preexisting and created groups   The group practice might have existed prior to its affiliation with a health plan, or it might be created for the purpose of contracting with a health plan. The preexisting group might agree to an exclusive commitment to a given health plan, but it is probably more inclined to continue to function as an independent group, providing services to the plan and retaining fee-for-service patients. An independent group might provide services to more than one HMO.

A created group practice is more likely to have an exclusive arrangement with an HMO, and not to have service arrangements outside the beneficiaries of the health plan. Kaiser Permanente's group model, for example, is a created group that is exclusively committed to the Kaiser Health Plan. Although physicians are employed by the Permanente Medical Groups, they have no commitment outside the Kaiser Health Plan.

Advantages and disadvantages   Group-practice models have many of the same advantages and disadvantages as staff models. They might have a physician panel that is small and perceived as being restrictive by the plan beneficiaries. They also require considerable investment in time and capital to develop practices in new markets. However, due to increased flexibility in income sharing, they have demonstrated the potential for increased productivity.

Network Models

The network model is formed when an HMO links a series of medical groups to provide services to the beneficiaries of the health plan. The HMO initially might link existing groups but then create additional groups to fill in its provider system, covering gaps in services caused by increased enrollment or expanded regions. The groups in the network might initially be multispecialty groups, causing the HMO to encourage primary care physicians to form a group to fill a gap in its delivery system.

The participating medical groups typically are capitated for members assigned to it by the HMO. If outside referrals are needed, they are paid for by the group. The group would represent the HMO in a region and adopt some identity and standards of the HMO, but would function with considerable independence.

Advantages and disadvantages   The network-model HMO overcomes many of the disadvantages of a staff- or group-model HMO. Networks can be more quickly formed and expanded to cover wide geographic areas. They also require less capital investment and can build on the reputations and practices of the groups that participate. The disadvantage is that the participating groups might have different orientations, cultures, and management systems.

Independent Practice Associations (IPAs)

During the late 1970s and early 1980s, private physicians became more interested in HMOs primarily for defensive reasons—to protect themselves from the loss of patients. At the same time, federal funding to support capital costs of starting groups was being phased out. Because high developmental costs and diminishing federal funds made it increasingly difficult to develop staff-model HMOs, independent practice associations (IPAs) became more attractive.

An IPA is an HMO that contracts with an association of physicians. The association constitutes a separate organization for purposes of contracting, but the physicians in the IPA retain their independent offices and practices. The IPA-model HMO provides the greatest degree of autonomy for the participating physician, which has been both an advantage and disadvantage. The IPA becomes attractive to physicians because of its limited control over their practices, including both the business and clinical functions. However, because of the limited control over physician behavior, utilization management is more difficult.

Physicians join IPAs because they become threatened by the growth of HMOs, and this positions them for capitation contracts. They also join IPAs to retain the benefits of independent private practice.

Other Models of Managed Care

In the wake of the impact of HMOs, several other types of managed care entities were developed by insurance companies and health care providers. HMOs had an impact on the utilization of health services and the market for patients, and the traditional system had to respond in order to stay competitive. The increased competition caused traditional indemnity insurance plans to more aggressively control costs.

The percentage of the population enrolling in managed care plans increased in many communities to the degree that hospitals and medical groups were threatened and needed to seek arrangements with these plans. As the levels of utilization of hospital beds started a rapid decline, fierce competition among hospitals resulted. This enabled managed care plans to effectively negotiate deep discounts in hospital rates, sometimes below cost, as hospitals struggled to fill what had become excess capacity in many communities. These conditions produced such managed care entities as managed indemnity plans, preferred provider organizations (PPOs), exclusive provider organizations (EPOs), point-of-service plans (POS), and many others.

Managed Indemnity Plans

Managed indemnity plans grew rapidly in the 1980s, at the expense of traditional indemnity plans. They lack the financial incentives of transferring risk created by capitated systems, but competition with capitated plans introduced utilization management as a necessary means of controlling costs. Managed indemnity plans use the same types of external controls over the utilization of health services as HMOs do, by requiring that a utilization management company be notified whenever hospitalization occurs or is recommended. Notification may also be required for certain outpatient procedures. Insurance benefits are reduced for noncompliance with these requirements.

A utilization management company generally contracts to provide certification of referrals, hospital admissions, assignments of expected lengths of stay, and authorization for certain procedures through preadmission authorization and case management programs. Some utilization management companies specialize in catastrophic cases or workers' compensation cases.

Managed indemnity plans are often merely utilization review processes, but they have been effective in renewing the competitiveness of indemnity plans with HMO capitated models. They are considered to be "followers" in the process in that they are able to compete with capitated models in reducing utilization, but they have not led this process in communities where capitation has not already captured a significant percentage of the market. These plans provide an attractive option for many providers, but their ability to remain competitive will depend on the same external controls introduced by the HMO models. The managed indemnity models allow freedom of choice of providers, which is still highly valued by many providers and consumers.

Preferred Provider Organizations (PPOs)

Preferred provider organizations (PPOs) contract with insurance companies, or directly with employer groups, to purchase health services from a group of selected providers. Providers are chosen on the basis of their cost and quality positions, their reputations, and their willingness to participate. These plans are indemnity plans that offer financial incentives to beneficiaries—in the form of reduced deductibles or coinsurance—for receiving care from a designated group of providers. The preferred providers agree to offer discounts or all-inclusive rates in order to gain access to a volume of beneficiaries and potential patients.

These arrangements become more attractive to providers as the utilization of hospitals and other providers decreases. In addition, the volume of beneficiaries offered through PPOs increases the dependency of providers on these plans, because contracts typically include a large number of beneficiaries and enable the PPO to play one provider against another.

In reality, there are limited short-term cost savings to the insurance industry through PPOs, in that discounts of charges, sometimes below cost, do not in themselves reduce utilization and instead result in cost-shifting to other insurance products. This is the art of management under fee-for-service reimbursement, but it can become the "spiral of death" for providers, as they become more aggressive in competing for a smaller market. As an increased percentage of the market comes under managed care control, the issue of excess capacity of hospitals and specialists still causes stress and considerable change in the system.

As PPOs become more sophisticated, they start to assume risk on behalf of the insurance carrier and to introduce utilization controls and incentives similar to HMOs. Participating providers agree to accept the utilization-control mechanisms as part of the contract, which has a further long-term negative impact on utilization. Some health care plans with both PPO and HMO options find themselves to be increasingly in competition for the same market and to be providing many of the same services.

Exclusive Provider Organizations (EPOs)

An exclusive provider organization (EPO) combines many of the functions of an HMO with those of a PPO; it is typically initiated by an employer group to manage health costs of the corporation through utilization management and preferred capitation rates. The preferred capitation rates of an EPO result from basing them on actual risk in that corporation's employee population. The assumption is that the risk of the employee group is less than it would be if the plan were based on the broader system of community rating, an initial requirement of HMOs under the HMO Act of 1973.

Like the PPO, the EPO purchaser contracts with a preferred set of providers for discounts and acceptance of an aggressive set of utilization-review procedures. Unlike the PPO, the EPO has an exclusive relationship with a set of providers and limits the beneficiaries to that set of providers.

The EPO functions like a closed-panel HMO by requiring the exclusive use of the EPO provider network, but it is technically not an HMO and thus falls outside the regulations pertaining to experience rating as opposed to community rating. However, since the 1988 amendments to the HMO Act, which included new experience-rating provisions, much of the appeal of the EPO model no longer exists. Some industries are still experimenting with this model, but the restrictive nature of services provided to the beneficiaries makes it less appealing, particularly when equal cost savings can be achieved through more open models. Like many other models, the EPO introduced important concepts that caused the field to change and adapt, leading to newer, more creative forms.

Point-of-Service Plans (POSs)

The point-of-service plan is a hybrid benefit package that includes services provided through an indemnity insurance plan, a PPO, and a capitated HMO. The main attraction of this package is the flexibility to choose among the three options at the point where the service is consumed. The indemnity plan offers the flexibility of indemnity insurance to choose any provider for any service, but with a relatively high charge. The PPO restricts the provider panel and the utilization of services somewhat, but it offers cost savings through discounts. The HMO offers the option with the least cost but with the most restrictive choice of providers and services.

The POS plan was developed by IPA models as a strategic move against HMOs and other plans without access to an indemnity insurance product. It is marketed as a plan that offers total flexibility of choice to the beneficiary, while including a low-cost option. These plans have become very popular and have forced most HMOs to develop linkages with indemnity insurance companies to offer a POS option. The POS package also has been popular with employer groups that want to convert from indemnity insurance to a capitated plan. The employer can offer the POS as a plan that retains all of the advantages of the old plan with the additional options available under the HMO. This hybrid plan usually results in a strategy to increase the premiums, deductibles, and coinsurance of the indemnity plan in order to encourage beneficiaries to utilize the HMO. Under most POS plans, 65 to 85 percent of the services are chosen from the HMO option.

Mixed Models

Many of the evolving HMO structures combine two or more of the traditional models to take advantage of each of their strengths. This will become increasingly true as the competition for managed care organizations shifts from indemnity insurance and fee-for-service systems to other forms of managed care. More staff- and group-model HMOs are already contracting directly with individual physicians or developing IPAs to add an IPA element to the basic model. In addition, various IPA models are directly contracting with individual physicians to provide coverage to a specific region.

These mixed models can be understood by separating out their basic elements, but they are more complex, because many models are combined within one organization. In the future, these combinations will give rise to completely new forms of models. That is the dynamic nature of the managed care system.

Specialized Managed-Care Models

Managed care for specialized populations introduces variables that pertain to public financing and accountability, to health services provided outside traditional insurance plans, and to specialized technology for managing certain population groups. These special applications of managed care build on the basic models but are complex in detail and varied in their applications.

Medicare

Managed care for Medicare beneficiaries is a significant potential market, but one into which there has not been much penetration. According to one study, of the 33 million people eligible for Medicare, only 5 percent are currently enrolled in managed care contracts. Given the financial problems with the Medicare trust fund, there is an increasing interest in managed care as a possible mechanism for reducing the costs of medical care to this high-risk population.

The Medicare program is administered by the Health Care Financing Administration (HCFA), which sets the rate for payment based on a complex formula that includes such factors as population, age, sex, income, and institutionalized status. This rate, called the adjusted average per capita cost (AAPCC), is based on the assumption of spreading risk across the range of the elderly population. The rate is different for each area of the United States, depending on the demographic makeup, and is consolidated to determine the average payment rate.

Future potential   The limited appeal of the Medicare program for managed care firms is due primarily to the high administrative costs and the seemingly low AAPCC. However, it may be that the utilization patterns and utilization-review procedures used for general commercial plans might not be adequate when applied to this special and high-risk population.

The unique nature of managing Medicare populations is starting to produce a special knowledge base in HMOs. One experimental program enrolls very small population groups (100–300 people) of high-risk elderly and aggressively manages risk, instead of distributing it over a large population. The results showed utilization rates for this high-risk population at or below the elderly population as a whole. The specialized nature of the Medicare population clearly requires a different philosophy, set of skills, and management system from those used by commercial plans, and they need to be explored before launching into this large and growing market.

Medicaid

Managed care for Medicaid populations is another significant area with the potential for considerable growth. According to one study, there are over three million Medicaid recipients in managed care plans, which is only 14 percent of the total population receiving Medicaid funds. Due to increasing budgetary constraints and rising health care costs, there is growing interest in managed Medicaid plans.

State regulations   Medicaid plans are public financing systems provided through each state's Medicaid office. As a consequence, each state has its own set of regulations concerning eligibility, benefit requirements, and choice, making it difficult to generalize about these provisions. While variability is a desirable feature and characterizes private financing approaches, public financing introduces additional accountability mechanisms to assure quality of services and to account for the expenditure of public monies. These rules can be rigid, changing, and not always effective in producing the desired result. For example, the restrictive nature of utilization-review mechanisms prescribe how services will be utilized. In addition, most states that allow managed Medicaid plans require many services that are beyond those available in most private plans. This introduces additional administrative and clinical costs to managed Medicaid plans.

Future potential   Providing health services to Medicaid recipients requires a provider system that understands the values, culture, and behavior of this special population and is accessible to them. Most facilities and services that are designed for commercial beneficiaries will not be adequate to meet the needs of this population. Issues of transportation and communication need to be addressed, as well as patterns of consuming health services. This population has become accustomed to utilizing the emergency room as the most accessible service in the community, frequently delaying care until the disease has progressed.

States are increasingly developing managed Medicaid plans in which waivers of many of the previous regulations and restrictions allow them to reduce administrative costs and externally imposed rules on services utilization. These experiments and the large volume of eligible recipients give this area great potential for growth.

Behavioral Health

The area of behavioral health includes mental-health and substance-abuse services. It has a large chronic-care population, whose treatment is provided primarily outside the managed care system. Managed behavioral health is primarily available through specialty HMOs, most likely an extension of the historic separation of behavioral health from somatic medicine in both the private and public sectors. Behavioral health is considered by most practitioners and institutions in the health system as hard to understand and manage, and it is typically "carved out" of health plans or limited in coverage.

Behavioral health illustrates an important contradiction in assumptions made by managed care organizations. On the one hand, it involves specialized knowledge about diagnoses, treatment, outcomes, and utilization review, which supports the merit of treating behavioral health as a specialty service and developing specialized HMOs. On the other hand, it has been demonstrated that the effective management of behavioral health in the enrolled population can yield impressive decreases in medical care utilization. This suggests that behavioral health should be managed aggressively as a primary care service and as part of the integrated primary care system.

The current financing models of managed care encourage the continuation of the "carve out" of specialized services, risk assessment and distribution, and risk management. Frequently, specialized services need to be coordinated with public- and community-financed services that are not connected with, or understood by managers and practitioners in, integrated service networks. This situation might well change with the shift from financing-based HMOs to provider-based, integrated managed care systems.

The financing-based managed care models try to retrofit a traditional delivery system onto a reformed financing system. The behavioral health area is an excellent example of the contradictions inherent in this type of social policy approach. It will, in time, produce a more basic reform of the provider system, which will likely "carve in" behavioral health as an important primary care service.

Managing Utilization in HMOs

A fundamental part of the structure of an HMO, as well as managed indemnity models, is the development of a mechanism for managing utilization. The HMO, as the financing system, assumes financial risk for providing "all needed health services" to the enrolled population by accepting a capitation fee, and it must develop a system for managing that risk by managing utilization.

Changing Behaviors

Most utilization management is focused on changing behaviors of physicians, specifically their clinical decisions to refer, hospitalize, and perform costly medical procedures. The HMO has a difficult task of changing these behaviors, because the clinical decision-making process is structured to assure the independence of the clinician. The development of HMO models of managed care has resulted in changes to the structure of health organizations but not to the structure of the clinical decision-making process. In addition, most clinicians continue to be reimbursed for many of their patients under indemnity insurance and fee-for-service reimbursement, which reward high utilization behaviors.

External Controls

Thus, HMOs are left with the task of altering the behavior of clinicians by using externally imposed controls and incentives. This results in a range of sanctions on providers, usually imposed without precise information on their effect, and administrative processes for managing them. These processes are described as utilization management and are distinguished from utilization review.

Utilization review is a phrase used in a restrictive sense as a process for retrospective review of medical charts to assure quality and to control utilization. It evolved out of the Medicare program, which required hospitals to carry out retrospective medical-chart review.

Utilization management is a broader term and includes a range of external utilization-review mechanisms, including retrospective review. Utilization management can be seen as managing access to medical specialists and the utilization of hospital services, including emergency rooms. Since hospital services account for 30 to 40 percent of the costs in a managed care plan, much of which is not supported by demonstrated improved clinical outcomes, it is understandably an important area of focus. Restricting access to medical specialists is justified on the basis of excessive utilization of highly technical and high-cost clinicians for routine or less complex conditions. This argument is based on the assumptions of the cost of each clinical encounter, while the true cost for a managed care firm is the total cost of the entire clinical episode. Increased research is needed to document total cost incurred across the continuum of care.

Gatekeeper Structures

The gatekeeper concept consists of rules requiring patients to enter the health system at the primary care level, with the primary care physician (PCP) having the responsibility for making the patient assessment and providing the necessary care, if it is within the technical capacity of the primary care team. If a referral is needed, the PCP (or gatekeeper) has the responsibility for making it and for coordinating the patient's care with the specialists.

Controlling access   The gatekeeper concept is designed to control access to specialists by mandating the point of initial encounter with the system and by controlling referrals. This alters the structure of the clinical process, but only by controlling access and specifying the sequence of the referral process. It does not restructure the clinical decision-making process used by each physician at the point of the clinical encounter, nor does it integrate the clinical decision-making process between the PCP and the specialists.

The gatekeeper concept is found in all models of HMOs, including IPAs. Initially many IPAs tried to avoid this form of structure, because it restricts the use of specialists in the physician panel. Most IPAs now require a member to select a primary care physician and to seek all care through this PCP.

Reducing costs   The gatekeeper concept can properly be credited with reducing the utilization of specialists and of the costs resulting from the high utilization of high-tech services. Some economists have raised the issue that cost savings are based on the per-encounter basis and instead should be measured on an episode of care. The concern is that the PCP might choose a less aggressive course of treatment and require more encounters, even though each encounter might be less expensive.

The gatekeeper concept can also set up an adversarial relationship between PCPs and specialists, where the specialists feel complex cases are held too long by the PCP, or that adequate follow-up and reporting by the PCP are not provided to the specialists. Conversely, PCPs frequently report that they do not get appropriate feedback from specialists on procedures.

Disadvantages   Patients can become frustrated with the gatekeeper system, because they must go through their PCP to get access to specialists on follow-up visits. The degree to which this is required depends on individual plans, but it remains a built-in frustration with the gatekeeper concept. This is a particular issue when managing patients with chronic conditions. As HMOs become more experienced with the concept, they provide more flexibility on follow-up visits, allowing the patient to go directly to the specialist for a defined number of visits. However, this increases the difficulty of coordinating care between the specialist and the PCP, particularly if there is not an integrated information system to support effective information exchange.

Utilization Review

Utilization-review strategies include the review of hospitalization prior to admission (prospective review), during hospitalization (concurrent review), and after discharge (retrospective review). The reviews are carried out by the HMO's utilization management staff and constitute one of the major functions of this form of managed care organization. The staff consists primarily of nurses, includes other health professionals, and is accountable to the HMO's medical director. This function is occasionally contracted out to an external firm but is usually carried out by the HMO itself.

Utilization reviews have been the standard mechanisms for controlling hospital utilization in HMO models of managed care organizations. The aim of the review process is to assure that the care requested is needed, is provided efficiently, and occurs in the appropriate setting.

Retrospective review   The first two stages of utilization review occur before and during hospitalization. The third stage, retrospective review, takes place after the patient leaves the hospital. Retrospective review has been historically the primary form of utilization review required under third-party insurance contracts. The Medicare program, initiated in 1965, required this form of review to assure the quality and efficiency of hospital care paid for with public funds. It was as much an accountability mechanism as it was utilization review, to assure that billed services were provided and that provided services were billed. Currently, retrospective review provides profile information on diagnoses and procedures, subscribers, and provider facilities. Provider profiles include such information as out-of-area services provided, physician productivity, referrals, and inpatient procedures.

Retrospective review has developed from the review of individual charts and profile information on costs and utilization to include the use of summary data on outcomes, including costs and quality. This shift has been part of a movement to assess performance on the basis of outcomes and to better understand the relationship between costs and clinical outcomes.

Employer groups have developed the Health Plan Employer Data and Information Set (HEDIS), which provides outcome indicators of health status and satisfaction. Professional organizations such as the National Committee for Quality Assurance (NCQA) and public agencies such as the Agency for Health Care Policy Research (AHCPR) have also developed outcome indicators for assessing quality and efficiency of care. These outcomes provide valuable information on overall system performance, but they lack information on the relationship between process and outcome. (For details on quality assessment, see Chapter 3, "Quality of Care.")

Managing Health Benefits

Structure of Benefits

The benefits structure of health insurance plans has changed from fee-for-service programs to capitated models. Under fee-for-service plans, benefit inclusions were based on the assumption that only high-cost services should be included, because they were the ones that placed great financial risk on the individual. To the degree these high-cost services were characterized by infrequent occurrence, they followed the basic models of fire, theft, and casualty insurance plans, which were the models for developing indemnity health insurance. This rationale led to the exclusion or limiting of benefits for services such as home health care, nursing home care, and routine physical examinations that were considered elective or affordable by individuals and their families.

Under capitation plans, there is incentive to expand the range of benefits, particularly low-cost community-based care and prevention services. The rationale is to maintain the health of the population and to seek early intervention for medical services. The reversed incentives caused a shift in philosophy from distributing high-cost medical risk across a population to managing risk by maintaining the health of the enrolled population and utilizing low-cost primary care services.

Limitation of Benefits

Both indemnity and capitation health plans restrict benefits as a way of reducing risk and controlling costs. The exclusion of benefits covering preexisting conditions is an example of a policy that clearly has risk implications. The risk implications of some other services are not so clear. Under capitation, a policy to restrict benefits based on high unit cost might be logical when considering the individual service, but such a policy might increase costs when considering the entire episode of care as a whole.

Benefit restrictions might result from the inability of the health plan to manage utilization in a specialty area they do not understand, or where they might not otherwise have the capacity to manage the risk. One example is behavioral health (as discussed on page 81), where services are carved out and managed through specialized HMOs. This strategy might be successful in controlling risk, but it also neglects the interdependencies among services that can lead to increased utilization of some services as a result of restricting benefits of others. The area of behavioral health is a good example of where the utilization of medical services can decrease if behavioral health is effectively managed. Dealing with health services as distinct entities is a contradiction of the assumptions about overall health maintenance inherent in managed care.

Co-payments and Deductibles

Co-payments and deductibles transfer some risk by having the patient share in the payment for services and by providing incentives to reduce utilization. Indemnity plans have historically used this as a strategy, and it has been proven effective in controlling utilization and transferring costs.

In contrast, capitated managed care plans originally structured their benefit packages on the principle of full benefits, without deductibles or co-payments. A full-coverage basic benefit package was regarded as part of the accepted principles of managed care. The HMO Act of 1973 reinforced that belief by prohibiting deductibles and restricting co-payments.

However, HMOs have gradually adopted co-payments and deductibles as a means of reducing utilization. Managed care firms have been cautious in their use of deductibles and co-payments for primary care because visits to primary care physicians are encouraged to prevent more costly use of specialized medical services. Co-payments and deductibles in managed care are similar in their purpose as indemnity insurance, but the incentives under indemnity insurance to defer care or to seek more expensive institutionalized care are reversed under managed care.

Managed care plans limit their risk of incurring a major loss due to a very high-cost procedure by reinsuring the risk with an insurance company that deals in high-risk areas. This stop-loss provision is a standard way of providing benefits to cover these procedures, while limiting the risk exposure of the plan.

Provider System Models—Future Potential

The provider system models—hospitals, clinics, nursing homes, rehabilitation units, and community-based services—are increasingly positioning themselves to assume risk under capitation contracts. These models will allow providers to benefit financially from managing risk, as well as from providing health services. This will give clinics and other facilities increased strategic control and greater potential profitability.

The challenge for provider-based managed care systems is to develop the capacity to manage the risk they assume more effectively than the competition. Some provider institutions are already organizing to form integrated health systems, which offer some potential for managing care. They can take the lead in coordinating the many services that are currently available but unorganized within the community. They might also provide the structure within which the clinical process can be reengineered and managed. The internal management of the clinical process has the potential for greater effectiveness than externally imposed controls and incentives. These internal models are only starting to evolve and are slow to develop, because they require a fundamental change in the structure of how the clinical function is carried out in the delivery system.

Altering the structure   Financial models of managed care differ, because they use external incentives and controls to change the behavior of clinicians, but they do not fundamentally alter the structure of the clinical decision-making process. Financial-based incentives and controls cause changes in the health care field and affect health organizations in various ways. For example, more physicians are joining medical groups, hospitals are consolidating, and hospitals are integrating with medical clinics to form integrated health systems.

Within these integrated systems, however, the fundamental structure of the clinical decision-making process has not been altered. The incentives have been altered in an attempt to change the behavior of physicians to reduce utilization of hospitals and specialists. Under provider system models, the structure of the clinical decision-making process itself will be altered as the means of managing care. The nature of this change will be more difficult to implement, but it has potential for increased effectiveness and greater acceptance by clinicians and provider organizations.

In order for provider organizations to assume and manage risk, they will have to develop internal structures for managing care at the point of clinical encounter and across the continuum of care. Traditional organizational models and structures will not be effective. There is need for a fundamental change in the structure of the clinical process and the development of systems to manage that process. Managed care will then move from being just a reformed financing system to a reformed health-care delivery system.

Levels of structure   Provider-based models of managed care can be understood from the perspective of three levels of structure within the organization. At the most basic level is the clinical encounter, where a physician interacts with a patient. This level has historically been removed from organizational control or influence, and is based on the principle of freedom of the patient and the physician to choose a course of treatment mutually agreed upon. This relationship has been subjected to external controls and incentives, but it has not been fundamentally altered. Provider organizations are now developing structures to alter this relationship as the basis for more effectively managing care.

The next level of structure within health organizations is the clinical process. Historically, the structure of the clinical process has been dependent on the specialized skills of numerous health professionals, where each knew what competencies the others had and involved them in the care based on the needs of the client. This relationship can be described as a loosely structured pattern of professional relationships within which care was provided.

At the highest level of organization structure is the institution, historically single institutions working together in some loose relationship. Increasingly the institution is becoming an integrated health system made up of a number of organizations. There has been considerable activity to organize physicians, to combine hospitals, and to integrate physicians with hospitals. This restructuring has been driven by changes in the health care field and in financial schemes, but it has done little in itself to alter the structure of the clinical process or the clinical encounter.

Managing the Clinical Encounter

The clinical encounter in medicine has been defined and structured by the health professions based on the assumption that individual clinicians and patients interacting in a doctor-patient relationship must have the freedom to diagnose the illness, and to select and follow a course of treatment. Historically, all health organizations have been structured so as not to interfere with this relationship.

Early attempts of physicians to form medical groups and accept salaries resulted in conflict with state and local medical associations, and occasional revocation of their licenses to practice. This set of values about the structure of the clinical encounter has been deeply embedded in the culture of health professionals and health organizations.

Evaluating process and outcomes   There is a growing body of evidence on the relationship between the clinical process and outcomes. This relationship is supported by scientific evaluation derived from randomized controlled trials (RCTs). The Columbia Registry of Clinical Trials constitutes the first attempt to systematically report the effectiveness of information as a clinical intervention. This registry currently provides the most detailed inventory and analysis of information interventions and their effectiveness in changing physician behavior. It not only reports the trials but also assesses the level of scientific support for the analytic methods.

The process of physicians using clinical guidelines is not systematically developed in most provider organizations, and their use, and the documented changes in clinical outcomes, are only now starting to be reported. The relationships between process and outcomes often are presented as clinical practice guidelines and are becoming available through computerized clinical decision-support systems.

An example of one report on a clinical process and its outcomes involved a study of cesarean sections carried out in a population, which revealed that the rate varied from 11 percent to 39 percent. Further analysis identified a range of factors that explained this variance, such as distance from a tertiary care center, type of health care benefit package, convenience of the physician, number of physician years in practice, and the physician's presumed knowledge about the clinical effects of vaginal deliveries versus cesarean deliveries. Were the high cesarean-section rates related to improved quality or reduced cost? The report showed that high cesarean-section rates do not necessarily relate to high quality or low cost. In fact, lowering the rates in some instances improved quality and decreased costs. The major question is how can cesarean-section rates be lowered, that is, how can the behavior of physicians and patients be changed?

Using clinical guidelines Traditional external controls and incentives provided by financial models would increase preadmission authorizations, alter financial incentives, and increase the utilization-review processes. Under a provider system model, a group of physicians might get together, review the scientific evidence, and decide under which conditions cesarean sections would be used; the physicians would then agree to adopt these guidelines as standards of practice for their clinic. Physicians would decide together, as an organization, how they would practice medicine, and then invest in the information systems needed to support this decision process. Physicians might use computers to provide clinical decision-support rules to guide their decisions. These decision rules are regarded as guidelines and not as prescribed procedures or "cookbook medicine," as they are often labeled.

The evidence is that these decision support processes are effective in changing behavior of clinicians, if they are presented in a way to provide systematic, timely, and scientific information and if there is organizational expectation and accountability for the highest quality outcomes. Since practice guidelines based on the best scientific evidence are consistent with the manner in which clinicians are trained, these guidelines can be incorporated into the culture and behaviors of quality provider organizations.

Internal controls Changing behavior within the organization (internal restructuring) is potentially more effective than imposing controls and incentives from outside. External controls are costly to administer, confrontational in nature, and inflexible to individual situations. They replace professional judgments of clinicians with institutional rules. External incentives and controls are unnecessary if internal controls are developed and managed. This approach could provide a potential competitive advantage for those organizations that are able to develop and utilize them to manage care. To do so, the organization would have to assume risk to provide the incentive to change behaviors.

Notwithstanding the focus on facilities and organizational health care, it is important to remember that the bulk of clinical care is still provided in the individual physician's office. Integrating these separate offices into managed care networks will remain the ultimate challenge.

Managing the Clinical Process in Facilities

Clinical encounters are defined as the relationship between individual health providers and individual patients. These encounters are linked together across health professionals, across organizational units, and across organizations to form an integrated clinical process. Historically, this process was "structured" by professionals based on their awareness of other health providers, their beliefs about the capabilities of other providers, incentives to use other providers, and the needs of the patient.

Hospital-based clinical guidelines   Although traditionally not structured to support an integrated clinical process, hospitals are addressing this issue through the development of clinical case managers and by structuring clinical processes through clinical pathways and guidelines. Case managers are responsible for coordinating care among the professionals and departments within the hospital, and for linking care in the hospital to an external setting through discharge planning.

Hospital-based clinical guidelines are written protocols that prospectively define the pattern of care to be followed and the role of each member of the caregiving team. These protocols require health professionals to meet as members of a team, define the expected and preferred course of treatment for each day of hospitalization, specify drugs and other procedures to be administered, and describe the involvement of each member of the team.

Clinical protocols embed the knowledge of managing the clinical process in the institution and not in individuals. They provide written descriptions which can be tested against clinical outcomes, and subsequently reviewed and changed to reflect new evidence on the relationship between process and outcome. They provide a framework for advancing the science of clinical practice and for institutionalizing it to assure that the most effective outcomes are achieved at the least cost.

Hospital-based clinical protocols are a step forward in the science of managed care. It is understandable that these developments are taking place in hospitals, in that they are within a single administrative unit and are the centers of managerial, economic, and technological power in the health system. However, the focus of managed care is to manage the clinical process beyond the hospital and across the continuum of care, which includes hospitals, clinics, nursing homes, home care, hospices, and other community-based services. The key to increased cost savings in managed care, in fact, is maintaining individuals in the home and the community, not managing them more efficiently in the hospital during the acute episodes.

Integrated guidelines across facilities   Managing care across institutional boundaries employs the same concept as managing it within the hospital, although it is much more difficult to do. Case managers can be used to provide the basis for communicating among professionals and institutions, for coordinating services provided and for assessing outcomes. Without a structured setting, however, it is up to professionals to structure and manage the interdisciplinary team. Frequently, more than one team becomes involved, each dealing with a different aspect of the continuum of care and each headed by a different professional. For example, nursing case managers interact with social-work case managers, which raises the issues of coordination, communication, and control. In addition, the knowledge base is contained within the person of the various professionals, rather than in the institution, which causes problems when there is turnover. This makes it difficult to document the relationship between process and outcome.

The project control technique called *critical pathways* can be applied to managing care across institutions, as well as within a hospital; it can also integrate institutional care with community-based service. In chronic care, critical pathways become complex, not only because they cut across a number of different institutional settings, but because they frequently involve a number of different clinical conditions. Chronic care patients frequently have multiple health conditions and risks that must be coordinated and managed. The challenge is to manage multiple pathways for chronic care patients and to integrate these pathways into an overall coordinated health plan; this concept is termed *integrated pathways.*

Chronic care solutions   Integrated pathways of care provide the means for interdisciplinary coordination of care, which is a basic premise of managed care. If the pathway is applied in an acute inpatient setting, the team leader might appropriately be a nurse. If the pathway is applied to a chronic care patient, representatives from a number of professions might form and function as a team, with no single profession dominant. The multiprofessional team focuses on which services will achieve superior outcomes for the patient at the least cost, with each professional contributing his or her specialized knowledge. While conflicts over professional turf and control have no place in managing care using integrated pathways, in practice the challenge is to implement and manage this method.

Integrated pathways also embed in the organization the knowledge of the relationship between the process of care and the outcomes. By altering the process and relating process to outcome, the science of managing care can be advanced and applied to other settings.

Therefore, the power of critical pathways in managed care is for managing chronic conditions. The difficulty will be developing the knowledge base, supporting information systems, and getting professionals to work in interdisciplinary teams. That is why the acute-care hospital setting has taken the lead as the setting in which most current work on critical pathways is being carried out. The payoff for managed care firms will be in managing chronic care. It will be difficult, but the providers able to do so will have a distinct competitive advantage in the market, by achieving superior outcomes at lower cost. In addition, integrated pathways can replace costly and less effective external controls and incentives.

Integrated Health Systems

Consolidating health institutions into integrated health systems is one of the major developments in the health system today. Major themes of this transformation are consolidation of hospitals, integration of hospitals and medical clinics, and acquisition by acute care systems of community-based service institutions. Consolidation is bringing about large regional and national systems that seem to have as their goal the ownership of the full continuum of health services.

The concept of an integrated health system that represents the dominant model under development is hierarchical in nature with vertical decision, coordination, and control structures; it duplicates the traditional structure of single health institutions but is now regional in nature. There is an expectation of increased coordination of services within the integrated system, because all factors of production are owned by the same corporation. In reality, the divisional units are typically under separate management and frequently have separate missions and strategies. The structures of this model are familiar to managers, which is no doubt part of their appeal; they also present effective strategies for acquiring new organizations, because new acquisitions are given a degree of identity and autonomy.

However, current regional health-system models are not the most effective as structures for managing care. Their design is based on traditional assumptions about how health services are organized and delivered, and they tend to reinforce traditional assumptions about health professionals and clinical decision making.

Many current integrated health systems have done little or nothing to restructure the clinical function within the integrated health system. Institutions are integrating, but the clinical process is not being integrated within them, frequently remaining entirely separate with separate management support systems.

Integrated systems that have a strong regional concept and strategy might not be inclined to develop a community-based integrated health system. The integration and coordination of clinical services under managed care is a very local activity. Regional systems tend to be concerned with expanding services within the region and not integrating them within the community. Acquiring additional medical centers in a region or expanding the region of operations have greater strategic priority than integrating community services into a continuum of care for patients with chronic conditions.

Models of integrated health systems can be assessed by their ease of implementation and management and the degree of control they provide over the clinical function. The key consideration is the degree of control over unit cost, utilization, and quality necessary to assume risk and to accept capitation contracts. Examples of some models for current integrated systems are described below.

Clinic Without Walls

A clinic without walls consists of independent physicians forming a group without the sale of the assets of each independent practice. A clinic without walls establishes a new corporation and contracts with physicians to provide such administrative services as marketing, billing, personnel, and insurance payments processing. The group can contract with a health plan to provide health services, which makes it similar to an IPA-model HMO. The physicians would then agree to a set of external controls and incentives similar to an IPA.

Advantages and disadvantages   This organizational model is easy to create, provides considerable autonomy to individual physicians, and is flexible, allowing physicians to join or leave the group without severe financial consequences. Strategically, it is easy to start and expand and can yield short-term financial returns from increased administrative efficiency.

However, advantages to individual physicians are potential disadvantages to the organization. Physicians have limited loyalty to the organization and little long-term commitment to the group. There is little control as to which physicians are included in the group, and a very limited ability to change the practice patterns of physician members. There is the possibility that the group will contain too many specialists, and that physicians will participate in multiple groups. There is also a possibility that high-quality physicians will leave to join more formally structured groups or groups that are more efficient and of higher quality.

Future potential   The potential is very limited for a clinic without walls to develop internal structures for managing care or managing risk, so these models will remain as "stage of production" models at best. Whether they will be able to compete with more highly structured models is a question, and thus their long-term viability is an issue. They might be effective models for remote areas, or for offering only selected or specialized services.

Physician-Hospital Organizations (PHOs)

A physician-hospital organization (PHO) is created by forming a new corporation, constituting a joint venture between a hospital and a group of physicians, typically members of the medical staff of a hospital. The existing clinic and hospital organizations remain, but together they form a new entity. The physicians might join as individuals or as members of a clinic. To provide capital for the new organization, each member of the venture commits funds, typically 50 percent by both the hospital and the physicians. The PHO functions in its own right but usually has representation from the parent corporations through interlocking directorates, that is, board members who serve on both the parent-unit and the PHO boards.

Reasons for forming a PHO are varied; initially they might serve a single purpose, such as jointly developing a new service. Once the PHO has responded to the organizing purpose, it frequently will broaden its scope and develop other products. Typical activities carried out by PHOs include administrative services for physicians, owning and operating ambulatory care centers, contracting with an HMO, and initiating an HMO.

Membership   Membership in a PHO can be open (for example, to the entire medical staff) or closed and selective. Initially the PHO might be open as a strategy for gaining support and then closed, resulting in increased selectivity as members are admitted and retained. The problem with an open PHO is that it might result in the wrong mix of physicians for potential managed care contracts, or in the unwanted retention of physicians with records of marginal productivity or quality. In other words, open and nonrestrictive PHOs might increase their acceptance by the medical staff but decrease their effectiveness in managing care. Therefore, in order to be effective in managing care, PHOs need to restrict membership and create a culture of high quality and efficient performance.

Future potential   The PHO brings physicians into a single organization structure, but it does not necessarily provide greater integration of services. There is potential for building management systems, such as information systems, to support the increased integration of services. PHOs will more likely use their buying power to get better prices on information systems than to create organizational structures that will integrate information more effectively. Even if integrated information systems are developed, there is not great potential for PHOs to actually develop clinical guidelines and integrated pathways as structures for managing care. The attraction of PHOs for physicians is that maximum autonomy is retained by the physicians. However, this autonomy is built into the structure and the culture of the organization and is difficult to change. The attraction of PHOs for hospitals is that they provide a patient flow to hospitals with empty beds.

PHOs are currently viewed primarily as transition models and as a strategy for moving to other models with more autonomy, financing capacity, and control over utilization patterns. PHOs are effective in bringing two important groups of providers to the table and developing the ability for them to work together. To do more will require more structure than is provided in a PHO. However, the threat of competition and increasingly constrained resources will provide external motivation for continued development of this form of partnership.

Management Services Organizations (MSOs)

A management services organization (MSO) is a corporate entity with ownership of the hard assets (building, equipment, etc.) of a medical group, which are then typically leased back to the group. The group gives its exclusive commitment to the MSO but retains its identity as a professional corporation and its control over clinical decision making. In a managed care contract, the medical group receives payment and is subject to the controls and incentives of the health plan.

The purpose of MSOs is to consolidate the assets of the physicians and hospital into one organization. This enables the MSO to invest in the strategic priorities of the corporation, such as integrated management systems, information systems, office space, and medical equipment. However, there might be limitations on the level of capital access, depending on the financial position of each party. The MSO can also invest in recruiting and strategically placing medical staff and other health professionals.

Advantages and disadvantages   The governance of the MSO is complex, with the hospital, MSO, and medical group each having its own board of directors, usually with interlocking members. There is greater potential in an MSO for developing an integrated strategy between physicians and the hospital than with a PHO, because of greater investment in and commitment to the MSO as well as greater resource and strategic control. There is limited ability to develop effective clinical guidelines and integrated pathways as systems for effectively managing care, because the organization is structured for the purpose of allowing clinical decision-making autonomy. Thus, the MSO is a new organization model structured around a traditional concept of the independence of individual clinical decision making. However, like the PHO, this structure and culture inhibits the development of effective systems for managing care.

Ownership Models

Ownership models include single corporation models and equity models owned by the physicians themselves. Each model has the same structural relationship between the organization and the clinical function, although financial incentives are different. If clinicians have an equity ownership in the organization, there might be increased commitment to maximizing the performance of the organization itself.

Ownership models have been traditionally considered the ultimate in organizational control over the clinical function, because physicians are employees of the organization. The assumption is that the employee status serves to align individuals with organizational goals. In actuality, the structure of traditional staff-model organizations is built around the autonomy of the clinical decision-making process. Clinical decisions are still based on individual judgment of physicians, guided by the profession. The organization develops incentives and controls for changing physician behavior, but it does not alter the structure of the clinical decision-making process.

Staff models   Staff models have been competitive with physicians practicing independently under fee-for-service insurance, which earned their reputation as efficient delivery models. Now they must compete with new emerging models of managed care, which might challenge them as inherently superior. Typically, staff-model HMOs are not structured to facilitate the development and use of clinical guidelines and integrated pathways as systems to manage care. In fact, because physicians are salaried, there might be greater resistance to organizational control over clinical decision making.

Equity models   Equity models might alter the incentives of physicians to manage care within corporate guidelines and protocols. They might be more inclined to subordinate their individual autonomy as professionals to a set of professional or corporate standards and protocols. It does not mean that the clinical function is subordinated to a financial objective. It means that individual decisions by the clinician are tested against the protocols developed and adopted by the clinical staff of the organization. These protocols are based on the relationship between clinical process and health outcomes using the best scientific evidence. If equity models of managed care can produce high levels of commitment from clinicians to restructuring and managing the clinical decision-making process, it might position them effectively for the future.

Managing the Health of Populations

All capitated systems provide incentives to invest in maintaining the health of the enrolled population, but there have been wide variations in the level of actual investment. There are several factors that seemingly influence the level of investment in health maintenance. First, the stability of the enrolled population in the provider panel will influence the investment in wellness. If there is a high degree of turnover (or churning) of the enrollment, there is less incentive to invest in health maintenance. Second, if price competition is still being determined in a community based on achieving greater efficiencies in the delivery of medical care, there will be little long-term investment in wellness programs. Once the efficiency of providing medical care has been achieved, the pressure on price will shift the competitive battles to the health of populations. This is an important policy issue for the strategic development of managed care organizations.

Managed care has been described as the degree to which an organization assumes responsibility for maintaining the health of an enrolled population. Thus far, this chapter has focused on improved management of the clinical process to achieve maximum health outcomes, and the degree of control an organization assumes over that process. This is the current orientation and goal of much of the health delivery system. There is less attention on investing in prevention services in order to maintain the population in the state of maximum health. This will be the next strategic shift of the provider system, because ultimately risk will not be managed by providing health services more efficiently but by maintaining the population in a health state. This takes the health system out of its traditional realm of hospitals, clinics, and nursing homes and into communities, culture, and behavior.

Assessing Risk

Managed care organizations have the task of assessing health risk of the enrolled population based on the factors of health status, age, employment, community, and lifestyle. Assessment is made to determine the level of health risk and to translate health risk into financial risk. This financial risk is used to set rates for the enrolled population.

Historically, insurance companies used actuarial analysis to estimate the health risk of the population. Managed care organizations attempt to enroll a population of sufficient size and composition so risk can be spread across a large population base. The assumption is that for every high-risk or unhealthy person in the population, there should be low-risk, healthy individuals. This traditional insurance assumption has given way in some health plans to a straight calculation of risk, setting a rate based on the risk and managing risk through prevention programs and the control of clinical-services utilization.

As discussed on page 80, the management of small, high-risk populations is characteristic of an experimental program that enrolls small groups of high-risk frail elderly. Risk is managed not by distributing it but by managing it through prevention and primary care.

Fostering Healthy Behaviors

Fostering healthy behaviors is a relatively new area for medical care providers, having focused historically on illness and medical services. State and municipal public-health agencies have served this function in the health system. There are several issues raised as managed care organizations venture into the domain of fostering healthy behaviors.

Effective maintenance of the health of populations requires an understanding of how health behaviors and attitudes can be changed to maintain the highest level of health possible. This requires an understanding of the social, cultural, and psychological context of individual behavior and their relationship to health status. It requires, in addition, an understanding of the role of a range of community institutions in providing human services. This is new territory for most health providers and will require new types of staff and programs to be effective. The problem is made more complex by the variability of social context in U.S. society, including the special applications of the Medicare and Medicaid populations.

Future Challenges

As managed care organizations move into the domain of health promotion and disease prevention, they will have to become knowledgeable about maintaining the health of the public and to forge new relationships with public health agencies. The boundary-spanning roles for all health organizations will be dramatically expanded, including information exchange and services integration. Coordination among organizations within the private sector and between private and public providers will have to be greatly expanded in order to effectively manage care. (For a description of some of the guidelines and objectives developed by the U.S. Department of Health and Human Services to foster health promotion and disease prevention for the year 2000, see Appendix B.)

Currently, managed care organizations can be placed on a continuum based on two defining factors. One is the health delivery system and the degree to which the provider organization structures and manages the clinical process. At the low end of the managed care continuum, provider organizations might use financial or other incentives to change behaviors of providers; at the high end, the organization might structure and manage the clinical process.

Another factor is the degree to which the health of populations is effectively managed through the emphasis and quality of effort given to health maintenance. At the low end, patients retain the responsibility for independently managing their own health risk and of accessing and utilizing health services; at the high end, all services necessary to maximize the health status of a population are provided. The operative word for understanding managed care is the *degree* to which care is managed. Managed care thus becomes an organizing principle and not a classification of a certain type of organization structure.

Finally, it must be recognized that the organization of health care in the United States is in transition. Which aspects of the current system will be retained, which discarded, and which modified will be tested and debated in the months and years to come. It is hoped that what emerges as the final product will provide high-quality, affordable health care sensitive to all the population's needs.

Chapter 5

The Computer in the Medical Office

Introduction   99
General Principles and Operational Techniques   100
Good Computer-Related Work Habits   107
Computer Networks   111
Configuration of Office Computer Systems   112
The Computer-Literate Asset to the Practice   119
The Future   120

Introduction

It is difficult to imagine a doctor's office in the 1990s without a computer system. In the 1980s computer systems began to appear in medical offices as innovative physicians realized what such systems could do and how much they could improve the efficiency of billing and scheduling. Though many of the early computer systems provided years of dependable service, technological advances and software enhancement enabled offices to buy computers that were faster than the ones initially purchased, as well as programs that could do more and more of the administrative tasks. Whereas electronic scheduling of appointments and computerized billing of insurance claims were initially described as new features, they are now routine components of virtually every medical management system.

As business management components became routine in the design of medical management systems, the health care system itself began to change. In the late 1980s and early 1990s, it moved further away from a fee-for-service environment in which a physician provided a service for which the patient was ultimately financially responsible toward a system of medical care in which reimbursements are determined by the institutions and organizations that pay the bills. Third-party payers gained greater influence, which allowed them to determine what they were willing to pay for services, and to literally revamp the system, changing it from provider-determined, fee-for-service care to care that is "managed" by the organizations who pay for it.

Managed care itself is in transition (for details, see Chapter 4, "Managed

Care"). Provider organizations compete for patient enrollees, negotiate reimbursement plans for providers (doctors, hospitals, allied health services), develop contracts and payment schedules for individual doctors and groups, and merge with one another. Yet providers must be paid for their services, and their computer systems must be capable of billing and tracking payments.

The result is that software for the medical office continues to undergo dynamic changes as the demands for comprehensive capabilities continue. A medical office billing system must be able to handle many different fee schedules based on contracts that a doctor has with any one of a number of third-party payers. When this payer is the government, through Medicare and Medicaid, the system must be flexible enough to deal with regulations and formats specific to individual states. (For details on billing procedures, see Chapter 10, "Financial Management.")

There is also an ongoing effort to develop improved software that will allow patients' clinical records to be stored electronically. This task is extremely complex, since standards of data entry must be developed, and an entire subindustry is evolving to deal with hardware requirements, means of entering data, and communication systems specific to medical records. At some point, this newer technology will merge with the business-related office management system. (For details on medical records, see Chapter 9, "Health Information Management.")

As technology continues to develop, computer hardware comes and goes; new products enter the market and then rapidly become antiquated. As the health care system moves toward some settled uniformity within the world of managed care, software will respond to the changing demands of the evolving health system as well.

The only certainty that exists in the application of computers to the delivery of health care is that it is going to continue to change.

You and other medical office staff will see many changes in the systems you use over the years. It is important, however, to have a basic understanding of office computer systems and also to reach a comfort level that will allow you to grow with the inevitable changes you will encounter as times goes on. Programs and technology are going to continue to change, and you will need to adapt as they do.

General Principles and Operational Techniques

Your Responsibility to Your Employer

This chapter is not intended to teach basic computer skills but rather to concentrate on computer techniques and applications within a medical office. If you do not know the function of a keyboard or the difference between hard drives and floppy diskettes, you could benefit from a course on the basic concepts of operating a computer. You really only need to know a little about computers themselves to be an effective part of the medical office team.

However, a word of caution is necessary to those who are knowledgeable about computers. Computers are not infallible, and from time to time glitches in programming appear. Perhaps a particular printer is not working, or the tape backup system is not responding to the backup command. In such situations there is often a degree of temptation for computer-knowledgeable employees to attempt to correct the situation on their own.

Support services   The best solution, however, is to call the support service of the software and hardware vendors who sold the system to the medical practice. You should not, under any circumstances, alter the configuration of the system or the program without their guidance. Alteration of a complex system by someone who lacks a complete understanding of the millions of lines of code required in today's programs may cause a great deal of damage, or even loss of data. Therefore, even if you are computer-knowledgeable, call the vendor support service; they will be delighted to have your help as they walk you through the steps necessary to correct the problem. If they can correct the problem by controlling the system themselves using telephone lines and your system modem, they will be pleased to have you on the other end of the line. If communication problems develop, or if something must be done manually to correct the problem, your expertise will be very helpful.

Security passwords   Always remember that the information contained within a medical office computer system is the property of the practice. To intentionally manipulate the financial or medical records is an illegal act. Many medical practices have had experiences wherein an employee discounted (or eliminated) charges for services rendered to a friend, altered the day's receipt reports in order to embezzle funds, or altered payroll data.

This is why many medical office computer systems use security passwords. When you are employed by a practice, you may be given a password that allows you to access certain elements of the computer systems' functions. The password you receive may restrict you from accessing higher levels of activity—for instance, billing, or generating financial reports. As your position in the organization advances, you may be given passwords that allow you higher levels of security clearance. You should not, under any circumstances, share your security password with any other employee in the practice.

If you are ill and other employees must replace you for the day, let them use their own security password, or have someone with a higher level password perform the work which would normally be your responsibility. Otherwise, you may find yourself in a position of having to defend yourself about questionable activities performed by someone using your password.

Security passwords are issued for a reason. To guard against illegal activity, some security systems allow your employer to know who used a particular workstation, and at what time the alterations of a particular file were performed.

The American Medical Association is also concerned with the need for computer security and has published guidelines on its position, as shown in Figure 5.1.

The Purpose of a Medical Office Computer

What do appointment books, insurance forms, recall notices, monthly bills, referral letters, form letters, lab reports, memos, files, and index cards have in common? Paper. Paper requires filing, tracking, and accessibility. Since what appears on paper was placed there by human beings, there is always the risk of error and misfiling.

Computers can accomplish each of these critical functions, memorize and file the information, and provide instant accessibility to the data exactly as it was entered. The concept of the completely paperless office has been

Fig. 5.1   AMA Position on Computer Security

1. Confidential medical information entered into the computer should be verified as to the authenticity of its source.
2. The patient and the physician should be advised about the existence of computerized databases in which medical information concerning the patient is stored. Such information should be communicated to the physician and patient prior to the physician's release of the medical information. All individuals and organizations with access to the computerized data bank (and the level of access permitted) should be specifically identified in advance.
3. The physician and the patient should be notified of the distribution of all reports reflecting identifiable patient data prior to distribution of the reports by the computer facility. There should be approval by the physician and patient prior to the release of patient-identifiable data to individuals or organizations external to the medical care environment. Such information should not be released without the express permission of the physician and the patient.
4. The dissemination of confidential medical data should be limited to only those individuals or agencies with a bona fide use for the data. Release of confidential medical information from the database should be confined to the specific purpose for which the information is requested and limited to the specific time frame requested. All such organizations or individuals should be advised that authorized release of data to them does not authorize their further release of the data to additional individuals or organizations.
5. Procedures for purging the computerized database of archaic or inaccurate data should be established, and the patient and physician should be notified before and after the data has been purged. There should be no commingling of a physician's computerized patient records with those of other computer bureau clients. In addition, procedures should be developed to protect against inadvertent mixing of individual reports or segments thereof.
6. The computerized medical database should be on-line to the computer terminal only when authorized computer programs requiring the medical data are being used. Individuals and organizations external to the clinical facility should not be provided on-line access to a computerized database containing identifiable data from medical records concerning patients.

Fig. 5.1 *(continued)*

7. Security:
   a. Stringent security procedures for entry into the immediate environment in which the computerized medical database is stored and/or processed or for otherwise having access to confidential medical information should be developed and strictly enforced so as to prevent access to the computer facility by unauthorized personnel. Personnel audit procedures should be developed to establish a record in the event of unauthorized disclosure of medical data. A roster of past and present service bureau personnel with specified levels of access to the medical database should be maintained. Specific administrative sanctions should exist to prevent employee breaches of confidentiality and security procedures.
   b. All terminated or former employees in the data processing environment should have no access to data from the medical records concerning patients.
   c. Involuntarily terminated employees working in the data processing environment in which medical records are processed should be removed from the computerized media data environment.
   d. Upon completion of a computer service bureau's services for a physician, those computer files maintained for the physician should be physically turned over to the physician or destroyed (erased). In the event of file erasure, the computer service bureau should verify in writing to the physician that erasure has taken place.

(Reprinted by permission of the American Medical Association)

a goal since the inception of affordable computer technology. While medical offices are still far from being completely paper-free working environments, there are many types of medical office information that can be stored on a computer rather than filed on paper.

Noncomputerized office   Why are computers so useful in medical offices? To answer this question, follow the scenario below, which might have described a hypothetical but typical patient visit to a doctor's office in the 1970s, when there were very few computerized medical offices. Telephone receptionists worked then (as many do today) with conventional calendars and scheduling books.

An imaginary patient, Mrs. Lotta A. King, is divorced, and her ex-husband is responsible for her medical bills. She works five days a week to support herself and her child. She has decided to see her doctor because she has had general discomfort in her joints for three weeks.

When Mrs. King places her call to request an appointment, she must first tell the telephone receptionist whether or not she has previously been seen as a patient in that practice. If she has, the receptionist looks to see if Mrs. King has any outstanding balance due from her previous visit, since an overdue balance must be satisfied before she can be seen again. The receptionist must go to the accounting records or card files, find Mrs. King's records, and review the account. Since it is possible that the practice has several patients with the same name, the receptionist may have to confirm the Social Security number or address that appears on the record when she returns to the telephone. Once it has been established that an appointment can be made, the receptionist checks the schedule of the doctor Mrs. King wishes to see.

Since Mrs. King has a job, she specifies that she can only be seen on certain days and between certain hours. Furthermore, she states that she must be able to leave the doctor's office by 4:30 P.M. to pick up her child at the day care center.

The receptionist must next determine how much time to allot to Mrs. King's appointment with the doctor. Since Mrs. King is an established patient, the receptionist inquires about previous visits, and the conditions for which Mrs. King has been examined. Mrs. King feels that her problem is somewhat sensitive and prefers not to tell the receptionist why she needs to see the doctor. Once again, the receptionist puts the telephone on hold, and goes to retrieve Mrs. King's medical file from the chart rack. Looking at the doctor's notes from the last visit, the receptionist sees that the doctor asked Mrs. King to have a blood test and return in two weeks—an appointment she did not keep.

The receptionist reminds Mrs. King of the suggested test, and asks her to be prepared to have it when she comes in. The receptionist now manually looks through the appointment book to find available appointment slots that meet Mrs. King's schedule. Having confirmed a date and time, the patient's name, home and work telephone numbers, and reason for the appointment are written in the scheduling book (in pencil, in case the patient cancels the appointment and the appointment slot can be given to someone else).

At the beginning of each day, a list or day sheet is prepared for the doctor, indicating who is coming in and at what times. Notes may appear beside each patient's name giving the reason for the visit, past diagnoses, account balances, or any comments that might be important for the doctor to know. On the date of Mrs. King's visit, the receptionist includes a note beside her name informing the doctor that Mrs. King has recently been divorced.

Such notes are useful since it is difficult to keep track of the personal lives of all the patients in a busy practice. Questions from the doctor that seem innocent, and almost perfunctory, can cause problems. For instance, the doctor would not want to ask how a patient's mother was doing if she had died two weeks before and the doctor had not been notified.

Some older patients resent being addressed by their first names—especially if they are older than the doctor. A note reminding the doctor and staff members to use Mr. or Mrs. before the patient's name may be helpful. Some unmarried women are sensitive about being called Miss, and do not appreciate the assumption that they are married which accompanies the inappropriate use of Mrs. before their surname.

The doctor may not know that a particular patient has had financial problems, so a note describing the situation may result in special consideration when determining the fee for that day's visit.

Therefore, an alert secretary or receptionist can use comments on the day sheet to keep the doctor informed and avert embarrassing moments for everyone.

After examining Mrs. King, the doctor writes the findings and recommendations on the patient's chart, indicates the diagnostic and procedural codes for billing, and notes when the patient should return for follow-up. Once written down, the paper containing the information is returned to the receptionist, who makes out appropriate requisition forms, puts the chart aside for future billing and insurance form completion, informs Mrs. King of the charge for that day's visit, collects and records the payment, or flags the chart for invoicing. A follow-up appointment is then made, and a note placed in the schedule two days before the return visit to remind someone to call Mrs. King to confirm her upcoming appointment.

Mrs. King reminds the receptionist that her ex-husband is responsible for her medical expenses, so the receptionist must adjust all the papers and files to indicate that Mr. King is the "responsible party" with respect to billings, and to record his address, work and telephone numbers, and other pertinent demographic information.

Many steps have been omitted in this precomputer-era scenario, but it is apparent that a lot of manual labor went into organizing, filing, writing, retrieving, and recording medical and administrative information before, during, and after Mrs. King's visit to her doctor. In addition, after her visit there were invoices to write out and send, insurance forms to complete and submit (and resubmit if payment was denied). Payments received in the mail had to be recorded and financial records updated. At the end of the day, the total financial receipts (including payments in the office and those received in the mail) had to be tallied, prepared for the doctor's review, and deposited in the bank.

Today's computerized office   The job of a medical assistant greeting Mrs. King in the fully computerized office of today is entirely different. Consider the following current scenario.

As an established patient, Mrs. King's demographic information has been entered into the computer on a previous visit. By entering one or two letters of Mrs. King's last name, the receptionist quickly searches a displayed list of names beginning with those letters. If more than one patient has the same name, another touch of the keys allows quick examination of each name to see which has the appropriate Social Security number, age, or address to identify Mrs. King. Another keystroke or two allows a quick review of any past balances due, and previous diagnoses.

When Mrs. King explains which doctor she would like to see and what dates and times she can come to the office, the receptionist needs only to specify the doctor, dates, and desired times by entering them in the computer. The next available time slot that satisfies all of the prerequisites appears on the computer screen. Another keystroke, and Mrs. King's name appears in that appointment slot. Her telephone number is readily accessible from this screen or may appear beside her name. (Some systems automatically remind the staff to call and confirm upcoming appointments, or automatically make the calls themselves using prerecorded messages and voice-recognition technology.)

At the beginning of each day, the computer prints a day sheet which displays the patients to be seen, the doctor who will see them, the appointment times, and any other information that the form is customized to show. Comment fields (with notes from the medical receptionist) can be included on the day sheet, and may contain those all-important reminders to the doctor about Mrs. King's divorce, her financial difficulties, and the test she neglected to have done. The day sheet can also show past diagnoses and balances due if the doctor wants to see this information at a glance.

When Mrs. King's visit is over, the docter circles the diagnosis and procedure codes on a computer-generated sheet and notes when Mrs. King should return for a follow-up visit.

When Mrs. King arrives at the front desk to check out, the receptionist enters the diagnosis and procedure codes in the billing screen for Mrs. King. The computer has been programmed to properly identify each code for the appropriate diagnosis and procedure, as well as the fee for each service entered by code. If multiple fee schedules are part of Mrs. King's insurance plan, the system knows which to use. It also knows that Mrs. King's ex-husband is the responsible party, and that the bill goes solely to him. (The "responsible party" feature of the computer system also insures that bills are not sent to children or employees when it is the parent or employer who is responsible for a bill.)

If the doctor is "accepting assignment"—that is, any payment received from insurance is regarded as payment in full—the computer knows not to send a bill to Mrs. King. If Mrs. King's managed care program requires that she make a co-payment for her visit, the appropriate amount shows as payment due from her at the time of her visit. The system also prints a receipt or summary of account for Mrs. King's records.

When the time comes for bills to be sent out, all outstanding balances are identified and forms printed for the appropriate insurance payer. If the payer accepts bills submitted electronically, the computer sends bills by telephone modem, eliminating the need for insurance forms and mailings. Some systems also update each account automatically when payment is received, a feature called *electronic remittance.* This is a useful feature; otherwise it is necessary to manually break down the portions of a large single check received from an insurance company to allocate the payments for each patient and then to enter the information in each patient's payment file. With electronic remittance, the computer's records are automatically updated for each service included in the check. (For details on billing, see Chapter 10, "Financial Management.")

At the end of the day, the computer system prints a report showing the names of patients seen, diagnoses and services performed (in total and by each doctor), the amounts charged, payments received in the office and in the mail (in total and by each doctor), a list of checks received with their check numbers, and cash received. It may also print a bank deposit slip with an accurate total to be deposited.

As seen in this hypothetical example, almost every step described for Mrs. King's appointment in the precomputer era of manual paper processing can now be efficiently performed by computers in seconds, with minimal effort and an extremely low incidence of human error.

Most, if not all, inaccuracies in a computerized medical office are related to human error. The computers themselves are rarely the culprit when errors occur. Most mistakes can be traced to inaccurate data entry or improper technique used by the operator. Therefore, it is important to have a basic understanding of how computers work and how to interact with them with confidence, accuracy, and innovation.

Good Computer-Related Work Habits

Basic Rules

There are a few basic rules to follow when you work with office computers, as described in the following paragraphs.

Food-free zone   Do not drink or eat near your computer or its keyboard. As an electrical device, many keyboards are shorted out by fluids spilled into them, or rendered inoperable by crumbs that can accumulate between the keys and their underlying electrical contacts.

Operating distance   Try to stay at least 24 inches from the front, and 48 inches from the back and sides of computer monitors. Computer monitors emit electromagnetic waves, which is more of a problem with older models; in recent years, manufacturers have produced monitors under strict low-emission guidelines. While it is not completely certain that electromagnetic waves in the range of those emitted from monitors are harmful, there have been studies that suggest they may be related to depression, spontaneous miscarriage, leukemia, and other specific disorders in situations of prolonged exposure. By staying 24 inches from the front, and 48 inches from the back and sides, you will be out of the electromagnetic fields and have no reason for concern.

Keyboard height   Keep keyboards at typewriter-stand height, not desktop level. Typewriter-stand height is 6 to 8 inches lower than a conventional desktop. Using a keyboard at the lower height diminishes the risk of wrist problems such as carpal tunnel syndrome and repetitive stress injuries. If you work at a conventional desk, ask your employer to install a keyboard tray; these inexpensive platforms fit under the desktop and slide forward when in use. A keyboard placed on such a tray can be used with less extension of the wrists, and will therefore make working with your computer much more comfortable, and safer for your wrists and hands in the long run.

Activation sequence   If you are using a personal computer for your office work, turn your computer on after the peripheral devices (such as printers, monitors, and modems) are turned on, and turn it off before these devices are turned off. When the computer is turned on, it checks to see what devices are connected to it; they will only be detected if their power is on when the computer goes through its start-up check.

Surge protection   It is always wise to have your computer connected to a multi-outlet power strip with a surge protector, or better yet, an uninterrupted power supply device. Multi-outlet power strips with surge protectors are relatively inexpensive and enable numerous electrical devices to have access to electrical power with a single switch. The built-in surge protector protects all of the connected units from sudden upward or downward surges of electrical energy that are associated with lightning storms or power losses; these surges can be damaging to computers and cause loss of data.

Uninterrupted power supply units are more expensive but well worth the money. The computer server is connected to the unit, which is then connected to external power. These units guarantee that the power to which the computer is exposed will always be constant, no matter what happens to the main power source. If lightning strikes, or if the power drops out completely, the computer will keep operating and not be exposed to upward or downward surges.

Lightning storms   Immediately save what you are working on, and turn the computer system off during lightning storms. This is suggested even if you have an uninterrupted power supply unit in place. The most dangerous time for a computer to be exposed to sudden change in power is when it is writing data to the disk (that is, saving information). Data is constantly being saved during the course of daily operations. If a surge hits at this time, the data is vulnerable to damage or loss.

Dot-matrix printer   If you work with a dot-matrix printer, do not turn the paper position roller knob to reposition the paper while the printer is on. Dot-matrix printers keep track of the position of the paper at all times. The printer must know what line it is on relative to the top of the paper in order for the printout to be properly aligned on the paper. If you want to advance the paper, learn how to use the Line Feed and Page Feed buttons, which allow you to make positional changes without turning the power off. If you want to position the printer heads at the top of a new page, just turn the printer off before manually turning the roller knob and repositioning the paper. When you turn the printer on again, it will think it is starting at the top of a new page.

Disconnection sequence   Never disconnect power or turn the computer off without going through all of the necessary steps to exit from the program you are working in. Many programs must organize data and save files when you leave the program entirely. Turning the system off before it has a chance to get organized may mean that your data may not be saved and readily available when you next use the program.

Accuracy When entering data, remember that computers are very literal and that your attention to accuracy is critically important. Below are two examples that illustrate the possible effects of inaccurate data entry.

In one situation, Mrs. MacDonald comes into the office for her second appointment. She is an established patient, and her billing information is already in the computer. You enter her name as *McDonald.* Since the computer does not differentiate patient names on the basis of sound but only by the exact spelling used, it thinks you have just entered another new patient named *McDonald* instead of *MacDonald.* On the next visit, you enter *Mac Donald* for the patient's name; to the computer, the inserted space in the name is another character. Now there are three accounts for the same patient, three sets of data with differing visit dates, and three bills that will be generated to the same address. Mrs. MacDonald will not be happy.

In another example, a check is received from an insurance company representing payment for three different visits by a single patient, two visits with one doctor and a third visit with an associate doctor. Being rushed, you forget to allocate the payments for each visit to the corresponding doctor and just credit the entire amount to services performed by one doctor. At the end of the day, the computer printout that indicates the total amount of money received for the day will still match the number of dollars ready for deposit. The two doctors, however, have not been credited accurately for income they each produced. Consistent errors of this type could have an effect on the doctors' business relationship, and on their individual incomes—especially if they perform services in a managed care environment. Persistent errors of this type are not likely to be tolerated.

Backing Up the Computer Data

If you have been given the job of performing data backup each night or of being certain that automatic backup has occurred, you have been given the most vital assignment within the organization—one with the highest possible degree of responsibility. Do not treat this assignment lightly, for the consequences of performing it improperly may be devastating to your employer and to your future within the organization.

Computers are quite hardy, but things can occasionally happen that destroy all of the information they contain. Fire, floods, hurricanes, lightning, and power surges are obvious examples. Computers can also be stolen. In addition, a computer-knowledgeable staff member who tries to "fix" a problem can actually make it worse, so that the data is irretrievable. Whatever the cause, loss of the data can spell disaster. Here are some rules to follow if you are designated to perform computer backup.

Responsibility Never rely on someone else who may be uncertain of procedures to do the backup. You are the responsible party. Personally train another employee to do the backup properly, and check the backup tapes they produce if you are not able to do the backup yourself.

Verification   Verify every backup tape after it has completed its backup cycle. The verification process will go through the data on the backup tape or diskettes and compare it with the data on the computer's hard drive.

Cycle   Remember that it is not necessary to back up the entire hard drive every night, only the files that have changed have to be recorded. (Some practices use backup cycles that last for much longer than necessary because they back up the entire program.) The backup feature within the program itself will usually be configured to perform backup in a certain manner and it should not be necessary for you to provide instructions. However, if the system takes an extraordinary amount of time to perform a backup cycle, it may be backing up files that need not be included. In such cases, speak with the vendor's support technicians to see if they can reprogram the backup feature so that only the essential files are backed up.

Frequency   Some argue that the entire hard drive should be backed up at least once a month. This is the safest approach; however, the actual program itself can always be reproduced and provided by the vendor. It is only the data that is related to your individual practice that needs protecting, and these are the files that must be backed up without fail.

Be certain that the most current backup tape (or set of diskettes) is removed from the office every night. The only backup tape that is physically in the office should be at least two days old. Set up a diary in a scheduling book that will account for every backup tape (or set of diskettes), indicate who performed the backup, and describe the whereabouts of each tape. If you follow this pattern carefully, the practice data will be protected.

Record   Most practices perform a backup at least once a week, but it is probably safer to do it every other day. Place a different color-coded label on each tape—Monday could be red, Tuesday blue, Wednesday yellow, etc. Then use a colored marker to identify each day in your backup diary with its corresponding color. Record the name of the person who did the backup, and note the location of the tape stored outside the office. Using this technique, the tapes can be cycled weekly, since there is no problem with recording over (and replacing) data that is one week old; there will be at least four other backups. In the worst-case scenario, only four days of data will be lost if the oldest tape is the only one that is intact.

Safeguard   Newer technology (such as client-server operating systems) allows for retrieval of data that has been lost through "on-the-fly" backup features. Currently, however, the majority of medical practices must do their backup manually. An additional safeguard is to hire an outside source to call your computer by modem every night and back up your data to their computer. This is the most foolproof method of preserving data.

Saving Your Work
When you work with the office computer program that manages the day-to-day operation of the practice, it will probably be designed to save the informa-

tion you enter every time you perform a function. The information is immediately saved on the computer's hard disk so that it will be preserved even if there is a power failure or if someone accidently turns the system off. Other programs that you may use may not provide this safety feature, so it is a good practice to save your letter or other material frequently as you work. Once you give it a file name, the newer version will be written to the hard drive, replacing the last one, each time you save it. If the power goes out, you will always have access to the last (and most recent) version of the letter you saved. The same principles apply to other types of work in payroll programs, accounting, or desktop publishing programs.

Computer Networks

A network is any system in which more than one computer shares, and works with, the same information. In a medical office, more than one person may need to perform different tasks on the computer at the same time. Each of their computer workstations is therefore part of the office system network. Once someone makes an entry or alters a file, that work is immediately available to anyone else who is working at a workstation in the network.

A medical practice with several satellite offices may have the computers at the peripheral offices networked into the main office system via a telephone-line communication system.

The type of network used within a particular office depends upon the operating system for which the software program in use is designed.

Operating Systems

Computers are nothing more than mechanical and electrical devices that are told how to react to instructions. There are different types of basic instructions that dictate how the internal components of the computer work together to produce the results you need; these are called *operating systems.* Operating systems are built-in programs that tell the computer how to communicate with its monitor, and what steps to go through for internal checks when it is turned on. Operating systems also determine how the computer will process information.

Certain programs will work only with specific operating systems. Macintosh programs, for instance, will not run on IBM DOS-based computers without specific additional programming capabilities to allow one of the two types of operating systems to recognize and work with the other. Because operating systems determine the environment that the computer works in, it is important to know which operating system your computer has.

DOS and UNIX   One type of operating system is DOS (disk operating system), the system used most frequently with IBM personal computers. Since there are many clones of IBM computers, there are different forms of DOS.

Another operating system is UNIX, used with large or specialized networks. There are other operating systems, but DOS and UNIX are the two most commonly encountered in medical offices.

CPU   In every network a central computer acts as the brain center of the system; this is called the *central processing unit* or *CPU*. It is also referred to as the *server* since it must service the workstations (or users), providing them with information and saving information for them. If the CPU does all the work, and each terminal simply sends in and receives data and instructions, the terminals are called "dumb" terminals. This is the type of network most frequently encountered with UNIX-based operating systems.

If each workstation actually processes information and sends it to the CPU, each of these workstations must be actual computers. These are called "intelligent" terminals, and are frequently encountered in DOS-based networks. A developing technology known as client-server systems provides the capability for UNIX- and DOS-based networks to interact.

Interrelated networks   The importance of computer networking goes far beyond its impact within a particular medical practice. The emergence of managed care as the primary mode of third-party payment has been accompanied by the need for practitioners to retrieve and report information about their patients and the results of treatment. As managed care organizations have become increasingly influential, dictating the terms by which practitioners are reimbursed for services, physicians have merged practices and formed groups such as independent practice associations (IPAs), preferred provider organizations (PPOs), and physician-hospital organizations (PHOs).

When many practices merge, there is often a need for each practice to contribute data from its medical database to a common computer system. Thus, a network of networks is formed. With practices using a variety of operating systems, establishing a common communication link among their computer systems may be a large task, but technology is rapidly evolving to allow varying systems to "talk" to each other.

Configuration of Office Computer Systems

The actual physical layout of an office computer system depends on many factors. Each office has a different floor plan and work patterns that are specific to the doctors and staff. Patient-flow patterns through the office differ for every practice and are dependent on the specialty of the practice. Larger practices with many doctors and a business manager have different financial management needs than a small, single-physician practice. All of these considerations, and many others, determine where terminals, printers, scanners, or other accessories should be placed.

Location

The first thing that must be considered in determining the location of the office computer-system server (or CPU) and the computer terminals is the location of the server itself.

Server   The server should be located in a spot accessible to the cables and wires from terminals around the office, printers, modems, telephones, and electrical power. Wherever possible, cables from terminals and power and telephone lines should be run within the office walls, so that people will not be stepping over or around them in their work areas. There should also be enough room to maneuver around the server, since someone may be working there performing a backup or transmitting files by modem. As with all computers, the server should be well-ventilated (do not put other appliances or equipment on top of it), and in as dust-free a location as possible.

Servers are often left on all the time. It is really not necessary to turn them off, particularly if certain activities will occur after office hours. A doctor may wish to communicate with the system from home, or electronic claims transmission may be scheduled to occur during the night. Keeping the unit on at all times does it no harm. What can harm the unit, however, is dust.

Dust problems   At the back of the computer is a small fan which runs at all times when the computer is on. It is designed to keep the transistor boards and the computer's power supply cool. A frequent cause of problems is that the fan becomes clogged with dust and is then unable to adequately cool the computer's internal components. It is a good idea to take the case off the computer every six months or so, and vacuum accumulated dust from the fan and the inside of the unit; this is particularly important if the computer is located on the floor or under a desk.

Extra cable   Once the location of terminals or workstations is determined, be certain that additional cable is left outside the wall at the point where it connects to the workstation, so that monitors and computers can be moved around. The extra cable can be coiled up and hidden if there is too much of it. The same is true of the cable at the server site.

Printers   Place dot-matrix printers away from areas of congestion and high employee concentration. These units are loud and annoying when they print long reports or pages of claim forms. Laser printers, which can be used for word-processed items, correspondence, and desktop publishing, can easily go in a private office, but there may be limitations on how far they can be physically separated from the computer to avoid signal loss.

Working Conditions

Terminal and workstation location will vary, based on the needs of the organization and on individual work habits. Some general principles apply to most offices, as described below.

Number of terminals Most practices that use electronic appointment scheduling require at least two terminals in the reception area. It is very taxing for the staff member responsible for appointment scheduling to also handle incoming calls, patient inquiries, and appointment scheduling alone. The best option is to have at least two staff members assigned to this task, or to have the incoming calls directed to those who are assigned to these duties.

Keyboards Keyboards should be placed at typewriter level (not at desktop level). Retractable keyboard trays can be mounted on most desks and are useful in helping to avoid repetitive stress injuries to the hands and wrists (see also page 107).

Chairs Chairs should provide good back support. A large number of chair designs specific for people working at computers are commercially available.

Monitors Glare deflectors for monitors are useful to reduce eyestrain. Be wary of those that claim to reduce electromagnetic fields, most do not. As previously stated (see page 107), it is wise to stay at least 24 inches from the front, and 48 inches from the back and sides of computer monitors to minimize exposure to electromagnetic fields. Be aware of these distances, and avoid working for prolonged periods within these ranges.

Eyeglasses People who require bifocals tend to tilt their heads back in order to read their monitor display information. After a period of time, this can be quite uncomfortable and cause neck pain. Graduated lenses are useful for those who can tolerate them; they allow you to focus within a wide range of vision instead of the restricted fields of near vision provided by conventional bifocals. Another alternative is to have glasses or bifocals made which place you in focus at your specific working distance from the monitor, and at conventional writing and reading distance. Before buying such glasses, be sure to measure the distances at which you work, and inform the examining eye doctor of your needs.

Screens that magnify the images displayed by monitors are helpful for many people who have difficulty reading small print on the screen.

Computer Terms

In addition to the information and terms used to describe computer systems and networks, there are specific terms that are helpful to know when discussing computers. The following paragraphs define some of the more common of those that can be applied to medical office computer systems.

Hardware Examples of computer hardware include the computer itself, the monitor, the printer, and any internal electronics or transistor cards.

Software Software includes information and programs that are loaded into the computer for it to do its work. A program is designed and written to perform exact and specific steps every time it is called upon. It will always perform the same functions. The user simply changes the information supplied.

A type of software that is designed to be used by many different users with the permission and encouragement of the manufacturer is called *shareware.* The features of shareware may be designed to be teasers to entice a user to buy additional products of the manufacturers.

Menu A menu presents a series of choices from which to choose the task the computer will be instructed to perform. Menus may fill an entire screen vertically, or appear across the top of the screen in a horizontal configuration (called a *pull-down menu*). When an item in a pull-down menu is selected, additional choices may appear, from which the desired task to be performed is selected. Menus or lists of choices that appear when a single key is pushed are called *pop-up menus.*

DOS DOS (disk operating system) is the set of commands that tells the computer how to operate, where to find information, and how to process information. The term *DOS* has come to be used interchangeably with Microsoft's MS-DOS—the operating system most frequently encountered on personal computer systems, especially those made by IBM.

There are several categories of DOS commands. Those that DOS carries out on its own are called *internal* commands. DOS also consists of a set of specific commands that can be entered from the keyboard to allow the user to instruct the computer to perform certain functions; these are *external* commands.

By using external DOS commands, for example, you can manually tell the computer to move a set of data from one area of memory to another. You can tell it to take all of the data off a diskette and prepare the diskette for new data. You can instruct it to perform a backup of your practice data, and copy all of the important information it keeps on the hard drive to a tape. However, your office software program probably has menu items that you can select to accomplish some of these same tasks with just a few keystrokes.

Drive Mechanical drives are the computer's sensory and motor apparatus for receiving and recording information. They ingest and store data. The term *drive* refers to the spinning motorized device into which diskettes are inserted, or the internal hard disk that records and holds data.

Often a computer's various memory compartments are referred to as drives. They may be hard drives, which store large amounts of information on internal disks, or floppy drives which also record (save) information on removable diskettes.

The floppy diskettes are inserted into slots to put them into the drive for the computer to read. They are used to transfer information between computers and to store information in a portable memory mode to be reentered into the computer when needed. Hard drives are generally internal to the computer (although external hard drives and detachable hard drives are also available). By convention, the mechanical floppy drives for IBM and clone computers are labeled Drive A and Drive B. If you only have one, it is Drive A. The internal hard drive is labeled Drive C.

Diskettes (Disks)   Diskettes, also referred to as disks, are removable and portable. Diskettes contain program information, files, and data. IBM and clone computers commonly have two sizes, 5¼-inch and 3½-inch diskettes. The smaller diskettes have greater data storage capability and a hard protective cover. The larger flexible diskettes are more fragile, and a great deal of care must be taken not to touch the disk surface or bend the diskette; this variety is seldom used today. Diskettes are often referred to as *floppies* whether or not they are physically soft or hard.

Directory   Directories (also known as folders) are like drawers in a file cabinet. They are given names to allow files and data that pertain to a specific program or subject to be kept in the same directory. For example, the internal hard drive *C:* may store several programs that you need to use, such as programs for word processing, accounting, and office management.

A directory named *WordProc* (upper- or lowercase letters can be used) could contain all of the word processing files. You might call the accounting directory *Acct,* and the office management program *OffMan.* You can call your directories whatever you like. (Some programs create and name their own directories when you install them.) In addition, there may be directories within directories (folders within a section of the drawer).

RAM   Formally known as *random-access memory,* RAM is the computer's internal workstation. The program instructions on a disk use the operating system to tell the computer how to process information and where to find it.

When a given program is called up, the operating system looks to the designated disk drive, finds the program, and loads it into RAM. When the operator keys in data, the system looks to the program in RAM to see how to handle it, and processes it in RAM. The system then displays the result on the screen or writes it onto the disk for storage (or does both). If the computer is not commanded to store the data, either by the user or by the program, the data remains in RAM, which makes the information vulnerable to loss.

Prior to the late 1980s, the maximum amount of RAM that DOS could work with was 640,000 bytes, or 640K. That meant that the size of the program that the computer pulled off the drive to put into its RAM to process information was quite limited. Very large programs, and large amounts of data could fill all of the available RAM, and the system might not have room to work. Since the programs themselves began to require larger and larger files, newer computers needed more RAM to handle them. Expanded or extended RAM gets around this problem. All the RAM that you may need is available on relatively inexpensive systems, and you can add RAM to computers quite inexpensively.

ROM (Read Only Memory)   ROM is information that can be read by the computer but not altered or added to. ROM is the basis of currently developing systems that store huge amounts of data (such as textbooks or encyclopedias) on a laser disk or other medium for retrieval only.

Byte   A byte is a piece of information (or one character of data) and the basic unit by which a computer converts the presence or absence of an electronic current to informational form using binary coding. The term *byte* is important only to help you gauge memory capacity terms and capabilities for informational storage.

One megabyte (or *meg*) is roughly one million bytes of information; 3½-inch diskettes can store up to 1.4 megs. First-generation computers with hard drives had 10 megs of storage; now drives of 500 to 1,000 megabytes (1 gigabyte) are standard. Optical drives use light energy to store even more massive amounts of information. Data-storage technology advances very rapidly, and there will undoubtedly be many more means of storing greater amounts of data in the near future.

A busy practice with three or four doctors should be able to store its office management system programs and data on a 500-megabyte to 1-gigabyte hard drive. If the software also stores clinical records and images (such as X-rays, electrocardiograms, color pictures, or ultrasound images), a great deal of additional storage space will be needed. When sound files are used (such as digitalized voice recording, etc.), enormous amounts of storage capabilities must be added to the system.

However, older, slower machines with less storage capacity are still good for functions that do not require a lot of high-speed calculation and information retrieval. They are excellent for word processing, and can be purchased inexpensively. Combined with a laser printer, they can generate very professional correspondence copy and graphics.

Megahertz   This unit of measurement indicates the speed at which the computer processes information. For situations that require complex calculations or working with large databases, faster is better.

Imagine, for instance, that a patient is waiting on the telephone while you schedule an appointment using the electronic scheduling capability of your office computer system. While you are making the appointment, the patient asks if a check sent in by mail last week arrived. Such a situation is one in which you will greatly appreciate a fast-response computer. Using a few quick keystrokes to rapidly display the information will make a big difference in your response time, and allow you to continue on with your appointment scheduling work. If you must wait five or ten seconds for the computer to display the requested information, and the same amount of time to return to the scheduling screen, before long you will not want to answer such questions from patients because of the inconvenience associated with waiting. This could then lead to unhappy patients who feel that their concerns are not being addressed.

Mouse   A computer mouse is a mobile, hand-held device that moves a pointer around the screen and selects command options when a button is pushed on its surface. A mouse is used in place of the cursor keys (arrows) and the Enter key on the keyboard. A mouse pad is used as a surface upon which to move the mouse.

Many people find that their wrists become sore when working with a mouse for prolonged periods of time. If you experience wrist pain, look for a mouse pad with a wrist rest. Properly supporting your wrist should alleviate any discomfort you experience in using these convenient devices.

Modem   A modem is a device by which computers communicate over telephone lines. There are now wireless modems that work like cellular phones, allowing portable computers to communicate from any location. A fax modem has the additional capability to receive fax transmissions and to send computer-generated faxes. It cannot be used to send copies of existing paper documents unless an image scanner is an accessory attached to the computer.

The speed with which data within a file is transmitted and received by modems is determined in bits per second or bps. Early modems communicated at a slow 1200 bps. Conventional fax machines communicate at 9,600 bps. Currently, 14,400 bps is the recommended minimal speed, but 28,800-bps modems are available.

It is important to remember that two computers communicating by modem will have the speed of their communications determined by the slower of the two modems in use. So, if you have a 28,800-bps modem, but Medicare accepts only 9,600-bps transmissions, your electronic billing will occur at 9,600 bps.

Certain files are extremely large, and therefore can take a lot of time to be transferred by modem. An X-ray image, for instance, may take more than one minute to transfer to another computer, even with relatively high-speed modems on both the transmitting and receiving ends.

Means of transfer of information that do not use conventional telephone lines are available, and greatly enhance the speed of data communication between computer systems. Asynchronous Transfer Mode (ATM), cable, and digital systems are rapidly developing technologies that will greatly impact the information highway in coming years.

Memory-resident program   When a computer is turned on, certain programs are automatically loaded into RAM to tell the system how to work. Every time a memory-resident program is added to RAM, more work space in the computer is lost, limiting the size of programs that can be used. Here, expanded or extended RAM comes to the rescue. Programs such as Microsoft Windows manage large amounts of extra RAM space, and track programs running simultaneously. Since Windows, in this case, is orchestrating the operation of many programs at once, it creates a multitasking environment. This allows you to make an appointment at the same time that you call up the patient's financial information to the screen.

The Computer-Literate Asset to the Practice

Once you become "computer-comfortable," you will start to appreciate and enjoy the endless capabilities afforded to you by personal computers and commercially available software. Many doctors are aware that valuable functions can be performed by computers in the office, but fail to see their full potential. By exercising a little imagination, and by spending a small amount of time in becoming experienced with a variety of software programs, you can become an invaluable asset to your medical organization. You can also save thousands of dollars for your employer, and generate additional income for the practice through your efforts. A medical office staff member who is imaginative and comfortable with a personal computer can become an important resource for the practice.

The following paragraphs describe just a few examples of what you can do with a computer for the organization.

Word Processing and Desktop Publishing Programs

Patient information sheets   Enhance the practice image by redesigning all patient information sheets (such as sign-in sheets; medication instructions; pre- and postoperative instructions; directions to the office, hospital, or outpatient surgical center; and referral letters). Make them look highly professional in appearance, and they will contrast favorably with the typewritten, badly reproduced forms used by many offices.

Signature forms   Place all consent forms or forms requiring signatures (such as operative notes, discharge summaries, or forms that follow standard formats) in files in a word-processing program, thereby reducing the amount of time spent in transcription and dictation.

Newsletter   Produce practice newsletters for patients and referring doctors.

Stationery   Design and produce brochures, mailers, business cards, stationery letterheads, cards, and recall notices.

Personnel manual   Record and update the personnel policies manual as required.

Accounting Programs

Use specific software for payroll and accounting functions, and to generate checks, pay bills electronically, and produce accounting reports.

CD-ROM Programs

Compact discs that hold thousands of text pages make CD-ROMs useful for many reference tasks.

Maps   Produce maps using copies of CD-ROM material that can be included in practice letters of welcome or instructions, such as the following: "Welcome to our practice; here are directions to our office." or "Your date for surgery is _____; here is a map to our surgical center." or "Your appointment with your consultant physician has been made for _____; here is a map showing the best routes to his office."

Telephone numbers   Use data from CD-ROMs to obtain telephone numbers for private and commercial listings anywhere in the United States. This is useful for tracing patients who have left your area, or for locating services quickly. (Telephone numbers are also available through the Internet.)

Reference material   Reference material for pharmaceutical or medical literature is available on CD-ROM, as well as through the Internet.

Multimedia Programs

With multimedia programs you can design slide shows for medical teaching and promotional seminars, as well as educational slide shows for patients. Interactive instructions and preoperative information for patients can be enhanced by multimedia programs. This format can also be used for interactive instructions to staff members on job expectations, office policies, and so on.

Communications Programs

Networks   Through on-line services such as CompuServe or America Online, you can participate in networks to stay current within the health care industry. In addition, you can access reference material and citations through bibliographic databases such as Medline.

You can also exchange E-mail with hospitals, consultants, vendors, and other offices through the Internet. In addition, you can rapidly order supplies or replenish inventory through various network linkages.

The possibilities for applying commercially available, inexpensive software to your organization are literally endless, and limited only by your initiative and your imagination.

The Future

Managed Care

The trend toward managed care that became established in the 1980s will continue to grow and to have an enormous effect on the cost-effective operations of medical practices. As an employee of a health care provider, you must be ready to provide quality care in the most efficient manner possible.

Before the onset of managed care, office computer systems were required to maintain baseline demographic information on patients, as well as their insurance carrier information. Referring-doctor files, third-party carrier files, recall schedules, appointment scheduling, and billing were all important functions of the system. Patients were billed, or their balances submitted to third-party payers for fees determined on the basis of a facility or provider fee schedule.

However, managed care has altered those procedures. Physicians, groups, and·networks of providers now contract with HMOs and other third-party payers in their many forms. The medical office staff member is now responsible for accurately recording information specific to each patient's insurance plan, collecting appropriate co-payments at the time of the patient's visit, and allocating charges according to the particular managed care contract that applies.

In a system that is fully capitated (that is, all the patients are covered by per-member–per-month payment to the provider), it is almost unnecessary for the provider group to have a computer billing system. However, electronic appointment scheduling, recall notices, and other nonpayment related needs would still be necessary in a capitated system, even if actual billing would not.

Outcomes analysis   Because the shift in payment for services is away from the individual patient and toward third-party payers, those payers are looking carefully at where they spend their money. They want to know which of their providng physicians deliver the most effective care. For example, which providers tend to order more tests, or refer their patients to more expensive specialists? How many visits must patients with a particular diagnosis have with a particular doctor in order to bring the problem under control? The result is that providers—physicians and hospitals—are under constant scrutiny from third-party payers as well as patients.

In order to assess a medical practice's performance, there has to be data to analyze. If the office computer system is not going to be used for billing in a capitated system, it will be used to a great extent for performance or outcome analysis. The person who will play a pivotal and essential role in collecting and entering necessary data will be the medical office staff member.

The level of expertise and basic knowledge of medical terminology required to perform this work can therefore be expected to rise steadily in coming years. The information that you are asked to collect will be essential to the survival of your organization, and will have to be reliably and accurately entered into the computer system.

The Paperless Office

Another future change, based on the need to reduce expenses and operate more efficiently, will be to reduce the amount of paperwork associated with patient encounters and administrative work within the office. While there has been talk of the "paperless office" for almost as long as computers have been around, this goal is still far from actually being implemented in today's medical practice.

Innovations   There are many products available that allow physicians to enter their clinical notes into the computer system by converting them to electronic files. Printed information can be scanned into the computer like an electronic picture, and recalled when needed. Voice-recognition technology allows doctors to speak into a microphone to enter information. Doctors can carry an electronic touch-pad which stores their written notes. Clinical information can be entered using bar-coded labels and scanners to read the codes.

The ultimate goal of all such systems is to reduce or eliminate paper and to enhance communications. Once a clinical record is in an electronic file, it can be transmitted anywhere in the world through a computer network, accessible to anyone who needs it (with appropriate security in place to protect the privacy of medical records). Computers can easily fax a patient's electronic record to another doctor, send images, such as X-rays and electrocardiograms, or print a hard copy of the record if needed.

Today, however, the problem remains that there are many disparate systems used in medical offices and hospitals; there is also little standardization of criteria for entering clinical data in specified formats. Work is being done to establish standards, and to allow differing types of computer systems to "talk" to each other, so there should be a great deal of progress toward a truly paperless environment in the next decade.

The Role of the Medical Information Technologist

What do future changes mean to the medical office staff member?

One change could be that the medical secretary of today will more aptly be called the medical information technologist of tomorrow.

These staff members will be essential in collecting and entering demographic data at each patient encounter. They will also be critical to the process of outcome analysis because they will collect clinical data and make certain that it is accurately recorded. They will need to know more than how to use a computer keyboard to enter and retrieve information, since they will also be scanning in images, sending computer-generated faxes, and transmitting files.

A medical information technologist will need to have an excellent working knowledge of medical terminology and an understanding of clinical treatment patterns. While some software programs already contain internal capabilities to be certain that procedural and diagnostic codes used for patient encounters are compatible, it will be the information technologist who is ultimately responsible for ensuring that coding is appropriately performed.

Practice performance and outcome analysis will only be as accurate as the data collected, and will only be possible if that data is properly entered into the practice database. With progressive development of electronic medical records systems and standardization of the manner in which clinical data is recorded, information technologists will be the on-site enforcers of these standards.

As providers continue to negotiate for managed care contracts, they will have to know the demographics of their patient base in order to estimate their ability to care for large populations of people at specific levels of reimbursement. This information will be based on the data collected by the information technologist.

These are exciting, evolutionary times in the transformation of the nation's health care system. No matter what the ultimate structure of the new system will be, computers and the medical information technologist are certain to be essential participants in the delivery of health care in the 21st century.

Chapter 6

Medical Office Components

Business Office Design   124
Clinical Office Design   130
Medical Office Personnel   141

As a health care professional, it is important for you to have an understanding of the design and components of medical offices, both within and outside the specialty in which you work. As you become more involved in the operations of the practice, you may have the opportunity to increase the efficiency of the office through positive changes in the facility at the time of a move, expansion, or remodeling.

All medical practices have both business functions and clinical functions. Since a physician's training and education emphasize the clinical side of the practice, it is not uncommon to see poorly designed business facilities. Physicians usually do not receive adequate advice when developing their offices, and they often underestimate the business needs. In addition, the increasing complexity in the business aspects of a medical practice (such as third-party claims processing and additional paperwork resulting from managed care programs) puts additional strain on a poorly planned business office.

Business Office Design

The business functions of a medical office occur in three principal areas:
1. Public areas (for patient reception and checkout)
2. Semipublic areas (for insurance processing and debt counseling)
3. Private areas (for accounting or transcription)

Since people staffing these areas often need to consult with each other, it is desirable to have a single business office where all the personnel and patient needs can be met. In a smaller medical office, these areas usually can be located near each other. The larger the practice, however, the more difficult it is to maintain proximity of all the business staff.

Reception Area
The receptionist is the host of the medical practice and generally the first person the patient encounters when visiting the practice. In smaller practices,

the receptionist also answers the phone and is the first person a patient speaks to. Just as it is essential for the office receptionist to have a friendly, courteous, and helpful attitude, it is also important for the reception area to be a warm, comfortable, and welcoming place for patients.

The receptionist's desk should be immediately visible to the visitor, which avoids confusion for first-time patients and provides a clear location to check in. The receptionist then can hand a new patient the necessary information form with a clipboard and pen. The receptionist should have visual access to all areas of the reception area in order to monitor patients and make sure no one is forgotten. Patients may enter the reception room without checking in, and it is important that they not be missed or overlooked.

Work space   The work space of the receptionist should include room for a computer, information material about the practice, a telephone, and writing area. The work space should be designed to enable the receptionist to talk on the phone without disturbing waiting patients. A counter at standing height should be available for patients to sign in. It is generally advantageous for the receptionist's area to be near the cashier or reappointment area so that these staff members can cover for each other. In small practices, the receptionist may play the role of the cashier and reappointment person as well. As a rule of thumb, the amount of space allocated to the receptionist's area should be 75 square feet for each person working in the area.

Waiting room   The size of the patients' reception or waiting room depends on the amount of seating needed; this relates directly to the hourly flow of patients through the office, as well as the number of exam rooms and subwaiting seats in the clinical end of the practice. In addition, extra seating should be considered if family or friends usually accompany patients or if the doctor commonly runs late.

Patients should usually be placed in exam rooms as soon as one is available; likewise, the subwaiting areas can be used. These procedures generally increase patients' perception of receiving prompt service and reduce the demand on the seating in the reception area. Finally, for emergency situations when the schedule falls way behind or there are an unusual number of guests accompanying patients, have some folding chairs available in a closet to accommodate the overflow.

Payment and Reappointment

After patients have seen a physician, they should be directed to the payment and reappointment area, preferably located on the direct path of the exiting patient and away from arriving patients. Ideally there will be an exit separate from the entrance, to facilitate patient flow. By having the same staff member handle both payment collection and reappointment, patients are served more efficiently. Adequate room should be allocated to provide privacy from others who are checking out.

Work space The cashier and reappointment work space needs enough room for a computer, telephone, and printer for printing receipts if another printer is not otherwise easily accessible. A counter at a comfortable writing height, with a 42-inch width is helpful for patients to write checks or make other types of payments. A drop portion of the counter for wheelchair patients should be provided if possible.

Like the receptionist's work area, 75 square feet for each person working in the payment and reappointment area is the recommended space allocation. In a smaller office, where one worker serves as both the receptionist and cashier-reappointment secretary, the layout should be designed to provide a separate counter for patients checking in and for those checking out. An example of a layout for the receptionist and cashier areas is illustrated in Figure 6.1.

Photocopy Work Area

With the high volume of use that copy machines receive today, ample space should be provided for a specific copier work area. In the medical office, the copy machine is heavily used for reproducing medical records, as well as for correspondence, newsletters, and information brochures.

In addition, a copier can receive heavy use from the receptionist and cashier for copying such things as patient insurance cards and information, charge and routing slips, and patient receipts. If it is not possible to provide the receptionist and cashier with easy access to the main copier, a small desktop copier is useful. If this is the case, allow space for the desktop copier when designing the reception and cashier area.

Work space The photocopy area should have a work counter five to six feet long for such jobs as collating, stapling, and other functions. A shredder should be available to shred all discarded copies—a recommended office policy, given the confidential nature of medical information. The area also needs adequate space for paper recycling as well as for other waste.

The copy area should be designed with acoustics in mind to minimize the disturbance caused by copier noise. It should not be near other work areas to avoid the temptation of unproductive conversation by the person waiting for the copy machine. Generally it is convenient to locate the mail equipment in this area, as well as a place to sort incoming mail.

A typical photocopy work area should be at least 36 square feet. Depending on the volume of mail and if the area is used to prepare statements for mailing, additional square footage is recommended, as well as additional counter space.

Medical Records Storage

Although more and more medical records are being stored and recalled electronically, the electronic chart is still in its infancy and a standard has yet to be developed. Currently, most offices rely mainly on paper records,

Fig. 6.1 Reception and Cashier Areas

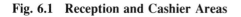

RECEPTION ROOM

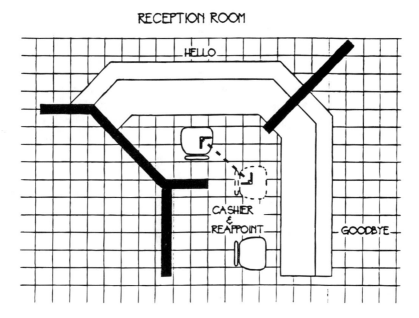

OR

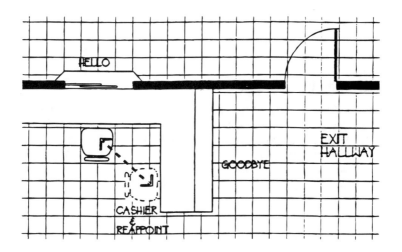

(Courtesy of Medical Design International, Atlanta, Georgia)

which require an accurate filing system and vast amounts of storage space. Even as offices change over to electronic records, they will have to deal with all the paper records of the past. It is likely to take many years before paper records are eliminated.

The method of storing and the location of the medical records should receive careful consideration. Traditionally, small practices allocate space for medical records near the receptionist. This enables the receptionist to pull the charts for the day's expected patients before the first patient arrives in the morning and to quickly retrieve charts for walk-in patients, emergency patients, and phone calls. In larger practices, this function becomes specialized and records are maintained by specific staff members. (For more details on medical records filing and storage, see Chapter 9, "Health Information Management.")

Credit-Counseling Area

It is important to have a semiprivate area to discuss financial problems with patients—to counsel those who are having trouble paying their bill or those who need assistance in understanding their responsibility versus their insurance's third-party responsibility. In a small practice the office manager usually handles this function. Larger practices may require a specific staff member to handle these tasks.

This credit-counseling area would preferably be near the checkout area so that if a problem occurs at checkout, the patient may be placed in the semiprivate area and patients without problems can continue to flow through normal checkout procedures. This counseling area may also be used to handle patients who have other problems and need to be counseled before seeing the physician.

It is appropriate for the counseling area to have a computer with access to patients' financial records, so that the employee handling the situation can call up the patient's account.

Office Management Area

Smaller medical practices generally have a key person in the business office who is responsible for the day-to-day management of the practice, participating in various business decisions and sometimes performing medical office functions. This key individual needs an office to conduct private phone conversations and meetings. In addition, certain confidential business can be performed there, such as payroll tasks, assistance with financial reports, and other private matters the doctors may wish the manager to undertake. As a practice grows, the office manager will normally spend more time managing and less time actually performing tasks within the office.

Larger practices generally need an administrator as well as assistant managers or department managers. An administrator usually requires a larger office for meetings with more people, as well as access to a conference room for larger meetings. In addition, large practices may need a number of small

Fig. 6.2   Administrator's Office

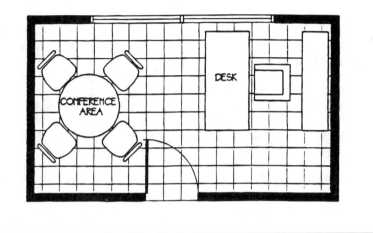

(Courtesy of Medical Design International, Atlanta, Georgia)

conference rooms that can be used by assistant managers and department managers to meet with staff, hold department meetings, and receive visitors. A suggested design for an administrator's office is shown in Figure 6.2.

Financial and Transcription Areas

Larger medical offices will need to dedicate space for other office personnel to assist in such duties as processing insurance claims, managing accounts receivable, and handling medical transcription.

Insurance   Insurance clerks or accounts receivable staff who become involved with counseling patients in person may need an office or at least ready access to a private area such as a small conference room. Otherwise, the work space could be a 6- by 8-foot "horseshoe," divided into three work surfaces. One of the surfaces could be shared with another insurance clerk, since insurance filers typically benefit from talking among themselves in order to verify such information as procedure and diagnostic coding, third-party reimbursement issues, and relevant contacts at the insurance companies.

Transcription   Medical transcriptionists generally prefer to be left alone and generally function best when they are in a comfortable, secluded area. Therefore, the transcriptionist space should be located away from the action of the office. Since medical transcriptionists need access to the medical records, if possible they should be located in an area near the medical records. Enough space should be allowed for the transcriptionist to have a computer terminal and printer. (For details on medical transcription equipment, see Chapter 11, "Medical Transcription and Correspondence.")

Clinical Office Design

The size of the clinical side of the medical office will depend on the size of the practice and its specialty. For example, the size of an exam room for an otolaryngologist might be as small as 90 square feet, whereas an exam room in a family practice where minor surgical procedues are performed would generally be about 144 square feet.

Having the right size and design of exam room is critical. An oversized exam room will waste expensive office space, whereas an undersized exam room will hinder the efficiency of the physician. Certain specialties have special needs for special rooms, such as a stress-test room for the cardiologist or an endoscopy room for the gastroenterologist, which further affect the design of the clinical office.

The clinical side of the medical office centers around the *exam module.* The exam module refers to the work space that contains all the rooms a doctor uses—the exam rooms, consultation room, doctor's area or office, and perhaps procedure room. The exam module should not be shared with other doctors simultaneously (several doctors could use the module in rotation, with staggered hours or days). Well-designed exam modules result in efficient patient flow and easy access for the physicians as well as the rest of the staff, as shown in Figure 6.3. Poorly designed exam modules hinder the physician's ability to work, create awkward patient flow, and slow the overall efficiency in the office.

Fig. 6.3   Typical Exam Modules

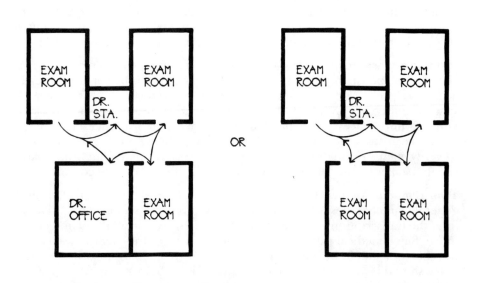

(Courtesy of Medical Design International, Atlanta, Georgia)

Exam Room

The exam room is the most critical area of the exam module and must be organized to directly support the physician, as well as accommodate the patient and staff. The exam room should be designed to allow the physician to conduct most of the exam with as little movement as possible. The room should also protect the patient's sense of privacy and confidentiality as much as possible.

Since most doctors prefer to approach a patient from the patient's right side, this should be kept in mind when organizing the exam room. Once the ideal layout of the exam room is determined, it can be replicated so that each exam room is set up the same; the physicians and staff will then know exactly where everything is located regardless of which room they are in.

Number of exam rooms There should be enough exam rooms so that a physician is never waiting to see a patient. In order to determine the number of exam rooms needed by a physician, add the average time spent with a patient to the average turnaround time—that is, the amount of time required for a treated patient to leave the exam room, the room readied for the next patient, and the patient prepared to see the physician. In specialties where the patient may need to undress (such as internal medicine), 15 minutes is usually allowed for the turnaround time; 8 minutes may be used for specialties where the patient does not need to undress.

Each physician needs one exam room plus a number of other exam rooms to use while the first one is being readied. For example, if a physician spends 5 minutes per patient and there is a 15-minute turnaround, the physician will need four exam rooms (5 minutes per patient × 3 patients = 15 minutes), so that exam room 1 is ready when the physician gets done with exam room 4. If there are only three exam rooms, the physician may be finished with exam room 3 (5 minutes × 2 = 10 minutes) before exam room 1 is ready.

The importance of having an adequate number of exam rooms available for physicians cannot be stressed enough. Since the physician is the most expensive part of the overhead in the medical office, the physician's time should not be wasted. On the other hand, having an excess of exam rooms in the office puts unnecessary pressure on the office overhead. Where there is a marginal situation, however, it is preferable to have too many exam rooms rather than too few.

Exam Room Attributes

Each medical specialty has specific requirements that affect the size and layout of the exam rooms.

Primary care In medical offices that specialize in general practice, family practice, internal medicine, or obstetrics and gynecology, the exam room is arranged in a similar way. The exam table should be accessible from both

Fig. 6.4   Primary Care Exam Room

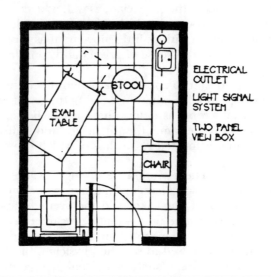

ELECTRICAL OUTLET

LIGHT SIGNAL SYSTEM

TWO PANEL VIEW BOX

(Courtesy of Medical Design International, Atlanta, Georgia)

ends and a side; limited access to the other side may be provided when the table is angled out from the wall. Visual access to the patient's changing area should be limited by the door. One or two chairs for dressing or for a family member are needed in the room. A sink, counter, and small desk area should be provided, as well as a stool for the physician that allows movement between the patient and desk area. The typical space allowance in a primary care exam room is 108 square feet, with dimensions of 12 feet by 9 feet. An example of a layout is shown in Figure 6.4.

General surgery   Where surgical procedures are performed in an office, a larger exam room or general surgery room is needed. The larger space allows for additional personnel and more equipment to be brought into the room when performing minor surgical procedures. A surgical room is generally 144 square feet, or 12 by 12 feet. The larger room allows access to both sides of the exam table.

Orthopedics   Although similar to a primary-care exam room, an orthopedic exam room is generally slightly larger, so that the physician can move around all sides of the exam table without having to turn the patient on the table. An orthopedic exam room is generally 114 square feet, or 12 by 9½ feet.

Pediatrics   A pediatric exam room is usually smaller than that of other primary care practices. Generally a bench seat is utilized for seating parents and siblings of the pediatric patient. The exam table may be placed against the bench and wall so that small patients can use the bench to get up on the exam table by themselves. The exam room should have a sink and counter/desk, but it should not have low cabinets that are easy for children to open. Make sure that supplies and sharp instruments are out of reach of young patients and their siblings. Generally a pediatric exam room is 96 square feet, or 12 by 8 feet.

Otolaryngology A small exam room is adequate for otolaryngology practices. Generally an exam chair replaces the exam table. Guest chairs are placed so that the physician can look at both the patient in the exam chair and the guest. Since otolaryngology patients need not undress for exams, privacy is less important than in other specialties. Some physicians do not close the doors in the exam rooms, but because of possible noise from the outer office, a pocket door may be appropriate. The size of an otolaryngology exam room is typically 90 square feet, or 9 by 10 feet.

Ophthalmology The exam room in ophthalmology is generally larger than in primary care practices, to provide space for specific equipment. An exam chair and instrument stand replace the exam table; typically an eye chart is projected onto a screen located at the rear of the room for use in eye exams. There generally is a sink in the room as well as a couple of side chairs for guests. The typical size of an ophthalmology exam room is 114 square feet, or 12 by $9\frac{1}{2}$ feet.

Doctor's Area or Station

In addition to the exam room, another important part of the exam module is the doctor's area or station. This is typically a small space for the physician to use between patients' exams to dictate notes, take telephone calls, check the PDR, look at X-rays, or complete other miscellaneous tasks. This area provides the physician with privacy without the need to leave the exam room module. Usually the area is a stand-up space with perhaps a stool for the physician to sit on. The typical size of a doctor's station is 36 square feet, or 6 by 6 feet (as shown in Figure 6.3.).

Doctor's Office

If the physician uses an office for consultations and considers it to be an integral part of the patient examination process, the office should be part of the exam module, near the patient flow. If the doctor's office is not used as part of the patient examination process, it may be located away from the exam module.

Some physicians do not use an office for patient consultations and in fact may share one with other physicians in the group. Other doctors have their offices designed to be used both as an exam room and as a consultation room. Therefore, the actual design of a doctor's office will depend on how it will be used.

Normally, the doctor's office is furnished with desk, credenza, guest chairs, and a bookshelf for the physician's library. A doctor's office is typically 144 square feet, or 12 by 12 feet.

Procedure Rooms

Procedure rooms for medical procedures done by the physician should be near or part of the exam module. Procedure rooms not requiring the doctor's presence, however, should not be part of the exam module. Procedure rooms are used for such purposes as stress tests, casting, or allergy testing. The office's need for a procedure room is based on the particular specialty of the practice, as described in the following paragraphs.

Cardiology   A large room for performing stress tests is part of cardiology practices. Generally this room is equipped with a treadmill, EKG machine, "crash cart," exam table, and chair, as well as the usual counter and sink found in an exam room. The room should be large enough for the treadmill to be placed where the staff can access the patient from both sides.

A stress testing room is typically 144 square feet, or 12 by 12 feet. A stress-echocardiogram room is slightly larger to accommodate additional equipment, and measures 192 square feet, or 12 by 16 feet.

In the cardiologist's office, and in many internal medicine offices, EKGs are typically done in the exam room. EKG equipment is mobile so it can be moved from one exam room to another and is generally stored in an accessible place, such as in or near the nurse's station.

A separate room may be provided for Holter-monitor and pacemaker checks, with space for computer equipment and a telephone. Although the room can be designed with enough space for the patient to lie down for application of the Holter monitor, this may normally be done in an adjacent exam room.

Orthopedics   Cast rooms in orthopedic practices are used to provide a special space for casting and splinting. Although a large, open casting area with several beds is sometimes used, this is less desirable than private casting rooms since it provides limited privacy for the patient. By batching cast rooms together and sharing a common storage area, the office is able to provide more privacy and comfort for the patient at only a slightly increased expenditure of space. A casting room provides space for an exam table, a sink with a plaster trap, and a counter. The space needed for a casting room is approximately 114 square feet, or 12 by 9½ feet.

Obstetrics and gynecology   A room for ultrasound procedures is quite common today in obstetrics practices. An ultrasound room includes an exam table for the patient to lie on and the ultrasound equipment, which is typically positioned to the right, near the head of the patient. The room includes a counter with a sink and plenty of open space to accommodate one or more family members, who are frequently encouraged to accompany the patient to this procedure. The minimum preferred space for an ultrasound room is 120 square feet, or 12 by 10 feet.

Allergy For allergy testing that requires blood tests, a phlebotomy station is needed. An exam room or special testing room smaller than an exam room is used for skin testing.

A room to mix and store special medications for individual patients is needed in allergy practices. The mixing room should be large enough for a large counter, and it typically includes a sink on each side of the room as well as a refrigerator to store the mixed medications. The size of the refrigerator depends on the practice volume; an active allergy practice generally requires a large commercial refrigerator.

Allergy practices have a flow of patients visiting the office to receive treatment. Normally these patients arrive and go directly to the nurse's station for medication. Adequate subwaiting spaces should be provided to seat these patients who must wait and be monitored after receiving medications. It is preferable not to mix these patients with general patients in the main reception area. The nurse's station should have visual control of the subwaiting room in order to immediately identify any oncoming reactions. A subwaiting room usually allows 18 square feet per seat needed.

Many high-volume allergy practices benefit by separating patients who receive routine allergy medications from the routine office patients. This could include a separate entrance directly into the medication area, particularly useful at times when the treatment area becomes congested.

Dermatology Medications are generally dispensed in dermatology offices. These need to be kept in a controlled and secure place and administered by appropriate medical personnel. There may be a small pharmacy room near the patient checkout area or as part of the checkout space. State and local regulations may govern special conditions for this service.

Dermatology offices may also provide cosmetics dispensing. This requires a visually screened area where patients can sit at a counter with a mirror and good controllable lighting. In or near this area are storage cabinets for the cosmetics.

If ultraviolet treatments are administered, space must be provided for this service. Typically a room of approximately 80 square feet is required for this space.

Plastic surgery Plastic surgery offices should have photo rooms placed between exam rooms so patients can go directly from the exam room into an adjacent space for the photographic documentation process without getting dressed. The photo room will have controlled lighting and a backdrop. The room generally measures 70–84 square feet, or 7 by 10–12 feet.

A consultation room for making presentations to the patient is necessary for a cosmetic plastic surgery office. This room will contain computer equipment and a camera to photograph the patient and digitize the result into the computer. Computer programs can create images showing patients how they would look if certain specific features are changed in certain ways.

The consultation room should contain counter space for the computer and audiovisual equipment and a place for the patient and staff to discuss different treatment options. Enough space should be provided to make the patient feel comfortable and not crowded or pressured.

Ophthalmology Ophthalmology practices may have a variety of special needs; many provide contact lens service. Inventory of contact lenses may be stored in a small lab. Contact lens fittings are done in a refraction "lane." An instruction area should be provided to teach the insertion and removal of the contact lens; the patient needs a mirror in front and a sink at the side. A counter should be provided to hold a supply of solutions; an inventory of solutions can be stored in nearby cabinets or shelves.

Many ophthalmology practices have an optical shop as part of or adjacent to the medical office. An optical shop requires display space for frames, a minimum of 150 square feet. An optical lab needs a minimum of 120 square feet. Counter space must be provided for fitting, dispensing, and storage. The size of an optical shop can range from 200 square feet to a few thousand square feet for a large operation. The optical shop may be set up as a self-supporting space and may have different hours than the medical practice in order to compete with other such businesses.

Space may be needed for diagnostic testing, such as fluorescein angiography, A- and B-scans, and fundus photos. Diagnostic tests may be done in small rooms or equipment can be grouped into larger rooms. If more than one technician is going to be using the various equipment, a single-room approach is not efficient since one technician may end up waiting for another one to finish with a patient. With separate diagnostic rooms, approximately 64 square feet, or 8 by 8 feet, is needed for each room.

Automated visual-field rooms usually measure approximately 56 square feet (or 7 by 8 feet), with the field machine placed against one wall and the patient facing it. Field machines that require a patient to sit on one side of the machine and the practitioner on the other would need to be wider, approximately 8 by 8 feet.

Urology A procedure room to perform cystoscopies is necessary in urology practices. These rooms need a treatment table, counter with sink and desk, and room for the cystoscope. In some cases the room may be equipped with radiographic equipment for X-ray cystoscopy. The room should adjoin, preferably with direct access, a toilet room. The cystoscopy room measures from 120 to 144 square feet unless equipped with radiograph equipment for X-ray cystoscopy, in which case approximately 180 square feet (or 12 by 15 feet) is appropriate.

Otolaryngology Otolaryngology practices have audio booths to test patients' hearing. These are either single booths, which hold only the patient being tested, with the technician's control area outside, or double booths, which hold both the patient and technician. In any event, soundproofing the booth is essential.

Gastroenterology   Gastroenterologists need a room for endoscopies, with space for an exam table, counter and sink, and an adjacent toilet. The endoscopy equipment is placed on the counter or on a cart. The room is usually designed so that the patient is to the right of the physician and the equipment on the left and behind, with the scope feeding over the right shoulder of the physician. An endoscopy room measures 120 square feet, or 10 by 12 feet.

Colonoscopy may be performed in the office. If this is the case, extra space will be required for the patient's prep and recovery.

Upper endoscopy may also be performed in the office, in a similar space. Because of sterility needs, however, it is not appropriate to interchange the procedures in these rooms. Likewise, if the scopes are not cleaned in the procedure room, there should be a separate room for cleaning the different scopes.

Psychiatry   A psychiatry practice has different requirements from other practices. A psychiatrist's consultation office will reflect the style and personality of the physician, and it is common to have both a formal area and separate informal seating area. While it is desirable to have a view out, it is important that there is no easy view in from any pedestrian area. The size of the psychiatrist's consultation office will generally run from 180 to 240 square feet.

A larger room for group therapy sessions is also common in psychiatry. This room is generally designed so that patients are able to form in a circle for discussion purposes. Audiovisual aids may be available in this room. The size of the room is determined by the number of patients in group therapy sessions.

Many psychiatrists feel that it is important that patients coming in for counseling do not encounter other patients directly. As such, there will generally be a "back door" for patients to exit through without having to return to the front reception area. In psychiatry, the reception area may be designed to be more private than in other medical offices.

Oncology   Oncologists will have a treatment area for chemotherapy patients. This is typically an open area with recliners for patient infusions and adjacent chairs for the patient's family members or guests. Approximately 80 square feet per treatment area should be allowed for this area.

The nurse's station is located to maintain good visual control of the treatment area. Generally the treatment area is open to facilitate this visual control and to support communications between the patient and family members.

The oncology office may provide some isolated treatment rooms to facilitate patients in greater discomfort or those with more problems. An isolated treatment room may be something like a small bedroom. Again, visual control by the nurses is important in this area.

Patient toilets should be adjacent to the treatment rooms for the convenience of the patients.

Nurse's Station

Although the nurse's station is not part of the exam module itself, it should be in the circulation path used by patients coming into the exam module and be in a position to provide nurses with visual supervision of the exam module. The physician should not have to go to the nurse's station, yet the nurses should be readily accessible to the physician.

By strategically placing the nurse's station at the junction of two walls, it can serve as a "landmark" for patients moving through the office and can reduce the patient's feeling of being in a maze. A design for nurse's stations and their placement in exam modules is shown in Figure 6.5.

The nurse's station should provide a stand-up, public work area in the front as well as a more private sit-down area in the back where patient information is discussed.

Fig. 6.5   Nurse's Stations with Exam Modules

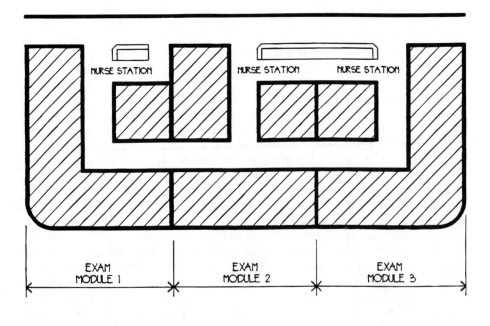

(Courtesy of Medical Design International, Atlanta, Georgia)

Phone nurse's area   Some medical offices, such as large pediatrics practices, use nurses to triage phone-in patients. The phone nurse or triage nurse needs easy access to medical records, as well as access to the physicians. This area may be part of the regular nurse's station, but it will need a telephone and space to keep charts. In larger practices where it is not possible to have the triage nurse near medical records, a system is needed to facilitate getting charts to the nurse quickly; this may require an "office runner." Since a physician may need to approve much of the advice the nurse is giving out, it is important that the triage nurse has ready access to the physician.

Laboratory Department

Many medical offices have laboratory facilities that range in size from an area for drawing blood to an area with sophisticated equipment for performing complicated tests. Most medical offices also send specimens to reference laboratories or hospitals for certain tests. Expanding federal regulations, such as the Clinical Laboratory Improvement Act (CLIA), Occupational Safety and Health Act (OSHA) regulations, and congressional legislation have made it more difficult for laboratories to be part of the physician's office. Offices that do have lab facilities include features described in the paragraphs below.

Venipuncture area   An area for drawing blood is equipped with a large chair with an armrest on each side, and a work surface nearby. If the venipuncture station is used by more than one patient at a time, the chairs are separated by a partial height barrier for visual privacy. The venipuncture station should be separated from the remaining portion of the lab.

Pass-through toilet areas   Handicapped-accessible toilet areas, equipped with a double door to pass specimens through, should be adjacent to the lab.

Lab area   The lab area itself, where specimens are tested, must be set up to comply with CLIA and OSHA regulations. These include rules governing separation of samples and reagents, calibration of equipment, general cleanliness, housekeeping requirements, and many other rules. A separate refrigeration unit, used only for the lab, should be provided in the lab area. The actual size of the lab will depend on the scope of test procedures performed and the amount of equipment required to perform these tests, as well as the practice volume.

The lab should be located so that patients have easy access to it. On a daily basis, some patients may visit the lab without a need to see a physician. Other patients will visit the lab in conjunction with a visit to a physician, or perhaps as a result of a physician ordering a test after examination.

X-ray Department

Many medical offices have X-ray departments, while a radiologist's entire office is virtually an X-ray department. Certain specialists, like orthopedists, may have expanded X-ray departments. There should be easy access to and from the exam modules to move patients back and forth. The X-ray department will generally consist of a number of support spaces in addition to the actual X-ray room.

X-ray room   An X-ray room is the place where the X-ray is taken. All workers in the medical office should be aware of X-ray hazards and know how to avoid unnecessary radiation exposure. The actual design and construction of X-ray rooms need to conform with specific requirements, as do the X-ray film processing and storage areas.

Dressing rooms   The X-ray department generally has small dressing rooms, particularly if the department is heavily used. This allows the practice's exam modules to be more productive by not using an exam room. Preferably the dressing room adjoins the X-ray room, to provide the patient with maximum privacy and facilitate the productivity of the department. At least one of the dressing rooms should be in compliance with the Americans with Disabilities Act.

Miscellaneous Areas

Drug and sample storage area   Many medical practices provide their patients with free samples of drugs, which have been given to the physicians by pharmaceutical companies. The office may also have drugs on hand to be used for injections.

Careful control of these drugs should be maintained in the office, including an inventory and lock system. If any of the drugs are considered controlled substances, a double lock system should be installed so that it takes two keys to open the cabinet. (See also Chapter 2, ''Health Law,'' for federal regulations that apply to the storage of controlled substances.)

Bathrooms   Medical offices generally have patient and staff toilets in the facility. These rooms must be handicapped-accessible with proper turning radius for wheelchairs, and include grab bars and accessible fixtures.

Conference room or library   Almost all medical offices have some sort of library, ranging in size from bookshelves in the physician's office to a separate library room. Most group practices have a conference room for doctors' group meetings, staff meetings, and meetings with visitors. Sometimes the room will double as a conference room and library.

Staff lounge   An area away from the patient flow should be provided for the staff to take breaks and have lunch. When the office is located in a large building, this area may be used in common with all the building's tenants. The staff lounge may include space for staff lockers, a refrigerator, counter and sink, and tables and chairs for employees to have lunch. There may also be a coat closet for employees in or near the staff lounge.

Storage space Medical offices need storage space for both medical and business supplies. Because of the high cost of medical space, offices often use remote storage space such as the building's basement or attic. Office workers should understand the office protocol pertaining to storage, location of necessary supplies, inventory control, and authority to use supplies.

Depending on the size and specialty of the practice, the medical office will include some or all the rooms described. Examples of designs for a small and a large practice are shown in Figure 6.6.

Medical Office Personnel

In addition to the importance of designing a medical office with the proper physical components, staffing the office with the necessary human "components" is equally important.

The size and type of personnel in the medical office will depend on the size of the practice. Medical practices range from solo practices with one physician and employee (although this is becoming rarer) to huge medical organizations such as the Mayo Clinic or the Kaiser Permanente organization. In larger organizations, there are more specialists within both the medical and the business sides of the practice, while smaller offices tend to employ more generalists.

For example, a large clinic has employees who do nothing but filing, while in a smaller clinic filing might be part of the receptionist's job. Likewise, a family practice physician in a rural setting may commonly perform or assist in the performance of surgery or obstetrical care, while in a large clinic surgeries may be performed by surgical specialists and deliveries by obstetricians. In the following review of clinical and business personnel, many of these positions may overlap, depending on the size and complexity of the practice.

Clinical Personnel

The primary function of the medical office is to diagnose and treat or recommend treatment for ill patients. The physician serves as the principal diagnostician and prescriber of treatment for patients. Physician assistants and nurse practitioners are the only two types of personnel that can support the physician in the area of actually making diagnoses or prescribing medications. The rest of the medical office personnel is nonetheless essential and can serve the medical practice in different ways.

Physician Since no treatment can begin until the diagnosis is made, the physician is the most important staff member in the medical office. The physician is responsible for identifying the ailment, the cause of the ailment, and the best treatment to cure the ailment. Physicians must have substantial formal education, pass rigorous tests, and have broad experience before they can practice medicine.

Fig. 6.6 Medical Office Designs for Small and Large Practices

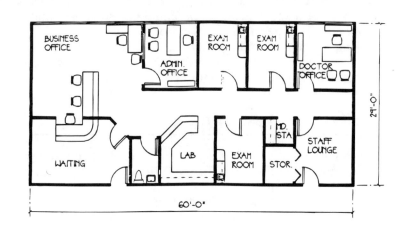

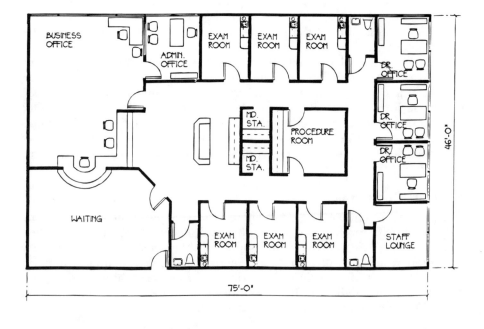

(Courtesy of Medical Design International, Atlanta, Georgia)

Physician assistant (PA)   In an effort to meet the need created by physician shortages, particularly in rural areas, the physician assistant (PA) program began in 1965 at Duke University. Today there are over 60 programs designed to train physician assistants to work with physicians, including the ability to diagnose ailments and prescribe medication.

The physician assistant studies some of the academic courses a physician does. The majority of PA programs end with a bachelor's degree, although master's-degree programs are continuing to grow. A PA completes a residency program, typically from 12 to 18 months, and some PAs may go on to work in a residency program that allows them to specialize.

The pressure on the health care industry to treat patients cost-effectively continues to encourage the use of physician assistants in the medical office. The PA can generally handle a substantial portion of the caseload with very little supervision by the physician. The physician, however, must at least review all of the PA cases; and the PA works under the protocols established by the physician. Physician assistants allow the office to handle many more patients per physician than previously was possible.

Nurse practitioner (NP)   Another response to the physician shortage in the 1960s was the nurse practitioner (NP) program. This program, like the PA program, has been enormously successful in allowing a medical practice to see more patients per physician. An NP may diagnose patients and prescribe medications, but must be supervised by a physician; the majority of patients seen by an NP will need only minimum supervision.

A nurse practitioner receives the NP designation after completing a four-year nursing program, becoming a registered nurse, and then receiving additional training that ranges from nine months to two years. Nurse practitioners have traditionally been trained in speciality areas such as pediatrics, obstetrics-gynecology, and internal medicine, but today they are becoming more involved in primary care. The demand for NPs will probably continue to increase as medical offices realize how useful they can be.

Registered nurse (RN)   A registered nurse is licensed by the state and has two to four years of formal education. Many registered nurses have a bachelor's degree in nursing, although this is not essential unless a registered nurse wants to advance into a nurse practitioner program. An RN is trained in a broad area of medicine to assist the physician in testing and delivery of treatment, and is qualified to perform services other assistants in the medical office cannot perform, such as giving injections and IVs.

Licensed practical nurse (LPN)   An LPN is similar to an RN, but without the same training; an LPN's academic training can be as short as one year. An LPN performs many of the duties an RN does in the office, and is also licensed by the state.

Medical assistant   A medical assistant may have formal training, typically through a nine-month program at a vocational school or other specialized medical training school. Some medical assistants receive all their training on the job by working for a medical office with an in-office training program. Medical assistants may become certified if they meet the criteria established by the American Association of Medical Assistants (AAMA) and pass its exam. The AAMA also has specialty certifications for those meeting designated criteria. These include concentration in either clinical or administrative duties; the professional ratings are CMA-C or CMA-A. Another professional group, the American Medical Technologists, offers the registered medical assistant (RMA) certification.

A medical assistant working in a small office may be expected to be skilled in both the clinical and the administrative sides of medicine. Normally, as a practice expands and more employees are hired, the medical assistant will focus more and more on the clinical side. The medical assistant's role will also depend on the other personnel of the office. For example, the medical assistant working on the clinical side of the practice will work in conjunction with the other professionals such as the RNs, LPNs, and technicians. The medical assistant will generally be able to assist in a variety of tasks from taking patient statistical data and medical history to drawing blood and assisting in lab testing.

Medical technician or technologist   The clinical side of a large medical practice may use technicians or technologists to assist in various clinical duties. Unlike medical assistants, who are generalists in the types of assignments they receive, technicians are usually specialized in a particular area. The following are examples of some different types of technicians.

X-ray technician   A radiologist employs X-ray technicians to assist in all of the various procedures performed in a radiology practice, from chest X-rays to CAT scans or MRIs. Other specialists with heavy utilization of X-ray technology, such as orthopedists, may employ X-ray technicians.

Laboratory technician   Laboratory technicians are commonly found in a pathology practice or an internal medicine practice with a large lab. A lab technician not only draws specimens but conducts laboratory testing and reports the results to the physician for diagnosis.

Other specialty technicians   Other medical specialties that use technicians specifically trained to assist in a particular category include cardiologists, who use technicians to assist with stress tests and EKGs; ophthalmologists, who employ specially trained technicians to assist in refractive examinations; and orthopedists, who might employ technicians to assist in such tasks as casting and cast removal.

The training of a technician varies; some technicians have minimal formal training and are trained on the job. Others come from educational programs and may be certified through their professional associations after completing the appropriate requirements, which generally include testing and continuing medical education.

Physical therapist and occupational therapist   Physical therapy relates to the rehabilitation of a patient's large motor skills, such as walking or using a wheelchair or walker. Occupational therapy focuses on the rehabilitation of small motor skills, enabling people to become more functional in their day-to-day living, such as cooking or using the telephone. Physical therapists and occupational therapists are generally employed by orthopedists or physiatrists and work together with the physician. Some orthopedic offices have physical therapy units to assist their patients in full recovery.

Other personnel   With the advent of the Americans with Disabilities Act, medical offices are expected to accommodate and communicate with patients who have various impairments, including language fluency. In many cities, medical offices may be faced with communicating with patients who do not speak English. Failure to have a method of proper communication for these patients can be disastrous. As a result, large practices may employ interpreters who are multilingual as well as individuals fluent in sign language. Smaller practices may have a staff member who is fluent in more than one language. They also may be prepared to handle the situation by having someone available on call.

Business Personnel

Just as the role of a staff member on the clinical side may depend on the size of the medical office, the role of the employee on the business side will likewise depend on the size of the office and the skills of the other workers. A very small office may employ one principal employee, particularly in its beginning stages. Although it is becoming increasingly rare to find the solo physician office with one employee, in the past this was the way many physicians started their practices. The following paragraphs outline some of the various roles that business employees play, recognizing that these roles often overlap.

Medical assistant   As mentioned in the section on clinical personnel, a medical assistant is generally trained both in the clinical and business sides of the practice. Typically, as a practice becomes busier, the medical assistant will become more involved in the clinical side of the practice and less involved in the business side of the operation. Some medical assistants, however, focus mainly on the business side of the practice and perform fewer of the job duties associated with the clinical side of the practice.

Receptionist   The receptionist is the person responsible for "receiving" the patient and whose principal role is to serve as a host. Since the receptionist is generally the first staff member that the patient sees when visiting the office, the receptionist should be trained to maintain a positive attitude at all times. A good receptionist may need to take the brunt of patient anxieties when the clinical staff is running behind and should be able to do so while relieving the patient of some anxieties and making the waiting patient comfortable. (For details on the receptionist's skills, see Chapter 8, "Human Relations in the Medical Office.")

Appointment scheduler   Like an air-traffic controller responsible for maintaining timely landing and departures from an airport, the appointment scheduler's job is to optimize the medical office's resources for smooth patient flow and efficient use of staff time, particularly that of the physicians, nurse practitioners, and physician assistants. The appointment scheduler is responsible for making patient appointments with the physicians and other medical staff or ancillary services.

The productivity of the entire office is affected by the appointment scheduler; a good one will schedule patients so that little if any of the provider's time is wasted, making sure that there is always a patient ready to be seen by the physician. A good appointment scheduler will also be aware of patient habits based on the practice experience, so that walk-ins and emergencies can be handled without disrupting the entire schedule and forcing patients to wait beyond their scheduled appointment time. An efficient appointment scheduler will work with the providers to make sure that the schedule has been optimized.

Bookkeeper or financial manager   The bookkeeper in the medical office may be responsible for one or more bookkeeping areas, such as accounts receivable processsng, accounts payable, and payroll.

The most important bookkeeping job in the medical office is managing the accounts receivable, the "blood line" of the practice. If the office does not have an efficient, accurate bookkeeping system and charge-and-payment processing system, cash flow in the office will be catastrophic.

It is also common for the medical-office bookkeeper to handle the accounts payable as well as the payroll. However, many offices use outside payroll management firms in an effort to reduce chances of payroll-tax deposit problems and for purposes of confidentiality.

In larger offices, the bookkeeping duties may be divided. A more experienced bookkeeper skilled in medical procedure terminology and diagnosis may be designated as the coding person. Since virtually all procedures must be coded in accordance with the Current Procedural Terminology (CPT) and the International Classification of Diseases (for processing third-party insurance such as Medicare and Medicaid), it is important to have knowledgeable people selecting the appropriate code. If a code is selected that is lower than the actual procedure performed, the office will be underreimbursed; if the code is higher, accusations of fraud and substantial penalties may result.

Sometimes a staff member is designated as an insurance clerk. These employees, although perhaps not coding experts, are responsible for making sure that third-party claims are filled out properly before being sent or transmitted, in order to avoid an immediate rejection by the third party. An insurance clerk will also monitor outstanding claims to insurance companies to make sure they are paid within 30 days or to contact the insurance company for follow-up if there are problems.

Collection is another duty frequently performed by the bookkeeper. In some cases, however, a designated person is assigned to be the collection clerk, focusing on accounts receivable from patients. This process includes the identification of delinquent accounts and a complete follow-up on the account until it is either paid or written off. (For details, see Chapter 10, "Financial Management.")

Medical transcriptionist The medical transcriptionist does all the physician's transcription for medical records. This person must have strong skills in typing and transcribing, as well as a broad knowledge of medical terminology. The medical transcriptionist also prepares reports and correspondence to other physicians involved in the patient's care. The work performed by medical transcriptionists is extremely important since the material they are transcribing is a critical part of the patient's medical record, documenting what the physician did and creating the history for future treatment for the patient. (For details, see Chapter 11, "Medical Transcription and Correspondence.")

Personal secretary Some physicians may employ a personal secretary to handle much of their business affairs. This is more commonly found in the office of a physician who is active in writing articles and textbooks, lecturing, and teaching. The personal secretary will assist the physician in these tasks, including screening the physician's mail and phone calls, flagging and making sure important mail is followed up, responding to routine mail, handling all sorts of correspondence, summarizing articles and other research materials for the physician, and transcribing lecture material and articles.

Office manager Smaller offices may have an office manager, who reports directly to the administrative physician. Generally, most if not all the staff then reports to the office manager. Larger offices may have an administrator to whom the office manager reports. Larger offices may also have a number of office managers or department managers.

In smaller offices, the office manager spends a portion of the time assisting in clerical duties. For example, it is not uncommon for the office manager to be responsible for preparing the accounts payable and payroll. As in larger offices, the office manager spends more time managing and delegates more duties. The office manager is typically responsible for dealing with personnel problems, wage scales, and employee reviews.

Administrator Larger medical offices have an administrator, who normally supervises the office managers. When an administrator has evolved, usually the physicians have delegated more of the decisions to the administrator. The administrator is normally involved in strategic planning and major decisions in the practice, including such things as the purchase of major equipment, annual budgeting, fee structure, negotiation of third-party contracts, facility planning, marketing, management structure, and personnel policies. Normally the administrator reports to an administrative committee of owner-physicians.

The Management Structure

All offices have a management structure; unfortunately, some have informal, poor management structures. A sign of a bad management structure occurs when employees are unsure who their boss is or feel they have more than one boss. This type of management structure usually evolves because it has never been thought out; it is usually found only in a smaller or solo practice. With a solo office, you can usually presume the ultimate boss is the physician. In a group practice, identifying the boss may be more difficult and there may be more than one boss. This occurs when there are really "separate" practices within the organization where each doctor has a certain amount of control over his or her employees.

Larger group practices will undoubtedly have a formal management

Fig. 6.7   Management Structure

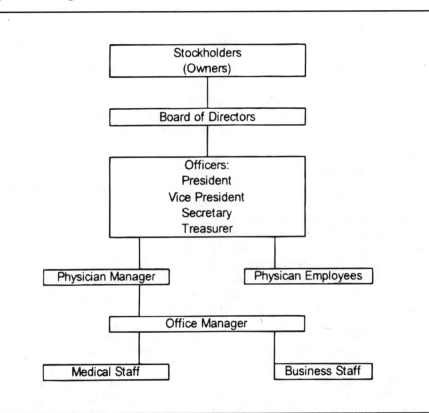

structure, since it is almost impossible to become large and successful without one. Today, most smaller offices likewise understand the benefits of having a formal management structure in place and keeping employees informed.

The preferred management structure of an organization will identify the chain of command, describing all job titles from employees with no supervisory tasks up to the president of the organization or owner. Illustrated in Figure 6.7 is a standard corporate flowchart for a small medical office. A more detailed flowchart can be expected to detail specific job positions and, in some cases, actual employee's names. In this way, employees know exactly to whom they are directly responsible. For example, both the medical staff (medical assistants, nurses, and lab technicians) and the entire business staff would report directly to the office manager. In this particular model, the office manager is empowered to hire, fire, and reprimand both the medical and business staffs. The office manager is responsible to the physician-manager, who in turn is accountable to the officers. The officers would generally be made up of other physician-owners. If the medical staff thought the office manager was making poor decisions, they could take comfort in knowing that the office manager was responsible to the physician-manager. (For details on medical office personnel, see Chapter 7, "Personnel Policies.")

In all medical practices, the physical design of the office is an important factor in the successful operation of the practice. However, equally important are the physicians and staff members who compose the human elements of the practice. When all components are working together, the result is an eminently successful medical practice.

Chapter 7

Personnel Policies

Introduction   150
Personnel Policies Manual   150
Recruitment of Medical Office Staff   153
The Hiring Process   156
The Working Relationship   161
Terminating the Working Relationship   165
Legal Requirements of a Working Relationship   169
Benefits of a Working Relationship   174
Death or Disability of a Physician   176
Conclusion   177

Introduction

Today's medical practice, and especially the small medical practice, is in the position of the small family farm that has been challenged and often replaced by monolithic corporations. Many specialty groups are merging into "mega-groups," and many hospitals are buying primary care practices to ensure bed occupancy at their facilities. However, many groups originally created for economic or political reasons are unraveling because of poor management, with more concern for the dollar than the practice of delivering quality medical care, more concern about equipment and systems than the people who operate them, and less attention to developing a practice or business philosophy.

Whether the medical practice is large or small, those who manage it should develop employment policies and philosophies that are reasoned and fair. The reasons are simple: effectiveness and liability. A physician is busy enough treating patients without having the added burden of being an office manager or employment specialist. If there are policies regarding hiring, termination from employment, and behavior while on the job—all in accordance with established employment law—the office runs more smoothly. In addition, there is less chance that a terminated employee might sue for an alleged violation of some real or perceived wrong.

Personnel Policies Manual

A written personnel policies manual is an essential tool for every well-run medical practice. Without such a manual, the practice is exposed to costly lawsuits, high employee turnover, and low employee morale, along with the subsequent obstacles to providing patient care. A personnel manual reduces exposure to litigation, clarifies expectations, helps to retain employees, and improves internal communications and employee morale.

Writing the Manual

There are many ways to develop a policy manual. One way is to create the text from scratch, using other medical-office manuals as a guide. A committee of staff members could determine what issues are important and work with the physician-owner to draft a set of policies. Sometimes a hospital human resources department will give advice; however, there are many areas such as federal wage and hour laws and health insurance requirements applicable to large employers that do not pertain to a smaller medical practice. Another approach is to hire a professional consultant to write the manual, developing it within your practice's parameters.

Whatever method is chosen, however, the medical office employees should review the draft of the manual before it is finished. This step often identifies problem areas of confusing language, and it can also reveal other topics that may need to be included.

Divide the manual into two separate sections: one for employee information, and one for benefits. The employee information section could contain the following information:

- Philosophy statement
- At-will or just-cause employment statement
- Working hours and definition of the workweek
- Employee classifications of exempt and nonexempt status
- Pay periods
- Ethics statement or policy for protecting confidential information
- Grievance policy
- Appearance or dress code
- Performance reviews
- Personal activities
- Open-access policy
- Termination or summary dismissal

The employee benefits section could contain information about the following:

- Paid holidays
- Paid vacation, sick-leave, and personal days-off policies
- Health insurance
- Life and disability insurance
- Dental insurance
- Bereavement leave
- Jury duty

- Emergency leave
- Pension plan
- Educational benefits
- Payment for mandated licenses or uniform allowance
- Reimbursement policy for company business expenses

Employment statement   The terms *at-will* and *just-cause* employment are terms in the employee information list that the office worker may not know. Generally, *at-will employment* means that employers can terminate employment whenever they want, without following some preset system of warnings or notices, as long as protected categories such as age, sex, religion, and pregnancy are not violated. Many at-will employers ask new employees to sign a statement that they are aware of these terms of employment.

Just-cause employment refers to written, established reasons how and why dismissal will occur. Since each state has different employment laws, it is always advisable to check with your practice's attorney or your state's department of labor to better understand the ramifications of either type of employment. In some states, just-cause employees have the right to a jury trial upon termination of employment.

Even if the employer has established an at-will policy, a terminated employee can file a wrongful discharge suit. Customarily, medical office support personnel do not sign employment contracts. However, a court may find that an implied contractual relationship existed if an employee handbook or policy manual contained statements that alluded to job security.

In an effort to appear friendly, some physicians or office managers might make statements such as "We're all family here" or "Most of our employees have been here a long time and will retire from here." An interviewing physician might say that the applicant could stay with the practice "as long as you do your job." An employee manual might state, "During a three-month probationary period employees can be terminated without notice; after three months permanent employment will be given." It can be argued that these statements imply permanency.

Open access   Another item under employee information with which office personnel may not be familiar is the reference to *open-access policy*. Passage of the Freedom of Information Act in 1966 and the Privacy Act of 1974, which applied only to employees of federal agencies, influenced the private sector to recommend similar open-access policies for employee records. There is little mandatory federal legislation in this regard, but many states have passed their own legislation. Some of the recommendations include the following:

1. Employees should be informed about what records are being kept and, upon request, be allowed to see and copy most of the material in their files.
2. Employers should not keep the arrest record of an employee or an applicant in the personnel file.

3. Personnel or medical records should not be released unless an employee gives written consent.
4. Employees should be able to correct or add to records that they feel are inaccurate, untimely, or incomplete.
5. Personnel records should be available only on a need-to-know basis to authorized users—such as a doctor seeking to inform a person of a possible medical problem; a law enforcement authority seeking information about home address or dates of attendance; a request for confirmation of employment, dates of employment, positions, or salary; a necessary protection of an employer's legal interest; a request pursuant to federal, state, or local law; or a request by a collective bargaining unit under the terms of a union contract.

If your practice's personnel files are closed, a change to open access deserves serious consideration. Again, contact your medical practice attorney before implementing an open-access policy.

Legal review   Once the draft of the personnel policies manual is finished and has been reviewed by the practice physicians and staff, it is advisable to have it reviewed by the practice attorney or a professional consultant familiar with employment law.

Why incur the expense of professional or legal review? Your manual might state something as simple as this: "Summary dismissal will occur because of any theft from the practice, patients, or other employees." That seems to be a straightforward and reasonable statement. However, if an accused embezzler, for example, were only fired and not legally prosecuted, the terminated employee could make a claim for wrongful discharge, asserting that the doctor was stealing from his own practice to avoid paying income tax and that when confronted with the allegation, the doctor fired the employee. A costly practice audit would occur in order to determine the extent of the loss. If the physician had not prosecuted the employee, who would be believed? Instead, the policy statement might better read: "Summary dismissal will occur when an employee is found guilty in a court of law for theft involving the employer, another employee, or a patient. The employee will be laid off from work until resolution and has the right to file for state unemployment benefits."

Updates   A personnel policies writer may wish to make the first try very basic and to update the manual every six months or so as issues occur. All manuals should be reviewed at least yearly. Updates should also occur as employment laws are created or changed. Be sure to date the manual and each change.

Recruitment of Medical Office Staff

Finding and Keeping Physicians
Medical practices, hospitals, and the private sector vie fiercely with one another to attract and keep qualified employees. To recruit a new physician to

your practice is not simply a matter of placing an advertisement in the want ads. Every week medical offices around the country are besieged by brochures offering high salaries in "ideal locations" to established physicians. These brochures are often sent by recruitment firms, hired at substantial fees by desperate clients.

Hospital recruiters   One possible source for new physicians is your local hospital's recruitment department. Hospitals are eager to bring new physicians on board, often offering "guaranteed incomes" if they refer the majority of their inpatients to that hospital.

However, many established physicians are faced with a dilemma when the new physician is offered a guaranteed income while they do not have such an arrangement. Further, in primary care, the amount guaranteed may be greater than that earned by the established physician. In addition, if the established physicians own a professional corporation, the hospital cannot pay the new doctor's salary because then the new doctor is not a corporation employee and cannot bill under a common provider number or the employer's federal employer identification number. (Note: Any joint venture between a newly recruited physician, a medical practice, and a hospital requires legal advice.)

Private practice inducements   Tactics that hospitals use to attract physicians can be used by private medical practices, such as offering a new physician "debt reduction." Physicians right out of residency programs often have substantial educational debt; the recruiting practice could offer a "signing bonus" for paying off, in whole or in part, the new physician's educational debt. Another inducement might be to offer a lower salary, but with the potential for generous quarterly bonuses based on work done.

Some physicians are reluctant to come into an unknown community. If they are married with children, they might have concerns about schools, spousal employment, and housing. A medical practice that is serious about recruitment might assign a staff member to assist in this effort by obtaining information from the local chamber of commerce, real estate companies, and board of education. Perhaps the recruiting physicians might offer a signing bonus as a down payment on a house. Whatever inducements are used, it is important to remember that the newly recruited physician must agree with the basic philosophy of the medical practice if the relationship is to be successful.

Recruiting Medical Office Support Staff

Recruitment of qualified support staff may be somewhat easier. Using proper methods of recruitment is the first hurdle for an employer to jump. For example, your initial employment ad must be bias-free.

Placing want ads   Few managers today would place an openly discriminatory employment ad unless the restrictions were clearly and unmistakably bona fide occupational qualifications. However, language that seems innocuous can be interpreted as biased. Consider this want ad: "Medical Girl Friday; no exp. necessary; high school grad; 17–20 years old in good health; file clerk duties."

Did you spot the flaws? There are certain terms that cannot be used in print without proving that each is a bona fide occupational qualification. The biased terms are shown below in italics:

- Gender: *Girl Friday*
- Physical condition: *good health*
- Age limits: *17–20 years old*
- Education: *high school grad.* A high school diploma is no longer a guarantee that someone can read and write; if the job requires English proficiency, say so in the ad.

Statements related to race, national origin, or religious preference are also prohibited.

Writing the ad Before writing your want ad, develop a job profile or job description listing the qualifications and characteristics needed to perform the job successfully. The job description requires a statement of what the job is and how the employee is supposed to do the work. The components clearly outlined should include the following:

- Position—title of the job to be filled
- Pay level—status of the position: entry level or "pay grade 3" if that system is used; exempt versus nonexempt status; salary range
- Reports to—name of the person to whom the employee will report
- Supervisory responsibilities—number of employees this person will supervise, if any
- Primary tasks—what the employee is expected to perform
- Skills needed—what the employee must know in order to perform those tasks; may include personal characteristics, even subjective ones, such as "friendly, willing to listen, or able to stand interruptions"

Guidelines for writing the ad Write a clearly worded description of the job with specific qualifications essential for performing the job properly; use standard abbreviations where possible. Consider the variety of presentations available by checking the want ads of your local newspaper. Call and get an idea of options and costs. An ad for a file clerk may not need to be as costly a production as might be used to catch the eye of a medical transcriptionist or a nurse practitioner.

Consider on what day or days the ad is to appear; customarily, Sunday is the day most employers run their ads. However, a midweek ad might also be productive.

Does the ad request a response to an anonymous post-office box number? Consider the alternative of having the applicant write directly to you; this tells the applicant that employees know of the open position, and it identifies the medical office openly.

Other Recruiting Methods

Do not rely solely on classified ads for finding applicants. There are other low-cost approaches useful in recruiting quality job candidates. One approach is networking between medical office staff and their peers. This is often far more effective than placing a newspaper ad. To get everyone involved, consider offering a bonus to a staff member who brings in a successful candidate. In addition, job fairs and local college placement offices are often excellent sources for candidates.

Hiring a worker through a temporary employment agency is another approach. This can serve as an audition for a successful permanent candidate. If the work the temp does is not satisfactory, have the agency send someone else; if it is satisfactory, ask the temp to become a permanent staff member.

Some innovative approaches to recruitment might include offering free child care, or flexible hours, or job-sharing. It is also advisable to have researched the salary ranges and fringe benefits of competitors to ascertain the marketability of the new position.

The Hiring Process

Contents of Job Applications

Whether hiring physicians or support staff, there are similar rules to follow. Once applicants are recruited, the first task is to review the contents of the job application. If the wrong kinds of questions are included, no matter how straightforward or innocent the intent, there is potential for a lawsuit. The following items in particular should not appear on the job applications: (1) date of birth, (2) arrest record, and (3) membership in religious or other social groups.

Never ask applicants if they have ever been arrested. This question is irrelevant unless there has been a conviction. You can (and should) ask applicants if they have ever been convicted of a crime if such a question is related to the work the person is expected to do. For example, you may ask applicants who are expected to handle money if they have ever been convicted of embezzlement.

For best results, the application should be divided into three parts: (1) work history, (2) educational background, and (3) personal information that could affect job performance. Work history and education are relatively clear-cut. Personal information is more problematic. Questions that pertain to job performance are acceptable. For example, applicants can be asked if they were ever convicted of sexual harassment or a violent crime. (Employers are not required to consider or hire a felon who could injure another employee.)

Avoid questions about an applicant's health or disability. However, questions about disabilities that would interfere with the applicant's ability to perform the job are allowed.

Your application form should include a statement that all applicants are required to sign. This might read, "I certify that answers given in this application are true and complete to the best of my knowledge. I authorize [insert the practice's name] to investigate all statements made on this application as necessary for reaching an employment decision. If I am subsequently employed, I understand that any false or misleading information provided may result in immediate discharge and/or legal actions."

Interviewing

Remember this rule of thumb during an interview: All questions must be job-related and must be asked of every applicant. For example, do not ask a woman, "Do you have adequate arrangements for child care?" Instead, ask all applicants, "Sometimes we have to work overtime; how do you feel about that?" Questions that require one gender to supply information not requested of the other gender are prohibited. Many states have publications available at no cost which outline permissible preemployment inquiries.

Interviewing physicians Other than the issues of legal versus prohibited questions, the process of interviewing a prospective physician will be considerably different and more complicated than interviewing an applicant for a staff position. The first discussions with a potential candidate may be very general and might be conducted by telephone. The recruiting physician should have the candidate's curriculum vitae in hand, along with a prepared list of statements and questions. The conversation might include details about the practice's needs, patient demographics, location, call schedule, participation (or not) in managed care, and the practice's mission statement or philosophy.

If both parties are still interested, an on-site interview might be scheduled, during which time the office and primary hospitals are visited. The recruiting medical practice will have to consider bearing the expenses of round-trip transportation, hotel accommodations, meals, and transportation within the city. Time spent courting a new physician is time spent not practicing medicine. If the budget is tight, it might be advisable to dedicate an entire day and evening to the process, with a complete itinerary provided so that the process does not have to be repeated.

Consider inviting the candidate's spouse, if one exists; there is no obligation to include a "significant other." The most satisfactory relationship between two physicians can be upset by an unsatisfactory relationship between their spouses; it is better to let them meet each other early in the process in order to avoid potential problems later. However, during the time that medical issues and business matters are discussed, it is generally accepted that the spouses are not present. The recruiting physician's spouse might accompany the applicant's spouse in a variety of activities geared toward the visitor's interests. All parties would then meet for a leisurely dinner to discuss general items and answer questions.

If the reaction seems mutually positive, a formal job offer can be verbally made with promise of a follow-up letter of intent and a job contract. However, the recruiting physician may need to wait before making a commitment until after discussions with a partner or an attorney, or until other recruits are seen.

Both physicians should try to be straightforward with each other. The candidate should be informed of the time frame when an offer can be expected. Conversely, if the recruiting physician has no intention of making a job offer, it would be best to inform the candidate that there are several other applicants to be interviewed before a decision can be reached. A brief follow-up rejection letter could include such phrases as "The position has been filled" or "I cannot make a job offer at this time."

Interviewing office staff   Medical office personnel have a variety of tasks to perform, and interviewing a prospective employee may be one of them. If it is your job, be prepared in advance for the interview. Set a time limit for each applicant of no less than 30 minutes; allow at least 15 minutes between applicants to make notes assessing each candidate. Try not to spend an entire day doing nothing but interviewing, because candidates' faces and qualifications tend to blur. If you have regular job duties essential to running the office and cannot interview during business hours, set aside time before or after office hours for interviews.

Many medical offices have office managers who are able to make hiring decisions within certain parameters predetermined by the physician-owners. However, many physicians insist on making the final decision, so there may be need for a second interview. Other physicians may insist on interviewing all clinical personnel with whom they will be working. Whatever approach is used, you as the initial interviewer should work out the logistics of all initial and subsequent interviews.

Select a location free from interruptions. Have all materials on hand for reference. Review the candidate's résumé and make note of any questions on a separate piece of paper. If the candidate is scheduled to be interviewed during office hours, give the name to the receptionist so that the applicant does not come into the office unannounced. People interviewing for employment are generally nervous and anything to put them at ease will be appreciated, especially later if they are offered a position.

As the interviewer, introduce yourself; offer a handshake to both men and women. Make some neutral remarks to put the candidate at ease and establish a nonthreatening environment. Sometimes refreshments are offered to the candidate.

The first formal requirement of the interview will be to have the candidate complete a job application. In this day of professionally prepared résumés, the job application allows you to compare the answers in person with those on the résumé. Sometimes, surprisingly, the replies will be totally different;

ask about them. Adopt a tone that reflects a desire for clarification rather than challenge or accusation. If the candidate becomes more nervous or perceives a threat, the interview will be nonproductive.

Ask the applicant to read the job description; then ask if there are any questions. As advised earlier, ask all candidates the same questions. Do not lose control of the interview by going off on tangents or allowing the candidate to do so.

When the interview has been completed, explain the process that you have established. Perhaps there are other candidates to interview. Perhaps a second interview will be set up immediately with the physician. Whatever the process, give the applicant the courtesy of a time frame when a decision can be expected.

It may be apparent early in the interview that you will not be hiring the candidate. However, do not abruptly terminate the interview; all time spent interviewing is good practice. Continue with the interview, and thank the candidate for his or her time and interest. Later, send a brief note explaining that the position has been filled.

Sometimes the perfect candidate will appear, and you will be tempted to offer the job on the spot. That is not advisable, as you will not have completed the process of checking references. Further, there are scenarios where an experienced candidate may recognize a novice interviewer's enthusiasm and use it to ask for a higher starting figure. All candidates should be interviewed so that you have a good selection pool from which to make a decision.

Checking References

It is essential to check an applicant's references in order to make quality hiring decisions. However, many past employers are reluctant to release the needed information. If the applicant has signed a statement authorizing a background check, you might fax that statement to the former employer. You could also send it by mail, with a follow-up phone call several days later.

No matter how adamant past employers are about not giving out information, try beginning the conversation with an assurance such as, "Anything you tell me will be kept confidential"; chances are good they will provide the necessary information. Have the questions you want to ask in front of you; these may include the following:

1. When was the applicant employed by you?
2. What was the applicant's title?
3. What were the job duties?
4. What was the salary at termination?
5. Why did the applicant leave your employment?
6. Would you describe the applicant as a team player?
7. Were there any problems with punctuality?
8. Will you share your record of absenteeism on the applicant?
9. Did personal problems interfere with work performance?
10. What work-related strengths did the applicant have?

11. What criticisms did you have of the work performed?
12. Would you rehire? If not, why not?

The last question on rehiring may produce the answer, "It is our policy never to rehire." If so, rephrase the question to say, "Theoretically, if you did not have that policy, would you rehire?" Listen carefully to the replies. Statements such as "I'd rather not answer that question," or shifts from spontaneous, easygoing answers to stilted ones may signal a problem.

In some areas of the country, a recruiting phsyician will just telephone the former physician employer. If that approach is used, have all relevant data on the physician's desk along with a list of questions you have prepared. They may not be used, but it will signal that there are real questions to ask and answers that are needed to make informed decisions. Physicians have been known to mislead other physicians deliberately in order to avoid having to pay unemployment compensation. More often, however, a physician may not be aware of the total employment history of a former employee and so, innocently, misrepresent that person.

Physicians' references   Checking a physician-candidate's references may not be a simple matter. The physician recruiter will have to be very candid in questioning. Questions should include a request for detailed information about malpractice history and any challenges to the candidate's licensure. Contact the National Practitioner Data Bank for up-to-date information (see Appendix B for details). Questions about compliance with CME (Continuing Medical Education) requirements should be raised.

Hospitals have forms that physicians must complete in order to obtain privileges. These are excellent tools for a recruiting physician to use. The time for finding out that a license has been suspended is before an offer is tendered, not when hospital privileges are denied. Court decisions, favorable or unfavorable, are a matter of public record. A malpractice insurance carrier may release that information to you as the recruiting office, especially if it is also your insurance carrier. A call to the state licensing bureau can confirm the validity and status of the physician's right to practice.

Written references   A caution about written references: beware, and never assume. A departing employee can easily obtain stationery and create a favorable reference. A call to the person who signed the letter may also be misleading. A written reference may have been given, but prose can be changed over a signature. Read the reference to the signatory and ask if that was the reference supplied. When references are obtained from physicians in charge of medical residency programs, it is unlikely that anything damaging would appear. Try calling those physicians and asking questions directly; they may be willing to say things over the phone, "in confidence," that they would be unwilling to write in a letter. It is not advisable for a support staff member or office manager to contact such a person; that is the responsibility of the physician.

Additional tips on checking references   If a position entails handling practice funds, call your practice's bonding insurance carrier; such carriers have extensive resources they may be able to utilize.

If a job applicant does not want you to talk to a specific person in the former office, ask why not. If you are told that "the office manager did not like me, I'd rather have you talk directly to Dr. X," you may be dealing with a problem employee. If a job applicant refuses to sign the statement authorizing your investigation, terminate the interview and tell the applicant that you cannot consider him or her for the position.

Be careful when you call a former employer that you are speaking with the right person; always get the person's name and title. It is not unheard of for a friendly ex-coworker to intercept a call.

Making a Job Offer

When the steps of interviewing, evaluating, background checking, and consulting with others are complete, it will be time to offer the position to the candidate of choice. The practice manager or physician may schedule a face-to-face meeting at which time the offer will be made, or a telephone call may be used.

If the offer is to a potential physician, a follow-up letter of intent might be used until an attorney can draw up a contract. There are a number of physicians who believe that a handshake is all that is needed. However, in today's legal climate, although hands may still be shaken, it is unwise to let it go at that. Check with your practice attorney for the recommended strategies when dealing with a contractual employee.

It is not uncommon for candidates, either support staff or physicians, to have several job offers. Ask what it will take for them to accept your offer. Weigh their answers and determine if their conditions are feasible. You might tell them that your offer stands until such and such a date and if they reconsider, they can call you. Sometimes their other negotiations hit snags and your offer appears as the best. Try not to limit yourself with inflexible rules when the immediacy of filling a position is vital.

The Working Relationship

Orientation

Once a new employee has been hired, the next step is to provide a period of orientation. Employees who do not feel comfortable in a new practice or who are not sure what their role is can quickly become discouraged and leave. Develop an orientation plan, which can be used to introduce new employees to the practice and how it operates. The plan could follow the steps described in the following paragraphs.

Introducing employees   If the practice is a large one, it may be more appropriate to introduce key employees. In some practices, the new employee is given a list of the people he or she is likely to be working with on the job. This list might include each person's name, title, responsibilities, and even some personal information.

Take the employee on a walking tour of the facility. In some offices, new employees are taken to lunch on their first or second day of work by their immediate supervisor or the office manager. This is another way of making the new person feel welcome and continuing the orientation process in a comfortable setting.

Outlining personnel policies   Give your new employee a copy of the personnel policies manual. Explain the office's policy on vacation time, absences, personal phone calls, pay days, and other key topics of interest to new employees. If there are any special rules that are unwritten and that you routinely enforce, now is the time to mention them. Unwritten customs such as Secret Santas or wearing costumes for Halloween can be discussed during this time as well.

Preparing the work space   Make sure the new employee's desk or work area is in order before the employee arrives. Check to be certain that all office supplies are stocked and that any training manuals are available.

Orientation checklist   Review the orientation checklist to be sure you have covered all the items that the new employee needs before moving on to the training stage. (See Figure 7.1 for a sample orientation checklist.)

Training

After orientation comes training. For some employees, this time will be very brief; for others it might take longer. Different practices have different ways of training an employee. Some have developed checklists of job skills, and before any duty can be performed without supervision, a new employee must demonstrate proficiency in certain skills. Where direct patient care is involved, such an approach is the most cautious. Other practices have their employees learn by doing. Some practices allow their new employees to work in gradually, while others have an immediate need for productivity.

Whatever approach is needed, it should be planned in advance, keeping in mind the limitations of other staff members. Few medical practices have the luxury of assigning one person to train new employees. If your office is one where it is a catch-as-catch-can situation, explain this to new employees immediately, so they are not intimidated by the confusion.

Motivation

One of the most important assets of a medical practice is a loyal, well-trained staff. To retain personnel, there must be incentives to stay that go beyond a fair wage. A high turnover rate is expensive in terms of disrupting patient care and time spent away from regular duties in order to recruit, hire, orient, and train new employees.

The key to motivation is good management. Much has been written on

Fig. 7.1 Orientation Checklist

Orientation Checklist

Employee _____   Date of Hire _____

Position _____   Orientation leader _____

1. Necessary documents

   a. Completion of I-9 form (required by the Immigration Reform and Control Act of 1986—this document is required by law to verify employment eligibility of anyone hired after November 6, 1986, and includes physicians.)

   b. Completion of federal, state, and local withholding forms.

   c. Completion of any required forms such as parking applications or emergency communication forms.

   d. Documentation of OSHA-required TB tests, HepB vaccines, etc.

2. Present key to the office and any restrictions that pertain to after-hours access.

3. Show where time cards are kept and if a time clock is used. Be certain that the employee is instructed in its use and rules.

4. Go over reporting requirements for absences.

5. Provide specific dates when employee becomes eligible for participation in group benefits:

   a. health insurance _____

   b. disability insurance _____

   c. life insurance _____

   d. pension plan _____

6. Give employee copy of personnel policies manual.
   Review with employee. Have employee sign and date manual to show she or he has been given a copy and understands that the manual does not constitute a contract. Also have employee sign statement of understanding that the practice is an "at-will" employer.

7. Discuss training period.

8. Tour of facility by _____

9. Introduction of immediate supervisor _____

10. Lunch plans.

11. Discuss accessibility to management.

qualities of leadership and management techniques, an office manager might want to purchase specific materials on these topics as a learning tool and as reassurance that the job is being done correctly. These books include some of the following advice to managers:

- Be accessible; do not always make employees come to you. Go to them periodically and invite them to share their concerns and comments.
- Be consistent; always follow through with promises.
- Delegate; do not micromanage. As staff members learn to handle increased responsibilities, their self-esteem improves and their worth to the practice increases.
- Use tact when criticizing. Never use criticism to intimidate or humiliate.
- Don't pass the buck. It is part of an office manager's job to assume responsibility when something goes wrong.

Give the staff recognition when they have done a good job. Feedback helps employees stay motivated. If employees do not know where they stand, they are apt to get discouraged. The feeling of being appreciated is a remarkable loyalty builder. When a practice goes through a difficult period, such as the termination of a key employee, it might be a good idea to give helpful employees special recognition at a staff meeting, thanking them for the extra effort. If an employee has helped to accomplish a practice objective of significant importance, that might be a good opportunity for a bonus.

Job evaluations   Periodic job evaluations are excellent tools to use to motivate employees. Generic job evaluation forms can be purchased from suppliers or practice consultants or they can be developed in-house. They need not be elaborate, and they can even be fun. For example, one practice used the format of report cards and gave them to each employee as self-evaluation forms; after the office manager completed her copy, she and the employees met for lunch and compared their results.

Job evaluations can be checklists or detailed narratives. The idea is to assess the employee's job performance and to solicit responses as to how the performance can be improved. If the need for performance improvement has been met, the evaluation can reflect the excellence of performance.

Whenever evaluating an employee, remember that it is easier to accept criticism if praise has been given first. There is merit to the approach of "You are doing such a good job with transcription, but by the way . . ." Whenever a written evaluation is given, be sure to retain a copy for the employee's files.

Always provide an avenue for the employee to object to any adverse comments. Sometimes the employee will need to take a copy of the evaluation and object to comments felt to be inaccurate. It would be appropriate to replace the original evaluation with the amended copy. The reviewer and the employee should always sign the dated document.

Pay raise   Another motivation tool is the pay raise. If a pay increase is to be given, it should be based on two factors: (1) the quality of the employee's performance, and (2) the financial situation of the practice. A suggestion for the percentage of pay raise is shown by the following scale:

Marginal to no improvement—0–1%
Above average improvement—2–5%
Significant improvement—6–8%
Exceptional improvement—9–10%

A wage and benefit statement is a useful tool that gives everyone a better appreciation of their true compensation (a sample statement is shown in Figure 7.2).

Terminating the Working Relationship

Reducing the Workforce

Not all terminations from employment come as a result of an employee's or employer's disenchantment with each other. With increased competition among the various health care providers and with ongoing government efforts to control reimbursement to physicians, many medical practices are reviewing the size of their workforce as a way to save costs and reduce expenses. This presents a dilemma. In a tight labor market, employers are forced to upgrade their pay scales as well as their benefits, yet market factors also mandate stringent control over expenses. It may then become apparent that a medical practice needs to downsize. Some practices are replacing any full-time employee who leaves with a part-timer; others are eliminating positions and laying off employees.

Medical practices in the private sector are usually not encumbered by legal restrictions that might apply to businesses dealing with union contracts. It is unlikely that a practice will need to continue benefits to an employee who is laid off. Such an employee may file immediately for state unemployment benefits.

The WARN Act

However, if your practice has more than 100 full-time, part-time, and on-call employees, it is covered by the WARN Act (Worker Adjustment and Retraining Notification Act), a federal statute in effect since 1989. The figure of 100 employees applies to the federal statute; however, some states have additional laws. For example, in Michigan, a payroll of 25 puts a medical practice under the state law; the number is 50 employees in Massachusetts, Maryland, Tennessee, and Hawaii.

Mass layoffs The WARN Act requires employers to give 60 days' notice in writing before a mass layoff—mass layoffs are numerically designated by law

Fig. 7.2   Wage and Benefit Statement

	This Year	Last Year
Wage and Benefit Statement for the Year _____		
Employee _____		
Gross salary	_____	_____
Social security (FICA) paid by practice	_____	_____
State unemployment insurance	_____	_____
Workers compensation insurance	_____	_____
Health insurance	_____	_____
Disability insurance	_____	_____
Life insurance	_____	_____
Dental insurance	_____	_____
Retirement plan contribution	_____	_____
Medical expense reimbursement	_____	_____
Travel reimbursement	_____	_____
Professional meetings/seminars	_____	_____
Dues and subscriptions	_____	_____
Parking fees	_____	_____
Uniform allowance	_____	_____
Day care expense	_____	_____
Tuition reimbursement	_____	_____
Bonus	_____	_____
Other: (paid sick days, paid vacation days, etc.)	_____	_____
Total Compensation	$_____	$_____

and also defined as one third of a workforce. However, in Michigan for example, the number is 25 employees, regardless of what percentage of the workforce they comprise. If your practice has several sites within a certain proximity, you must include all employees at all facilities in your calculations.

Even if you have a stable workforce and do not anticipate mass layoffs, you should learn about WARN provisions before catastrophe occurs. Consider the following scenario: You manage a five-physician OB-GYN office that is a professional corporation operating out of two sites within 100 miles of each other. Counting full-time and part-time employees and five physicians (in a professional corporation or P.C., the owners are counted as employees), there are 30 people. Since the practice is in Michigan, it is covered under state regulations. It is early spring and one facility is suddenly rendered uninhabitable by a tornado. In the same tornado, Dr. X and his family are killed and Dr. Y receives a serious injury, disabling him for several months. It is immediately apparent that you must lay off the 10 part-time employees who staffed the destroyed facility. Since this is one third of your workforce, the WARN provisions come into effect.

Layoff notice   Each worker must receive the layoff notice personally. In addition, the state agency that oversees retraining of dislocated workers must be informed; so must the mayor or county executive where the office is located. The notice may be delivered by mail, by hand, or in the employee's pay envelope. The notice has to be in the employee's hands 60 days before the job ends. Even with a catastrophe, you must continue to pay salary and benefits for those 60 days. Failure to do so or to comply with the regulations in the Act will create serious monetary penalties.

Are there any exceptions? The 60 days' notice is not required if the management could not be expected to know 60 days ahead of time that it was going to have to close down an operation. But with this scenario, you are not closing down, only laying off since you still have a facility open. As noted, it is important to know the provisions of WARN before a crisis comes.

Replacing Employees

If your medical practice is not covered under the WARN Act because it is a small office, and you decide to lay off full-time employees and replace them with part-timers, be sure to offer a full-time employee the option of staying as a part-time employee before you fill the position.

If you decide to get rid of a problem employee by terminating the job position and laying that person off, thereby circumventing charges of wrongful discharge and avoiding the unpleasant task of firing, be certain that a reasonable period of time passes before you "reevaluate" the need to create that position once again.

When you hire to fill that re-created position, it is wise to make it either full time if it had been part time in the past or vice versa. Make certain that the person filling the "new" position is at least as qualified as the person who was laid off; a more qualified candidate would be better. If the person who held the original job were really disgruntled, litigation about your strategy could occur. Failure to navigate the choppy waters of employment and labor law can drown you!

Employers' Rights

As constricting as the laws and regulations may appear to be, employers also have many rights at their disposal, if management takes the steps necessary to make the laws and regulations work for them. All the laws in the 50 states cannot deprive you of your right to fire substandard employees, at will, provided you back up your action with appropriate procedures protecting you.

Documentation   Carefully document the employee's performance and show that your grievances are justified. Keep a written record whenever the employee has been warned, disciplined, or given advice on how to improve performance. Never rely on having a coworker or supervisor back you up later. Documentation is the most effective weapon in any type of legal action. The following list describes what should be kept in an employee's file:

- Job application
- Performance evaluations
- Résumé
- Time records
- Wage and salary records
- Documentation of verbal warnings made to the employee

The Equal Employment Opportunity Commission (EEOC) requires employers with 15 or more employees to maintain records for six months or more on such actions as layoffs, transfers, and demotions. The Department of Labor requires employers to maintain wage records for two to three years. If you have required all employees to sign an at-will statement specifying that they may be terminated at the discretion of the employer, that should also be kept. This statement can be part of the personnel manual and should make clear your authority to terminate employment at will.

Personnel policies manual   Review your practice manual for language that could imply a contractual relationship. You may even want to include in your personnel manual the following statement, "This manual does not constitute a contract of employment." Instruct all those involved in recruiting not to make statements such as "Your only limit is your own ability" or "We don't hire, we adopt."

Litigation   This is a litigious society, and wrongful discharge suits are more common than in past years. The states with the most liberal laws (from the plaintiff's point of view) are California, Indiana, Massachusetts, Montana, and North Dakota. However, even in a high litigation state like California, the state has moved to limit damages while still allowing employee lawsuits to occur.

Even if you have taken all the precautions, have been a fair and reasonable employer, and have acted in good faith, you may be second-guessed by a jury. When you discharge an employee, you must have established that it is for just cause; then you have a good chance of winning any wrongful-discharge suit that might be brought against you.

Final Steps in Termination

When the time is at hand that you have to terminate an employee's working relationship with your practice, there are some nonlegal tips to follow.

1. Do not let the terminated employee stay in the office after termination, as computer and other forms of sabotage frequently occur. This may entail your walking the employee around the office while she or he collects personal belongings. You might offer the option of returning at a time when the office is closed and no other employees are around if you feel there is need to save face. However, if you elect this option, make certain your physician-employer is there as well for your protection.

2. Have the employee's final paycheck in hand. While you conduct your exit-interview, make certain that parking passes, keys to any equipment the employee might have, and keys to the office suite or building are collected. There may be documents that need to be signed: conversion from group to individual coverage on life insurance, or health insurance if COBRA is involved. All those should be completed before you hand over the final paycheck. If the employee is an hourly worker and you cannot figure out the pay ahead of time, be certain to explain to the employee when the final paycheck will be available.

3. Watch your attitude. Treat the employee with dignity. State the facts simply, as shown in this example: "It is the decision of the physicians that your work performance justifies terminating your employment. As you have been warned on multiple occasions, your failure to clean instruments properly and in a timely fashion has placed the doctors in an untenable position."

4. If the employee is being laid off for some reason not attributable to fault, you may want to call other offices to see if they have a position available. You might familiarize yourself with the state's unemployment benefits regulations in order to assist the employee. Anything you can do to help the employee is bound to be appreciated and will limit the bad feelings that might otherwise exist.

Legal Requirements of a Working Relationship

Federal Regulations

Some of the federal rules that affect your ability to hire and fire office employees are described in the following list:

- Older Workers Benefit Protection Act—requires that the worker and employer must reach agreement that meets the "knowledge and voluntary" standard. It stipulates guidelines for early retirement incentive plans.
- Family and Medical Leave Act (FMLA)—requires employers of 50 or more employees to give employees time off when they are ill or must assist in the care of an ill spouse, child, or parent, or if there is a new child in the family. Twelve weeks' leave per year must be given, though it need not be

paid leave. Medical benefits must be continued and the returning employee must get his or her old job back or one that is equivalent not only in pay but also in duties.

- Age Discrimination in Employment Act (ADEA)—prohibits discrimination against an individual 40 years of age and over where action is age-based.
- Occupational Safety and Health Act (OSHA)—regulates safety practices and hazards in the workplace.
- Americans with Disabilities Act of 1990 (ADA)—forbids employment discrimination against people with disabilities.
- Consolidated Omnibus Budget Reconciliation Act (COBRA)—requires employers of 25 or more employees to continue group health insurance coverage for terminated employees and their spouses and dependents for up to 18 months after termination (at the employee's cost), or up to 29 months in the case of disabled employees.
- Employee Retirement Income Security Act (ERISA)—provides rules on employee pension coverage and prohibits employers from discharging workers in order to stop them from getting pension rights, among other issues.
- Employee Polygraph Protection Act of 1988—forbids private employers from giving prospective employees lie-detector tests.
- Equal Pay Act—prohibits employers from paying one gender less than the other if they are working on jobs that require equal skill, effort, and responsibility, and if those jobs are performed under similar working conditions.
- Fair Labor Standards Act (FLSA)—sets wage and hour standards in the workplace.
- Pregnancy Discrimination Act—prohibits discrimination based on "pregnancy, childbirth, and related medical conditions."
- Title VII of the Civil Rights Act of 1964—bars discrimination based on race, sex, color, religion, or national origin.
- Rehabilitation Act of 1973—prohibits discrimination against the disabled by government contractors (if your practice participates in any way with Medicare, it could be considered a government subcontractor), requiring reasonable accommodation for handicapped workers.

This list includes only some of the federal laws involving employees and employers. There are additional laws, often more stringent, that are imposed by state legislation. Note: If any of the above issues is the basis for a decision to terminate employment, be sure to seek legal counsel before acting.

Publications detailing these regulations can be obtained, often free of charge, from your local office of the Department of Labor or from your congressman; the latter is an excellent source. You can also write the Superintendent of Documents, U.S. Government Printing Office, Washington, DC 20402, although there may be a charge for each publication.

There are additional legal requirements of a working relationship, among which are federal wage and hour regulations.

All practice managers must be familiar with the Federal Fair Labor Standards Act (FLSA). It explains the standards of minimum-wage, overtime and equal pay requirements, record-keeping requirements, and child-labor provisions. This Act applies to medical practices that have gross receipts of more than $25,000 per year or that have more than two employees.

Overtime

At one time many medical practices mistakenly believed that since hospital personnel were exempt from overtime because they were allowed to average the workweek for their personnel, so were physicians' offices exempt from the provision of the 40-hour workweek. However, exemptions from overtime are dependent on specific and clearly defined criteria under the Fair Labor Standards Act. These criteria refer to the two classes of employees in a medical office: exempt employees and nonexempt employees.

Exempt employees This category includes executive, administrative, and professional personnel, who are defined by specific criteria. For executives, these depend on a salary above a certain level, supervision of two or more employees, management of a department, the exercise of discretionary powers, and an allocation of no more than 20 percent of hours worked to activities not closely related to managerial duties.

To qualify for administrative status, the duties must be directly related to management policies or general business operations or to academic instruction or administration. Such personnel would work under only general supervision along specialized technical lines requiring special training, experience, or knowledge. Other criteria noted above that refer to the percentage of hours and salary level would also apply.

Duties of exempt employees The following are examples of duties that are managerial when performed by an employee managing a medical office or supervising other employees:

- Setting and adjusting pay rates and work hours
- Directing work
- Planning and distributing work
- Evaluating efficiency and productivity
- Determining work techniques

Nonexempt employees This category includes all other employees. The classifications of exempt and nonexempt are commonly ignored in medical offices, but unfortunately this can result in substantial legal and financial problems.

Job titles do not determine if an employee is exempt or nonexempt. Also, designating employees as salaried does not make them exempt. For example, registered nurses are exempt employees because they meet clearly defined criteria, having completed a formal educational process of long duration. However, a licensed practical nurse and a medical assistant with an associate's degree are not exempt, even when they perform the same work as an RN, because they do not meet all the criteria of an exempt employee. On the other hand, just because an RN is exempt does not mean you cannot pay overtime if you want to. Many medical offices feel that it is only fair to pay overtime to all nonowners if they work over 40 hours in a workweek. Two other examples of nonexempt employees are bookkeepers and transcriptionists.

Duties of nonexempt employees   Nonexempt duties might include the following:

- Performing the same kind of work as the employees supervised
- Performing any work, even though not like that performed by subordinates, which is not part of supervisory functions
- Preparing payrolls
- Performing routine clerical duties such as billing, filing, operating business machines, bookkeeping, or transcribing (An RN acting in the capacity of a bookkeeper or transcriptionist is no longer considered exempt.).

Salary versus wages   Many medical offices call all monies received by their employees "salaries," probably because it sounds more professional and after all, a medical office is a professional office. You can refer to wages paid by any title, but in the end you will have to calculate all nonexempt employees' reimbursement by establishing an hourly rate of pay in order to fulfill the requirements of the law.

Time records   To meet the overtime provisions, you will have to keep time records. These can be automatic time clocks, generic time cards, or record-keeping methods such as individual calendars. In any case, the employee—not the manager—fills in the number of hours worked each day and signs the document attesting to its accuracy. Without the employee's signature, the document is invalid.

Hours worked include all the time the employee is required to be in the office or on duty, even time spent waiting. Work permitted is counted as work time. The law says that management has the responsibility for enforcement. Announcing that no overtime will be paid or saying "If you come in early and start working, you won't be paid for that time" will not relieve managers of the responsibility to pay overtime.

Other Wage and Hour Requirements

Other provisions that affect employees are reviewed in the paragraphs below.

Offering a salary for a workweek that exceeds 40 hours   A fixed salary for a workweek longer than 40 hours does not discharge the statutory obligation to pay for overtime. Again, the issue is whether or not an employee is exempt.

Pay for foregoing holidays and vacations   In some instances, employees are entitled to holiday or vacation pay but work on that day. If they receive their customary rate or higher for their work on a holiday or vacation day, the additional sum given as holiday or vacation pay is excluded from the regular rate of pay.

Rest and meal periods   There is no law that says employers must give either rest periods or meal periods. However, many employees would not continue to work for a practice if such conditions of employment were not offered. Rest periods must be counted as working time if the employee is not completely relieved from duty and cannot use the time effectively for personal purposes.

A transcriptionist who is waiting for dictation to be finished and takes a break and reads a magazine is considered to be working because the employee is engaged to wait. However, if the transcriptionist, under the same circumstances, leaves the building to smoke a cigarette or run an errand, that would not constitute working time.

Holiday pay and vacations   Again, there is no law that requires an employer to give time off with or without pay. As a matter of good business sense, however, it is unlikely that a medical practice would not give employees Christmas or Thanksgiving off. Urgent care centers often must stay open on holidays and they must be staffed; a premium to the regular pay might be offered to attract employees but there is no legal requirement to do so. As with holidays, there is no law mandating vacation pay. Again, it is a business custom and not dictated by law.

Time off in lieu of pay   The overtime pay requirement may not be waived.

Docking pay   An employer may penalize an hourly or salaried nonexempt employee for excessive lateness. Employees should be warned that they will be docked one or two hour's pay for every hour they are late. The wage and hour law also says that an employer may double-dock in accordance with these three rules: (1) the deduction cannot bring an employee's pay below the minimum hourly wage; (2) the deductions must be made at the regular hourly rate of the employee, not the overtime rate; and (3) the maximum permitted weekly deduction is based on a regular workweek. Obviously, you cannot double-dock a part-time file clerk being paid the minimum wage.

Payment of overtime   Overtime compensation need not be paid weekly. The general rule is that overtime pay earned in a particular workweek must be paid on the regular payday for the period in which the workweek ends. If the correct amount of overtime pay cannot be determined until some time after the regular pay period, the employer must pay the overtime compensation as soon after the regular pay period as is practical.

Penalties   The Fair Labor Standards Act describes methods for recovering unpaid minimum and/or overtime wages owed to an employee. If an employee, current or former, files a complaint with a federal or state agency, that agency can legally audit your records. The name of the employee is protected. If the employer attempts to retaliate against the employee, there are heavy fines and penalties.

Benefits of a Working Relationship

In order to be fiscally effective and reduce exposure to malpractice occurrences, physicians must hire and retain qualified personnel. In order to attract qualified personnel who can deal with the sophisticated technologies and ever-changing health plan requirements, today's medical office must offer competitive wages and fringe-benefit packages. Some practices bypass the need to provide substantial fringe benefits by hiring part-time personnel, who do not qualify for the benefits received by the full-time employees. However, this strategy may be costly in terms of lack of commitment, which in turn can compromise patient care.

Fringe Benefits

If it has become apparent that your practice is not attracting qualified personnel, it might be appropriate to review the fringe-benefit package that you offer. Your ability to offer substantial fringes will be determined by your practice's budget and the labor market. Typical fringe benefits include the following:

- Paid vacations
- Paid holidays
- Paid sick days
- Paid personal days
- Health insurance
- Life insurance
- Disability insurance (short-term and/or long-term)
- Uniform allowance
- Tuition and/or license fee reimbursement
- Professional dues
- Pension plan
- Dental insurance

Personal days   Some medical offices have reviewed the policy of personal days off and determined that it is actually less expensive to close the office for a day and give employees an extra day off during a holiday period, such as the Friday following Thanksgiving, than it is to offer personal days off. Personal days are taken at the employee's will; their arbitrary nature can cause havoc within a medical office. Some medical offices have done away with sick days and personal days and have scheduled their offices to be closed after 12 noon on Fridays. This practice not only increases morale but also decreases the need to pay overtime.

Health insurance   This is a costly benefit. Whoever decides which plan to choose should call on several insurance agents to discuss their programs. Health insurance carriers have multiple products to sell. In order to qualify for group coverage without the requirement of underwriting and/or noncoverage for preexisting conditions, a medical office must have a certain number of participants.

If your practice is small and if the physician-owner is a member of a state medical society, insurance could be purchased through that group. There are other groups physicians can join in order to supply their employees with group rates; various professional associations also offer a variety of group programs for members.

There are many strategies medical offices can use to lower the cost of health insurance. They can pay the entire premium for their employees, they can pay a portion of the costs, or they can obtain the lowered group rate and make that available to employees who bear the cost of the premium. Some offices offer premium reimbursement when the employee is included on the spouse's insurance. Some insurance carriers will individualize a policy; for example, if all employees are not of childbearing age, the carrier may be able to reduce premium costs by not offering that particular benefit.

Life insurance   The majority of medical office personnel are women, and a number of them may be single. Life insurance obtained as a benefit of employment may be the only life insurance they have. For the older employee, it may bring a certain peace of mind to have life insurance as a benefit, while to a young woman starting her career, it may have little or no value.

It is important to review programs from carriers to see what is available at what cost. Avoid companies without proven track records. There are insurance companies that offer low-cost policies but who delay claims processing for six months after a death or who refuse to pay claims outright unless legal challenge is implemented. In order to more fully understand the details, write to your state insurance commission and ask for any materials available.

Disability insurance   If a premium for disability insurance is paid by the employee's medical office, monies received by the disabled employee will be taxable. If an individual pays the premium, the monies are not considered taxable income. Group disability policies for medical office personnel are becoming hard to find and are nonexistent in several states because of abuses. Generally, disability insurance includes a waiting period before benefits can be obtained, and a percentage of wages the disabled employee will receive for a specified period of time is tied to Social Security benefits.

The definition of total disability is important when considering one company's policy over another. If a physician were unable to practice medicine but theoretically could teach, this would not be considered total disability by a company that uses a conservative definition of total disability. A company that uses a more liberal definition might state "as long as the party is disabled from performing the duties of his employment." As with other insurance, costs can be reduced by having the employee pay the premium.

Wages in lieu of benefits   To some employees, a particular benefit may have no value; they would prefer an increased wage to a specific benefit. However, unless your office offers a "cafeteria" fringe-benefit program worked out by attorneys to ensure legal compliance, do not get involved in this practice. The federal government is giving increased thought to considering fringe benefits as taxable income, and it would only complicate matters to enter into this type of negotiation with employees. By networking with other offices of the same specialty and size, you can more easily determine what the standard fringe benefits are in your community.

Intangible benefits   What can a three-physician family practice do to compete with a ten-physician plastic surgery group? It is in this area that an office manager has a chance to be creative by offering informal or intangible fringe benefits of employment. For example, besides the ideas already suggested, one office orders and pays for pizza every Wednesday afternoon. Another office offers each employee and their family a free week of vacation at the employer's vacation home on a nearby lake. A third office rents a bus and driver, schedules a "mental health" day, closes the office, and takes all employees to a discount mall for a day of shopping.

   If a practice cannot compete with increased wages and comprehensive benefit packages, it can make the office an enjoyable place to work. Some potential employees might not be able to consider employment with your office because of their financial needs; however, there will be others who will be attracted to an office that offers recognition of personal accomplishment and other intangible benefits.

Death or Disability of a Physician

Fifty years ago, when a practicing physician died, the spouse or family would sell the medical practice—that is, the accounts receivable, the medical records, and the good will. Today, however, that procedure is uncommon although still utilized in dental practices. When a physician dies unexpectedly, many issues must be resolved, depending on the type and size of practice. In a large professional corporation, there will be preestablished death benefits and buyout clauses. In a small partnership or solo practice, however, the issues of "what to do" might be much less clear. It is advisable for medical office managers to have established a worst-case scenario replete with a checklist of who to call and what to do about existing staff.

   If it is a solo practice, issues will arise as to how to notify patients, the transfer of medical records, the storage of unclaimed medical records, accounts-receivable collections, accounts payable, termination of leased space, cancellation of existing benefits and insurance policies, notification to insurance carriers and the state licensing board, as well as the disposition of office furniture and equipment.

It is probable that the physician used an accountant who will be able to deal with the issue of taxes. Obviously, this is a time of great stress on all those involved with the physician's practice: the spouse and family, the patients, and the staff whose employment will be terminated. Often, some staff member will stay to close out the practice. Normally, this burden falls on the staff member who has the most familiarity with the financial aspects of the practice.

This staff member is well-advised to meet with the person legally responsible for the physician's estate (if deceased) or affairs (if disabled) and to negotiate an acceptable working agreement. This should include role and responsibilities, length of time required, remuneration, place of employment, and other specifics.

If desired, a practice can find help from practice management groups—management advisers that can provide expertise and personnel to assist in these matters. The medical society in your community or state can probably help identify such advisers. Since this will be a stressful time and a period of sadness and anxiety, it may be useful to have people working with and for you who are less personally involved and consequently more objective.

If the physician is disabled but still mentally competent, he or she will remain the decision maker and still be part of the health care team. If this is not the case, the person with whom you must work may hold the physician's power of attorney. This could be someone totally uninformed about legal or administrative matters, and your experience and knowledge will be critical in guiding the successful closure of the practice.

Conclusion

By educating yourself about the variety of employment laws, by establishing clearly written personnel policies, and by having a practice philosophy or statement that is fair and equitable, the physician and the medical office manager will be able to effectively provide patient care without the disruption and expense of litigation. If litigation does occur, by having documented employee performance and having followed sound business practices, the risk of financial disaster can be minimized.

Chapter 8

Human Relations in the Medical Office

Introduction   178
Patient Service   178
The Telephone   184
Human Relations among Staff Members and with Patients   195
Conclusion   200

Introduction

At no other time in history have human relations skills been more important to medical practices. Health care today is in a state of constant transition, brought about by economic factors, alternative delivery systems, and changing patterns of patient expectations. These factors have created an extremely competitive environment, and have resulted in the need for medical practices that are more attentive to providing "patient service." Having the technical skills needed to practice medicine is not enough to establish good relationships with patients. Patients have a right to expect physicians and office staff to be courteous as well as technically competent.

Today's patients have a choice of physicians, and they are choosing those who satisfy their wants and needs. Most patients are not knowledgeable enough to recognize when they are not receiving the best possible medical treatment, but they do recognize when their dignity has been respected and when they have received kindness, courtesy, and attention to their needs.

Patient Service

Human relations and patient service are the nontechnical sides of medicine. They include the bedside manner and the healing touch that help patients feel better, often improving their health regardless of the medical treatment. These are also the qualities that keep patients returning to a medical practice and referring others.

In today's realm of health care, patient service is not a choice, it is a core component measured by the National Committee for Quality Assurance

(NCQA), the accreditation agency for managed care organizations. Managed care firms often use patient-satisfaction data to determine compensation levels and physician performance. Without participation in managed care, the practice often has no access to patients, and without patients, the practice dies.

Indicators of Excellent Patient Service

The goal of patient service is to satisfy the patient's real as well as perceived needs. Real needs deal with essential aspects of medical care that everyone agrees are important. For example, a medical office should be clean, neat, safe, and staffed by technically competent physicians and ancillary personnel.

However, patients also judge their medical visit and form their overall opinion of a medical practice through sensory perceptions (such as sight, smell, taste, touch, and hearing). Patients in the reception or waiting room have time to observe and to form opinions about the quality of care they are about to receive. Their senses are heightened as they anticipate their examination or treatment. They are consciously and unconsciously recording their feelings about what they are hearing (staff or patient conversations, office music, television); seeing (office decor); smelling (odors from perfumes, lunch rooms, bathrooms); tasting (possible refreshments); and feeling (seating materials, drafts, air temperature, and their own pain or discomfort). In addition, patients are keenly aware of the personal interactions among the physicians and the staff members. Every sensory perception that patients have during their stay at the office creates an impression that either makes them want to return and to refer others or to go elsewhere.

In a practice that provides patient service, patients feel that they are valued by the doctor and staff and are important to the practice. Staff members contribute to these perceptions through their actions with patients and fellow employees.

Patient service is a mind-set, a positive attitude projected to every patient that sends the message, "We realize that you don't need this practice—this practice needs you!" This attitude consists of the following six characteristics: willingness, readiness, preparedness, responsiveness, attentiveness, and trustworthiness.

Willingness Willingness is a quality that cannot be taught. Physicians and staff members must believe in and practice the tenets of the Hippocratic oath and the AMA's Principles of Medical Ethics (see pages 2–3). These doctrines convey a genuine commitment to the profession and a willingness to help patients. The following examples illustrate opposite levels of commitment.

Willingness to help: "Mrs. Stevens, I'm glad you called. Tell me what happened so we can correct it for you."

Unwillingness: "What's this about."

Readiness   Readiness means that the physician and staff members are focused on their responsibilities to the patient, not on distractions such as personal conversations that are unrelated to the patient.

> *Readiness:*   Patient enters office, and goes to reception desk; receptionist ends conversation with other staff member in order to acknowledge the patient. "Good afternoon, Mr./Mrs. White" (to an existing patient).
>
> *or*
>
> "Good afternoon. Welcome to our practice; I'm Sue" (to a new patient). Wait for patient to give name, or ask, "May I have your name, please?"
>
> *Unreadiness:*   Receptionist continues conversing with staff member while handing a sign-in sheet to patient.

Preparedness   Preparedness means that physicians and staff members have the mind-set and materials needed for patient care. They have the training, tools, support, and authority to act appropriately for patients. A physician needs training (medical school and residency); tools (instruments, medications, equipment, and supplies); support (personnel); and authority (licensure) in order to serve patients.

Staff members also need training (specific to their job functions); tools (telephones, computers, office supplies, and equipment); support (assistance and feedback); and authority (empowerment to take certain actions) in order to properly perform their jobs and provide patient service.

Responsiveness   Most patients perceive their problems or requests as urgent, and they expect others to see them as urgent, too. The speed at which staff members respond to patients affects the rapport between them. Responsiveness includes some of the following:

- Answering the telephone within three rings
- Allowing patients to speak without placing them on hold or interrupting them
- Greeting patients immediately upon their approaching the receptionist
- Making eye contact with patients and using reinforcers (such as nodding your head or saying "yes, . . . I see . . . tell me more") to show attention to them
- Acknowledging the importance of the patient's situation, with a willingness to help as quickly as possible

Attentiveness   Attentiveness means that patients understand that they have not been forgotten, and that someone is taking action to solve their problems or to help them. Specific actions that show attentiveness include the following:

- Telling patients who telephone that their call will be handled quickly or transferred to someone who can help
- Giving patients a specific time or time frame when their call will be returned

- Calling patients to inform them of delays in lab test results to allay their fears and worries
- Announcing that the physician is running behind schedule and giving patients an opportunity to reschedule or offering them beverages, access to a telephone, or other compensation for waiting

Trustworthiness   Trustworthiness means that the patient can count on the medical practice and its staff members to do what they say they are going to do. It implies reliability, responsibility, and consistency.

Patient Service—Choice or Mandate?

Managed care organizations (MCOs) are now measuring patient satisfaction. Therefore, it is better for a medical office to find out directly from patients if there are problems than to find out from the MCO at contract-renewal time. The nonprofit National Committee for Quality Assurance (NCQA) seeks to improve the quality of patient care and health plan performance in coordination with MCOs, purchasers, consumers, and government agencies. A major undertaking for the NCQA was the development of HEDIS (Health Plan Employer Data and Information Set), a systematic method for measuring physician and plan performance. The organization is committed to making information about health plan quality available to all interested parties. Since individual physicians (providers) contribute to the overall performance of a health plan, the NCQA has developed questionnaires to survey enrollees' (or patients') firsthand experiences with providers of care. Patients are asked about their satisfaction with such areas as the following:

- Access to appointments in a timely manner
- Convenience of office location and office hours
- Friendliness and courtesy shown by physicians and staff
- Availability of information in office and by telephone
- Interest in and attention to patients' concerns and comments
- Explanations of diagnosis and treatment options
- Thoroughness, skill, experience, and training of physicians and staff
- Amount of time spent with physician and staff during a visit

Measuring Patient Satisfaction

Assessing patient satisfaction need not be a complicated process. Simply ask patients how they feel about the quality and service provided by the practice and what suggestions they have for improvement. This could be done by questionnaire, by telephone, or in person; the most successful patient-service surveys utilize a combination of all three methods.

Questionnaire   A patient-satisfaction questionnaire allows respondents to rate their visit on a verbal or numerical scale that goes beyond simple yes and no answers, enabling them to indicate borderline feelings. (For a sample questionnaire, see Figure 8.1)

Each questionnaire should be reviewed, with action taken to improve issues that are consistently rated less than satisfactory. Some offices survey patient satisfaction for a few weeks or months and then stop, assuming that if everything is satisfactory, things will continue to be satisfactory in the future. This a dangerous assumption. Since the key to patient service is consistency, measuring patient satisfaction should be an ongoing commitment, not a one-shot effort.

The best time to present the questionnaire to patients is at checkout. For example, simply say, "Mrs. Jones, here is a questionnaire that Dr. Brown would appreciate your filling out and depositing in the box by the door. It's our report card, and it lets us know what kind of a job we are doing for you."

Be sure to give the questionnaire to the patient on an attractive clipboard with a pen or pencil. For those patients who are too ill or tired to complete the questionnaire, give them a self-addressed stamped envelope and tell them they can fill it out at home. Some patients may feel burdened by receiving a questionnaire at each visit. For these few patients, staff members can simply say, "Mrs. Smith, each visit with you is separate and special to us. We just want to make sure that you are completely satisfied every time you see us."

There should be a covered drop box by the front door for depositing the completed questionnaires. Patients who wish to remain anonymous or who have written complaints are more likely to use a drop box than to hand a negative report to a staff member.

Telephone survey   Another way to measure satisfaction is to telephone patients, especially the ones who have not responded to their recall notices. The main purpose for calling is to check on them to find out if everything is all right. The secondary purpose is to uncover any reasons why they do not wish to schedule an appointment. If the reason has anything to do with dissatisfaction in the practice, staff, or services, you can assure them that the matter will be corrected and that they are highly valued by the practice.

In-person survey   Face-to-face encounters with patients can yield important information about satisfaction. Simply asking "Was everything satisfactory today, Mrs. Jones?" or "Do you have any suggestions on how we can improve our service to you?" will give the patient the opportunity to voice any dissatisfaction.

Attributes of Patient-Service Employees

Today's medical office manager must be a director of patient service. That means casting employees for the roles that they will perform for the benefit of patients.

To find staff members best suited to their roles, the job interview for new employees should focus on human-relations skills in addition to task-oriented skills. Open-ended interview questions can be used to uncover an applicant's

Fig. 8.1   Patient Satisfaction Questionnaire

Your practice logo and physician name(s) could appear here.

Setting Our Sights on Your Satisfaction!

We are committed to providing you with the best possible health care and personalized service. Please give us your frank comments and suggestions about your visit today. You can be sure that whatever you say will help us provide you with service that exceeds your expectations!

	Satisfied	Somewhat Satisfied	Somewhat Dissatisfied	Dissatisfied
1. Your telephone calls to our office were handled to your satisfaction.	( )	( )	( )	( )
2. You were greeted promptly and courteously by our receptionists when you entered our office.	( )	( )	( )	( )
3. Our reception area was comfortable.	( )	( )	( )	( )
4. Your doctor exhibited confidence and expertise in performing your exam.	( )	( )	( )	( )
5. The technicians exhibited competence and expertise in performing tests.	( )	( )	( )	( )
6. The exams were explained to you by the doctor and technicians.	( )	( )	( )	( )
7. You were treated with dignity and respect by all of our staff members.	( )	( )	( )	( )
8. The total time your exam took was reasonable.	( )	( )	( )	( )
9. Your questions about our fees and Medicare were answered to your satisfaction.	( )	( )	( )	( )

10. Will you recommend us to others? _____ Yes _____ No _____ Maybe
    Please explain if No or Maybe

11. How would you rate us? _____ Excellent _____ Good _____ Fair _____ Poor

12. How did you find out about us? _____
    If friend, patient, or doctor, please give name

Additional comments and suggestions _____

Thank you for taking the time to share your thoughts with us.

Name	Date and Time of Appointment

(Reprinted by permission, © 1993 Kim Fox)

attitude toward difficult patients with memory or comprehension problems, irrationalities, or physical handicaps. Examples include the following questions:

- What are your feelings about angry patients who use profanity to vent their frustrations? How would you handle such a patient who was making a scene in the reception room in front of other patients?
- How would you handle a patient whose ride has not shown up, and it is almost time to close the office?
- How would you handle a situation where your telephone is ringing, a patient scheduled for tomorrow is at your station arguing that the appointment is today, and your doctor is standing in the doorway asking you for a chart?
- What is your main strength when it comes to handling difficult people? Your main weakness?
- What gives you the greatest satisfaction from working with patients? Fellow employees? Doctors?
- Can you share any examples of situations where you helped calm someone down and helped solve their problem? What was the outcome for them? For you?
- Have you experienced any life-threatening situations or serious illnesses that you feel will help you relate to what a patient might be experiencing or feeling?

If a job applicant can hold up under the pressure of an in-depth interview and still make the interviewer feel comfortable, the chances are that this applicant may also be able to make patients feel comfortable. (For details on interviewing job applicants, see Chapter 7, "Personnel Policies.")

In the past, most medical practices have been more concerned with hiring employees who have prior health-related experience and task-oriented skills than those who have human relations or "people" skills. Today's medical office employee must excel at both task-oriented skills and human relations skills.

The Telephone

Nerve Center of a Medical Practice

The telephone is the nerve center of the medical practice. It is where images and first impressions of the doctor and the practice are formed. It is where appointments are made, relationships are established and nurtured, information is exchanged, referrals are converted to patients, and malpractice risk is reduced. The practice may be providing exceptional medical care and still be sending a negative message to patients or potential patients through the telephone. In the first critical 7–10 seconds of a call, the staff member gives the caller the impression of just how much the doctor "cares" for patients.

Telephone etiquette must be provided to all callers, since anyone calling the practice is a potential patient or referral source. This is especially true for referring physicians, whose staff members usually make the calls to coordinate care for their patients. These staff members have the power to change referral patterns. If they receive curt, insensitive treatment, are transferred too often, or are kept on hold for too long, they might call another practice or complain to their physician, who will then refer patients to someone else.

Increased use   The main problem with telephone service in the medical practice is that a receptionist's job description has traditionally included responsibility for the telephone. This worked when offices were small and patient loads were light. Today, however, many offices have reduced staff and increased patient loads, with the result that more duties are being performed by fewer staff members.

The impact on telephone service of overworked staff members juggling multiple tasks can be endless busy signals, numerous rings before answering, interminable and multiple waits on hold, and hurried treatment from an overworked individual. Unfortunately, some practices are resorting to automated touch-tone menu systems, thinking that this will relieve telephone congestion. However, nothing is more soothing to an individual than the sound of a warm, friendly, helpful human voice.

Successful service   Instead of resorting to expensive automated equipment, a practice-wide effort should be made to streamline the handling of telephone calls so that a positive image of the practice is projected with every call. Successful telephone service depends on the following:

- Positive attitude toward the telephone
- Adequate telephone equipment and number of telephone lines
- Distraction-free environment for managing calls
- Sufficient staffing and training
- Effective call-handling procedures
- Scripted responses to various calls
- Quality assurance system

Positive Attitude

Staff members need to regard every ring of the telephone as a patient-service "opportunity" instead of an interruption to their work. The approximate monetary value of each patient to the practice can be shown in return visits and referrals. Additional evidence to convince staff members of the importance of telephone service is to present the following facts, taken from business surveys:

1. A business usually hears from only 4 percent of dissatisfied customers; the other 96 percent just go quietly away.
2. A typical dissatisfied customer tells 8 to 10 people about poor service; one in five will tell 20 people.

3. Sixty-eight percent of customers who quit a business do so because of an indifferent attitude shown toward them by someone in the business.
4. The average business spends six times more money to attract new customers than it does to keep established ones.

Finally, ask staff members to compare the service given through the medical practice telephone with service-oriented businesses that they personally call. Ask them to share a frustrating occasion that caused them to hang up and to call another competitor; what were the circumstances of the call, and how monetarily important was their lost business.

Adequate Telephone Equipment

Telephone equipment need not be the latest, most sophisticated technology. This may be too expensive for most medical practices, and it is impossible and impractical to keep up with the rapidly changing technology in the telecommunications field.

What is important, however, is that telephone equipment have adequate features for efficiency and that these features be fully utilized. For example, it is a waste of time to physically track down a staff member for a telephone call when audible paging through a P.A. system or through the telephone itself is a feature available on all new telephone systems. On the other hand, you do not need to invest in expensive features that will probably never be used by a small practice.

Group practices with many physicians and employees may find it advantageous to purchase a system that enables a "switchboard operator" to answer, screen, and direct calls or to monitor telephone activity and special instructions coming from each telephone. Such systems have the capability of showing activity on a computer screen, and they allow for detailed reports on incoming and outgoing telephone traffic. In this case, an independent telecommunications consultant can save a medical practice thousands of dollars in costly mistakes through a proper needs-assessment plan.

Number of telephone lines   Years ago, Bell Telephone used the slogan "Keep Your Telephone Door Open for Business." Nothing shuts the door on appointments and patient satisfaction faster than an inadequate number of incoming and outgoing telephone lines. To help with this problem, telephone companies can conduct a "busy lamp" study to let the medical practice know the average number of busy signals coming from the practice lines in a given time period. This information can then be used to determine the number of published telephone numbers and rotary lines that are needed for the volume of calls received. For instance, insurance verification calls can occupy a line for a long time, causing busy signals for patients; therefore, a separate unpublished number could be reserved for outgoing calls.

Distraction-Free Environment

Full concentration on the caller is important. Patients and other callers can hear when someone is preoccupied or distracted, which can make them feel unimportant. Select an area away from the mainstream of office activity where telephone receptionists will be able to concentrate on callers in a relatively noise-free, distraction-free environment. Arrange the work space so that the telephone receptionist is not facing areas that may present visual and audible distractions.

Sufficient Staffing and Training

Telephone staff in office   Adequate staffing is essential to telephone service. Large practices may need to create a position called Telecommunications Coordinator or Telephone Professional or Telereceptionist. These titles give importance to the position and imply that the job involves much more than just answering the telephone. In smaller practices, all front-office staff usually handle telephones. However, this can lead to standoffs where it is uncertain just who will answer a ringing telephone. Although it is important for all front-office staff to be trained in telephone techniques, one person and a backup should be given the telephone as a primary responsibility. That person should also have secondary duties that can be immediately interrupted in order to answer the telephone within two or three rings.

A sample job description for a telephone professional is shown in Figure 8.2. The person selected for this responsibility should possess the attributes shown below:

- Maturity
- Empathy
- Patience
- Poise
- Tact
- Integrity
- Judgment
- Assertiveness but not aggressiveness
- Flexibility and adaptability
- Ability to handle various types of pressure
- Professional and caring manner
- Ability to create relationships with others
- Ability to accept criticism
- Dependability and responsibility
- Effective listening and communication skills

A staff member's duties may need to be reassigned or job descriptions may need to be reorganized so that those staff members most innately talented in communication and people skills become responsible for the telephone, where their skills can best benefit the medical practice.

Outside telecommuter   An alternative to hiring additional full-time employees to handle telephones is to use help from outside the medical practice, possibly through a "Telecommuter." A rapidly growing alternative to an on-

Fig. 8.2   Job Description for Telephone Professional

Job Description for: Telephone Professional

Reports to: Officer Manager

Major Responsibility: Since the patient's or caller's first impression of our practice is formed over the telephone, the Telephone Professional strives for excellence in communication. This is accomplished by creating a favorable impression of the practice and by being efficient, informed about the services of the practice, and responsive to caller's needs when answering, screening, directing, and returning calls or when taking messages for telephone calls.

Primary duties include:
- Answering all incoming phone calls
- Focusing on the needs of every caller regardless of the nature of the call
- Greeting callers using the standard phone greeting adopted by the practice
- Properly screening calls and transferring them to the appropriate person
- Conserving valuable human resources of the practice by properly screening calls and taking messages when appropriate
- Taking messages for calls as designated by circumstance or procedure
- Maintaining a log of all callbacks and insuring that patients receive callbacks on time as promised
- Insuring that messages are timely routed to the appropriate person
- Screening all incoming personal phone calls and handling them according to the policy for personal phone calls
- Reporting to management any problems with the telephone system
- Creating a favorable first impression of the practice through telephone contacts
- Responding to emergency situations requiring telephone assistance according to procedures established by the practice
- Providing management with statistics and logs collected from telephone encounters for use in practice management, marketing, and service improvement
- Using active probing techniques to determine patient satisfaction and unexpressed short-term and long-term needs
- Conserving valuable resources of the practice and suggesting to management ways the practice can save money without compromising patient care or effective communications
- Completing any paperwork, computer work, or tasks as assigned by management
- Any other duties as assigned by management

(Reprinted by permission, © 1993 Kim Fox)

site employee, this person works from home or other location with the aid of a computer, modem, telephone, fax machine, and other communication devices. The telecommuter can relieve telephone traffic in the medical office by scheduling or rescheduling appointments, checking on patients who miss appointments or do not respond to recall notices, creating and updating patient records, and other such tasks. If properly configured by computer, a telecommuter can even process insurance claims for the practice.

Training   Continued training in effective telephone techniques and human relations skills is what separates merely "getting it done" from providing outstanding service. Telephone skills and patient-service training come in a variety of formats, ranging from in-office workshops to audio- and videocassette training materials.

Effective Call-Handling Procedures

It is important to establish procedures for politely and professionally screening and handling the most common types of telephone calls. These include calls concerning appointments, emergencies, medication refills, records requests, insurance, collections, personal calls, and requests for information about a patient.

Written procedures should be word-processed so they can be quickly and easily updated with any changes. Written procedures also facilitate the training of existing, new, and temporary employees.

Scripted Responses

Telephone scripts are an essential part of telephone service. They enable staff members to rehearse answers to questions so that their responses consistently cover the most important issues. Without scripts, people ad-lib. Ask ten people how they would ask or answer a question or make a statement, and they will give ten different responses. To identify the most frequently asked questions, the staff can hold a brainstorming session and help write several scripts with the best answers.

Remember to include in your scripts the features, advantages, and benefits of your practice's doctors, staff, facility, services, and procedures. This helps differentiate your practice from others and tells callers what they can expect. Organize your scripts in a rotary alphabetical file or notebook, or on a computer (using a word or phrase prompt to bring up a specific script). The scripts then become a major tool in training staff members.

Telephone procedures handbook   In addition to specific telephone scripts, a medical office should have a telephone handbook of procedures. Having a handbook devoted to the telephone establishes its importance to the practice.

The handbook should serve as the practice's telecommunications bible, and it should be used in training every staff member on how to effectively use the telephone. The handbook should include the following guidelines:

- Answering the phone correctly
- Limiting the number of rings before answering
- Learning, using, and correctly spelling the caller's name
- Establishing rapport with the caller
- Putting a caller on hold politely and handling on-hold circumstances
- Transferring a call
- Screening different types of calls
- Documenting and routing a phone message
- Handling emergencies
- Screening personal calls politely
- Handling complex types of situations, such as irate, frightened, confused, anxious, or irrational callers
- Improving the skill of listening
- Using specific words and phrases to make callers feel valued

Quality Assurance

To insure that the telephone service receives continued attention, it should become part of the medical practice's quality assurance (QA) program. If the practice does not have a QA program the telephone is an ideal place to begin one. (For details on implementing a QA program in the medical office, see Chapter 3, "Quality of Care.")

QA is a method for insuring that actual performance and quality meet predetermined standards. For instance, a QA program can set standards for telephone service, such as answering the telephone by the third ring, not leaving a caller on hold for more than one minute without a status report, and using a scripted greeting specific to the office. The staff are then trained to these standards.

Follow-up questionnaires to patients and regular checks by managers measure actual performance against the standards. Any complaints from patients or deviations in the standards are then investigated by the manager to determine the actions needed to bring performance back up to the standards. As a key to ongoing quality assurance, the various aspects of the QA program are documented: the predetermined standards, the feedback from patients, the observations of actual performance, the actions taken to maintain the standards, and the changes or improvements resulting from the actions.

Resolving Complaints

It is estimated that seven out of ten complaining patients will stay with a medical practice if their complaint is resolved in their favor. Therefore, it is no surprise that staff members are usually most concerned about learning how to handle upset or irate callers. Here are some steps that can be taken to turn complaint calls from patients into positive results.

1. Office managers should have a positive attitude about using complaints to improve patient service.

2. Management should support staff members, not reprimand them, for information obtained from irate or upset callers.
3. Callers who take the time to call and complain should be valued for giving the practice the opportunity for improvement.
4. Every member of the practice should feel responsible for welcoming and resolving complaints.
5. Patients should be encouraged to voice their complaints and be assured that their suggestions for improvement will be carefully considered.

Turning complaints into opportunities   Irate callers want one thing, to be listened to, completely, while they finish their whole story. A staff member who is preoccupied with a patient or other tasks cannot provide this full attention. Therefore, irate callers should be transferred to someone, such as a manager or the practice administrator, who can give them full attention. If no such staff member is available, callers should be asked if they can be called back within a certain time period in order to receive the undivided attention they deserve.

Once undivided attention is established, the following 10-step guidelines and sample scripts can be used either over the telephone or in person to diffuse emotionally charged situations.

1. Empathize with the caller.

   "I can hear that you're upset. I'm glad you called."

2. Offer to help in partnership with the caller.

   "Let's see what we can do to work this out together."

3. Get the facts by asking questions.

   "I want to understand exactly what happened. Please tell me everything I need to know."

4. Don't interrupt; let the caller finish; reinforce with comments to show your attention to the caller.

   "Yes" . . . "I see" . . . "Um hum" . . . "Ah" . . . "Please go on."

5. Confirm what happened.

   "Let me make sure I understand what happened." (Paraphrase the caller's story.) "Is that correct?" "Is there anything else?"

6. Offer a solution.

   "I'll be glad to. . . ." (Tell specifically what you'd like to do to help them.)

7. Get the caller's agreement.

   "Is this agreeable with you?"

8. If there is no agreement, let the caller decide.

   "Mrs. Smith, what do you feel would be fair?"
   or
   "Mr. White, what would you like me to do for you?"

9. When agreement is reached, restate the action and a time frame for completion.

"OK, I'm going to . . . (state the action) . . . by 3:00 p.m. on Friday."

10. Ask for the caller's confirmation.

"Is this agreeable with you?"

There may be occasions when a staff member cannot stop to speak with an irate caller. The following reply could be used:

"Ms. Martin, I understand you're upset, and I really want to help you, but I'm not able to give you the attention you deserve right now. May I call you back in five minutes, and I promise to try to work this out with you then?"

If the caller refuses to be called back, transfer the call to another staff member who can help; be sure to explain the situation so the caller will not have to repeat the whole story.

Sample Script for Upset or Irate Caller

Most complaints from patients fall into several categories. The following sample script describes how to respond to an upset or irate caller.

Upset patient

"I got this bill from your office and it isn't right. You've overcharged me, and I want my money back or I'm reporting you to the insurance commissioner."

Receptionist

"I'm really sorry you're upset. Billing and insurance matters can be very frustrating. But I'm going to help you get this straightened out. Liz Smith is our insurance counselor, and I'm going to connect you to her so she can help you. Can you hold for a moment while I transfer you to Liz?" (Wait for response.) "May I tell Liz who is calling?"

Upset patient

"Yeah, I guess so. It's Todd Jones."

Receptionist

"One moment, please." . . . "Liz, I have Todd Jones on line 2. He's very upset about a bill. Can you take his call."

Insurance counselor

"Sure, I'll pick up line 2." . . . "Mr. Jones, this is Liz Smith. I understand you're having a problem with a bill. How can I help?"

Upset patient

"Well, I got a bill from your office for $125, and I don't owe a cent because Medicare was supposed to pay for it. This just isn't right! You people are trying to rip off us old folks. You can't keep your records straight, and we end up with the headaches!''

Insurance counselor

"Mr. Jones, I have your complete billing record right here in front of me. Let me verify this, it's Todd Jones at 400 West 2nd Avenue in Toledo? . . . Let me take a moment to examine that charge for you.''

Upset patient

"Yes, but you don't need a moment because I know I don't owe it!''

Insurance counselor

"Mr. Jones, many times this is as frustrating for us as it is for you. Let me assure you, I'm here to help you. You're very important to our practice, and I'll do whatever it takes to clear this up for you.''

Upset patient

"I'm sorry I'm taking this out on you. My wife and I have been so sick lately. It seems like all we get are bills, bills, bills.''

Insurance counselor

"Don't worry, Mr. Jones. I do understand your frustration, and I'm sorry you've had a hard time. . . . Oh, here's that charge. Let's see if I can explain it over the phone. If it's still confusing, I'll send you a note explaining the figures, and then we'll speak again when you have my figures in front of you. Is that all right, Mr. Jones? (Wait for agreement.) On August 11, you had in-office laser surgery on your right eye, for which Dr. Melville accepted Medicare assignment. The charge was $625, and Medicare approved that total. They paid $500, which was 80 percent of the total; that left a balance of $125. We sent a claim for that $125 to your supplemental carrier, and they denied it, saying your premium had not been paid.''

Upset patient

"Yes, we just couldn't pay it. And we can't pay any more bills either.''

Insurance counselor

"I understand your predicament, Mr. Jones, so let's see what we can do to work this out. Since you can't pay the full amount now, can you send us a small payment of $31 a month for the next four months?''

Upset patient

"I suppose so.''

Insurance counselor

"That's fine, Mr. Jones. You can ask for me from now on. I've made a note of our conversation so that I can help you with any future billing problems or questions. Now just so we're in agreement; You'll send us $31 a month for four months by the 10th of each month. Don't worry about the last $1;

we'll write that off for you. Your first payment will be due by the 10th of January."

Upset patient

"OK."

Insurance counselor

"Thanks for calling, Mr. Jones. We don't know if there's a problem unless you tell us. I'm really sorry about your hardships, and I hope things get better for you and your wife. Good-bye."

Effective elements The elements that made this call effective were the specific telephone procedures used by the staff members. As the first staff member to answer the telephone, the receptionist correctly followed these steps:

1. Listened intently and courteously
2. Told the patient exactly what action she was taking ("connecting to Liz Smith, our insurance counselor")
3. Asked permission to put the caller on hold for transfer
4. Announced to Liz Smith the patient's name and reason for the call, and verified that she could take the call

As the staff member most appropriate for resolving the patient's complaint, the insurance counselor used the following effective procedures:

1. Listened intently and courteously
2. Made the patient feel important
3. Empathized with the patient's feelings and predicament
4. Offered to help
5. Explained the situation without becoming hostile or defensive
6. Ultimately solved the caller's problem, with his agreement
7. Repeated the solution to confirm the patient understood it
8. Offered future help
9. Encouraged the caller to complain
10. Made notes of the conversation and kept a reminder of the first payment for follow-through

Complaints from patients can be used as opportunities to improve procedures in the medical office. What were the opportunities from this call?

1. The patient is telling the practice that he does not understand his bill. Therefore, the practice can improve its billing by enclosing a typed or handwritten explanation on the bill followed by a personalized closing such as the following:

> Mr. Jones, please call me if you have any questions about this bill. I'm here to help. 395-5888.
>
> Sincerely,
> Liz Smith
> Insurance Counselor

2. The practice can examine its financial counseling to make sure that the patient fully understands the charges, coverage, and personal financial responsibilities of any medical operation or action.

Evaluating Telephone Performance and Patient Service

Telephone performance and patient service should be included in regular employee performance evaluations. After setting the standards for performance by defining what a practice's telephone service should be, and giving staff members the tools and the education they need to do the job, an office manager can give them specific feedback on their performance. Praise or reprimand should be specific in order to be effective, such as the following example:

"Joan, you really put that caller at ease when you offered to stay with her until she was connected to the person who could help her. This showed her that she could count on you, and ultimately count on our practice! Good job, Joan."

This type of praise can be done privately, but it can also be done in front of other employees for an even greater motivating effect. In fact, studies show that it is more motivating for an employee to hear a fellow employee being praised for outstanding behavior than it is to receive a reprimand, so that a poorly performing employee will learn what it takes to attract praise and attention and will change behavior accordingly.

Human Relations among Staff Members and with Patients

The way that physicians and office staff interact with each other affects patient service. Staff members need to feel supported by the physician, managers, and other staff members before they can adequately support patients. Tension and infighting among staff members will negatively affect their ability to deliver superior care and attention to patients.

Physicians and managers should treat all employees with the same attention and respect that they expect the employees to give to their patients and to each other. An atmosphere that encourages open communication should be created so differences can be worked out before they become resentments. Staff meetings conducted on a regular basis will help bind the group together as a team.

Respect

Respect between doctors and staff members begins with how they address each other. Even if staff members are on a first-name or nickname basis with physicians outside the office, they should address each other appropriately during office hours. Physicians should always be referred to in the office as Dr. (last name). Using physicians' first names leads to using patients' first names, a practice that many patients find disrespectful.

Respect is also shown by the way doctors and staff members speak to and about each other; negative comments often cultivate resentments and biases that influence the entire office. When doctors and staff members are truly supporting each other, they speak highly of each other and handle misunderstandings face-to-face instead of behind each other's backs. Positive interactions among staff members directly influence and produce positive interactions with patients.

Sensitivity to the Sick

A new patient comes to the practice with a sense of insecurity. For older, sicker patients, this insecurity can be intense. Not only does the physical environment of the office need to be comforting and soothing, so does the psychological environment. The staff members create the psychological environment for the patients. Even though it is the doctor who provides patient care, it is staff members who create the impression of just how much the doctor cares for the patient.

Sensitivity to patients should become an integral component of an office policies manual; the following example is used by one practice in its manual:

> Negative attitudes and infighting affect how we present ourselves to our patients. Any behavior that is less than caring, understanding, attentive, and helpful is not acceptable in this office. Our main mission is to serve and support our patients, fellow employees, physicians, and anyone else who has dealings with our office.

Empathy   It should be stressed to staff members that sensitivity to the needs and feelings of another person is an attitude and a way of being. Sensitivity, empathy, and compassion are felt from the heart and cannot be taught. Medical personnel who have experienced illness, incapacity, surgery, near death, or the death of a loved one firsthand are more likely to be able to empathize with patients.

For those who have not experienced certain physical conditions or limitations, simulations can help create empathy for the suffering. For example, staff members can experience what life is like for a patient with cataracts by wearing a pair of glasses that simulate dim, blurred vision. Wearing a cast for a day or trying to go about normal daily activities from a wheelchair can simulate physical disabilities.

Patients are placed in unnatural situations and unfamiliar surroundings during their medical encounters. Conversely, for medical personnel, life-threatening problems are routine. Patients share intimate secrets with medical personnel. Conversely, medical personnel rarely, if ever, share intimate details of their lives with patients. Medical personnel need to remind themselves of these different roles. As they struggle to balance careful scientific analysis and limited time, they also need to remind themselves that a person with feelings, concerns, and fears occupies the body of each patient. Only then will they be able to connect on a personal, empathic level with each patient. Otherwise, patients can misinterpret a purely scientific approach to their care as detachment on the part of the medical personnel.

Practice Limitations on Patient Service

Patient service begins at the top, with the attitude and actions of the physician. Unfortunately, many physicians are feeling increasing pressures from changes in the health care system. Longer working hours, heavier patient schedules, decreasing reimbursements, and uncertainty about the future are creating enormous new pressures for many physicians. They are trying to figure out what to do and how to position themselves in the new health care marketplace.

Gone are the days of physicians hanging out their shingles and either succeeding or failing on their own merits. Now they have to think in business terms, about what contracts they can be part of. The result of these changes is that physicians may appear to be rushed, worried, or have less time to give staff members the coaching, reinforcement, and nurturing that many of them need. Tension emanating from the physician is passed down through the staff members and ultimately to the patients.

Today's practice manager or office administrator must be role models for communication and patient service. Many will need additional education or training in business or health care administration.

Practice managers must have coaching skills and open lines of communication with their physicians to be able to offer their understanding and support in the pressures they face. Only then can they minimize the negative impact of this stress on staff members or patients. They must be knowledgeable about the availability of computers and office automation to help their reduced staff become as efficient as possible to leave time for the human interactions of patient service. All this is not a quick or easy task for today's practice manager. It is an evolutionary process.

Examples of Patient Service

Situations calling for extra attention to patients occur daily in a medical office. Some of the most common are listed below, along with suggested scripts, words, and phrases that express patient service.

"Mrs. Miller, let me call a cab for you."
instead of
"You'll need to call a cab, Mrs. Miller."

"Thank you for calling Atlanta Family Care. This is Julie."
instead of
"Atlanta Family Care, please hold." (click!)

Walking beside patients to escort them to the exam room
instead of walking in front or way out ahead of them

"May I offer you (a telephone, a beverage, a quieter room, etc.) while you are waiting?" or "The doctor is delayed about 30 minutes due to emergencies. Can I do anything to make your wait more comfortable, or would you prefer to reschedule your appointment?"
instead of
"He's running about 30 minutes behind. You'll be called as soon as possible."

"Certainly, Mrs. Miller. I'll be glad to schedule your appointment, but my computer is temporarily down right now. May I call you back within the next hour? It should be up and running by that time."
instead of
"You'll have to call back. My computer is down and I can't get into the scheduling program."

Neat, legible patient forms and information sheets
instead of   crooked, spotted, blurred, hard to read copies

Providing printed medication instructions to reinforce verbal instructions
instead of   merely telling patients when and how much of their medication to take

Calling patients personally to remind them of their appointment
instead of   using an automated calling system

Words and phrases   Words that spell service include the following, with examples to show their use with patients.

please:	"Please tell me more about that, Mrs. Jones."
names:	"Hello, Mrs. Jones. This is Karen, Dr. Matthews' assistant."
how:	"How may I help you, Mrs. Jones?"
thank you:	"Thank you for holding, Ms. Brown."
understandable:	"That's understandable, Mrs. Curtis."
certainly:	"Certainly, Mr. Stevens. That won't be a problem."
glad:	"I'll be glad to call a cab for you, Ms. White."
help:	"How may I help you?"
happy:	"I'll be happy to see that you're called back by 4:00 p.m."
important:	"It's very important to me that we get this right for you, Mr. Wallace."
priority:	"I'm going to place a priority on this, Mrs. Smith."
spell:	"Can you please spell your name for me, Mr. Franklin."
appreciate:	"I appreciate your patience, Mrs. Crane."
considerate:	"That's very considerate of you, Mr. Harris, to be willing to wait until next week, but Dr. Breck said he'll be glad to see you tomorrow."
thoughtful:	"That's very thoughtful of you to ask about Marge's condition, Mrs. Jones."

promise: "I promise to call you just as soon as we receive your test results." (Note: Don't make a promise you can't or don't intend to keep.)

verify: "I'd like to verify some information with you, Ms. Green, to
insure   insure that your personal record is up-to-date."

pleasure: "It's my pleasure to connect you."

repeat: "Could you please repeat (that appointment/those directions) to me, Mr. Black, so I can make sure I communicated clearly."

Phrases that convey a feeling of professionalism and service to patients include the following:

"yes"
   instead of "yeah" or "uh-huh"

"Here's what I suggest you do."
   instead of "You'll have to . . ."

"He's with a patient at the moment."
   not "He's busy."

"I'll be glad to see if he/she is available. May I tell him/her who is calling?"
   instead of "Who's calling?"

"I'm sorry. Can you please repeat that?"
   not "Huh" or "What?"

"Our phone connection is weak. Are you able to hear me, because I'm having trouble hearing you?"
   instead of "I can't hear you."

"She's running an errand but will return at (when)."
   instead of "She's not in."

"I expect him back around (give a time frame)."
   not "He won't be back."

"Can you please tell me more about this so I can get you connected to the right person?"
   not "What's it about?"

"Here's what we can do for you."
   instead of "We can't/won't . . ."

"What would you consider fair in this situation?"
   not "I can't help you."

"The person who can help you is (name)."
   not "She doesn't handle . . ."

"May I call you back at (when)?"
   instead of "You'll have to call back later."

"May I call a cab for you?"
   not "You need to call a cab."

"May I take your number for quick reference?"
   not "Does he have your number?"

Conclusion

Patients are now being advised to take responsibility for managing their own health care by finding the right doctor, hospital, or insurance plan to cover their needs. Today's health care consumers are more astute than ever before. They have changed from passive to active consumers. Active consumers question the medical advice they are being given and leave providers who do not meet their medical as well as emotional needs. Today's medical practice must be patient-friendly and service-oriented in order to meet the emotional as well as physical needs of its clients. This will enable the practice to provide the type of care that service-oriented patients expect from everyone with whom they interact.

Chapter 9

Health Information Management

Components of Health Information Management   201
Collecting Health Information—Appointments   206
Patient Registration Information   210
Health Records Information—Format   212
Health Records Information—Content   217
Releasing Health Information   226
Using Health Information for Insurance Billing   233
Managing Health Information   237
Filing Systems   239
Health Records Retention   246
Health Records Disposition   250
Computer Use in Health Information Management   253

Components of Health Information Management

Health information management is the development, implementation, maintenance, and management of systems in order to capture, store, retrieve, and release patient health information effectively. Health information management is also known as medical records administration. The procedures and practices of health information management are similar in all health care settings, although the ones used in the medical office are less complex than those used in hospitals and large medical centers. Nevertheless, the goal is the same: effective and efficient management of the health information of the patients served.

Information is the basis for all decision making and planning, and the primary source of health care information is the patient's health record. Records management is commonly defined as the systematic control over the creation, maintenance, retention, protection, and preservation of records. The efficient and economical handling of records is the primary objective of any records or information management program.

The health information manager, nurse, medical assistant, and office manager all play significant roles in maintaining, retaining, protecting, and preserving records and the information contained within. The role of the health information manager is a critical one in health care facilities because the information handled is of a very personal nature. In addition, the absence or loss of needed health information may jeopardize appropriate patient care. Not only do health information managers serve as records managers, but they also use health information to meet the many needs of patients, physicians, third-party payers, and regulatory and accrediting agencies.

The Health Record

The health record is a compilation of knowledge and facts concerning the patient and the patient's care. It is an orderly report providing a total picture of the patient's health status. Subjective information such as the patient's complaint is supported by objective physical findings and diagnostic test data. The diverse information in the health record serves as a channel of communication between those involved in caring for the patient. What people forget, the record remembers. The health record identifies the following facts:

1. Who the patient is
2. What the symptoms and physical findings were
3. What care or procedures were administered
4. Who provided the care
5. Where and when the care was given
6. How the patient responded to the care

While there are many reasons to create and maintain health records, several primary purposes exist, as described in the following paragraphs.

Continuity of medical care   The physician examines the patient and records the findings in the patient's health record. These findings are the key to establishing a diagnosis. The physician may order different tests to confirm or augment the clinical findings. As reports of these tests are received, data is used to support the diagnosis. The physician then can plan a course of treatment for the patient that hopefully will result in the patient's recovery or improvement in health status.

Complete and accurate health records help a physician provide continuity in a patient's health care. Previous illnesses and difficulties that are recorded in the patient's record may supply needed information about the patient's current health. Diagnostic test results can be compared over a particular time period, along with the patient's response to treatment, so that future treatment can be adjusted accordingly.

Quality management   The health record can document the quality of care rendered by demonstrating the physician's use of current medical data and its efficient application to the patient's ongoing care. The record may be reviewed by the physician's peers to evaluate the appropriateness of the care delivered. Information in health records is used to determine the effectiveness of certain treatment protocols and to determine the incidence of diseases. Correlation of such statistical information may result in a new outlook on some phases of medical care and can lead to revised treatment mechanisms and techniques. The statistical information compiled from individual patient records can also be used for medical research and continuing medical education. (For details on quality management, see Chapter 3, "Quality of Care.")

Legal interests The patient's health record is also a business record and a legal document. Since there is dual ownership of the record—the physician or provider owns the physical property of the record, but the patient owns the information—the health record serves the legal interests of both physician and patient.

Physician's interest The physician uses the health record as evidence of services rendered. In a sense, the record is generated as a result of the "business" the physician performs. The record serves as documentation of the delivery of health care and may be used by the physician to support the bill sent to a patient or third-party payer. The record serves as legal evidence of the type of care rendered if a question is raised about its appropriateness or quality. The health record can be the most important evidence in any medical liability suit, regardless of the factual issues involved. Detailed office records ordinarily prevail with a jury, as opposed to a patient's recollections. Juries often assume that good records indicate good care, while inadequate records can imply substandard care.

Patient's interest The patient has a legal interest in the health record as well. Information about the care received by the patient may serve to substantiate a claim of damages sustained in a motor-vehicle accident or injuries sustained on the job for a workers' compensation claim. The patient may need documentation to support a claim for medical disability or Social Security supplemental income.

In a claim of ineffective or inappropriate care received, the patient may use the same record to file legal action against a physician or other health care provider. Patients' attorneys often use the argument "if it was not documented, it was not done" as the basis for a claim of inadequate or incomplete services rendered.

State and federal laws and regulations Laws and regulations specify that a record is maintained for each patient treated. The physician's office records also provide the documentation needed to complete various reports required by law—such as reports on violent crimes, child abuse, domestic violence, elder/aged neglect or abuse; reports on communicable diseases; and birth, fetal death, and death certificates.

Insurance and reimbursement Reimbursement systems, both private and governmental, require evidence of care rendered in order to justify financial reimbursement to either the physician or the patient. Prior approval of services, second-opinion requirements, and referrals of patients to other health care providers, such as specialists, are also required by many insurance companies and managed care organizations.

Physicians need detailed health information of the patients they serve in order to negotiate and maintain preferred-provider agreements and managed care contracts. The physician's productivity and collection rates are also well-served by complete, orderly, and legible health records.

Users of Health Information

Understanding who uses the information contained in health records is the first step to effectively communicating with them through the health record. Today the health record is important to users both inside and outside the physician's practice.

Health care providers   The health record was originally developed as a reference source for the physician's own use; today many medical professionals, organizations, and entities use it as well. Physicians create health records to document the nature and extent of each physician-patient encounter. In general, the record is used by the primary care physician to:

- Reference past encounters
- Record current patient evaluation and care plans
- Monitor patient progress
- Document the course of each episode of care

Other physicians and health care professionals use the record in the following ways:

- To communicate with other physicians and caregivers
- To promote continuity of care, particularly when another physician takes over part or all of the care of the patient
- To supply clinical data for research and educational purposes
- To provide a utilization and patient-mix database that can be used to evaluate or justify admittance to a medical group or health system

Physician's business office   The physician's business staff use the documentation in the health record in several ways to obtain payment for physician services. They may bill directly from a charge ticket, based on the encounter and its documentation. They may also bill directly from the health record. For example, when billing for surgical procedures, staff members routinely review the operative report or note, determine the procedures performed, and then assign codes for billing them. Documentation is used extensively for appeals and requests for reconsideration of payment. The quality, completeness, and specificity of documentation will have a significant effect on the payer's response.

Hospitals   The hospital or other health care institution uses the physician's documentation for several important purposes. The physician's dictated or handwritten history and physical examination reports, operative reports, consultation reports, progress notes, and other documentation are used by the hospital to assign diagnosis and procedure codes. The codes are used to formulate a specific diagnosis-related group (DRG) for billing certain payers such as Medicare, or they may be used alone to bill other payers.

When physicians couple their financial future with hospitals by joining physician-hospital organizations (PHOs), physician-hospital networks, or vertically integrated organizations, the ultimate financial health of each is interdependent because it is based on the documentation in the health records.

Third-party payers Insurers, HMOs, third-party administrators, Medicare, Medicaid, and other health care payment entities base their reimbursement on physician documentation, either directly through actual review of the record or indirectly by payment of coded services assumed to be substantiated by equivalent documentation. Most payers have a contractual obligation to their enrollees to pay only for services that are:

- Covered and payable under the patient's contract or benefit plan
- Medically necessary for the diagnosis and/or treatment of the patient's condition (that is, consistent with the diagnosis and provided at the most appropriate level and location)
- Actually rendered and documented
- Coded and billed as rendered

Now more than ever, the financial health and longevity of the medical practice depends on documentation patterns.

Managed care organizations Managed care organizations (MCOs) view documentation as a more valuable commodity than do other third-party payers. Because most MCOs are responsible for providing care (as opposed to simply providing reimbursement for it), they also share accountability for its quality and outcome. Until recently, most of the efforts of MCOs have been focused on reducing costs. Today these organizations are turning their attention to quality of care and outcomes measurement, based in part on review of data extracted from health records. Increasingly, the information gathered from physician documentation is matched with cost information and used for a number of purposes, such as the following:

- Identification of the most productive, high-quality physician
- Physician credentialing
- Physician contracting and retention
- Identification and implementation of optimal treatment patterns
- Marketing, strategic planning, employer contracting, and other issues
- Assessment of documentation for the quality of care

Managed care is increasingly a major component of health care delivery. As physicians and hospitals compete for contracts to provide care for thousands of people, current documentation will have a profound impact on the outcome of that competition.

Attorneys and the courts Attorneys and the courts use the health record for a number of purposes because it can represent legal proof of the quality of care provided. A health record can be admissible as evidence in court for several reasons:

- It is recorded by parties involved in the care of the patient.
- It is contemporaneous with the events that occurred in the course of that care.
- It is considered more reliable evidence than an individual's memory of the events at a later date.

A health record is the first and most important item a plaintiff's attorney will use to determine whether or not to bring a negligence or malpractice claim against a health care provider. Well-documented records will help juries make their decisions. Records with missing or illegible information can raise questions in jurors' minds regarding the standard of care or legitimacy of the records. A complete, accurate, and legible health record can be the best evidence to support a health care provider.

Government The federal Health Care Financing Administration relies on coded diagnostic procedures that hinge on documentation in order to determine payment to hospitals and physicians. Diagnosis-related groups (DRGs) and the resource-based relative value scale (RBRVS) are reimbursement mechanisms that provide a substantial proportion of the payments hospitals and physicians receive for patient services.

Each state government has considerable power in determining reimbursement for health care services through Medicaid. Some state Medicaid programs pay hospitals under a modified PPS (prospective payment system), and others use a flat rate or capitation. Physician payment arrangements vary widely as well.

As health care reform evolves, not only will dollars spent be more closely scrutinized, but decisions concerning the types of coverage offered will depend on the coded data provided for billed charges. Again, physician documentation through the health record plays a pivotal role in the reimbursement system.

Collecting Health Information—Appointments

Health information management begins with the collection of information about the patients seen in the office, through appointment scheduling, patient registration, and compiling health record forms. The first step involves the scheduling process.

Appointment Scheduling
The efficient scheduling of patients is a process that is critical to the success of the practice. Each practice must determine what type of scheduling system

meets the needs of the patients and the practice. Factors that are considered when scheduling a patient include (1) which physician will see the patient, and (2) how much time is needed for the visit, based on the patient's medical condition or reason for the visit. There are several different approaches to scheduling, including scheduled appointments, flexible office hours, and open office hours.

Scheduled appointments   Most physicians report they are more comfortable seeing patients according to a scheduled appointment system, which allows the physician and the office staff to know in advance the volume of work they are likely to experience in a day. Efficient scheduling requires an understanding of the type of practice and average time required to see most patients and the work style of the physicians.

Once a scheduling system has been implemented, the practice must make every effort to start on time and see patients according to the time promised for the appointment. Patients have been known to leave physicians who consistently keep them waiting an unreasonable length of time whenever they arrive for a scheduled appointment.

Flexible office hours   Flexible office hours often meet the needs of many patients and their families today. Health care providers such as family physicians, pediatricians, and others are turning to flexible schedules that coincide with many people's work schedules. Under this system, the practice is open at different hours during the week, to include early morning, evening or a combination of both. For example, on one day per week, office hours might begin at 7 a.m. and end at 1 p.m.; on another day, they might be from 1 p.m. to 9 p.m. On one or more evenings a week, the office might be open from 5 p.m. to 10 p.m. On other days, the regular hours of 9 a.m. to 5 p.m. would apply. In this manner, various options are available to patients and result in increased patient satisfaction.

Open office hours   With this scheduling pattern, the office is open at specific hours of the day or evening. The patients know they can come in to see the physician during this time period and realize they will be seen in the order of their arrival—a first-come, first-served approach. The practice does not have to be concerned about the problem of no-show patients as no appointments are made. This type of scheduling is used at "emergi-centers" or "urgi-centers," where patients prefer the convenience of simply stopping in at the physician's office on the way to or from work or whenever a minor medical emergency arises. Predicting the staffing requirements for an office with open office hours may be difficult at first, but most practices can predict the busy times and the slow times of the day and adjust staffing levels accordingly.

The Appointment Book

The appointment book today may be a paper ledger or a software program on a personal computer. In either paper or computerized formats, the appointment book needs certain basic features. It must be large enough to accommodate all members in the practice. It must allow for easy data entry, correction, and deletion of patient information. Access to software programs and retrieval of information may be based on date, time, patient name, or physician name. Pages in a book or images on a screen should allow viewing of one day at a time, one week at a time, or even one month at a glance. The appointment time slots should be suitable to the practice and be flexible to allow different time slots for different physicians within a practice. Scheduling in advance sometimes requires blocking off time periods when a particular physician is not available to see patients (such as days off, holidays, hospital rounds, or meetings). (For more on scheduling by computer, see Chapter 5, "The Computer in the Medical Office.")

Scheduling Guidelines

The scheduling system must be adjusted to meet the needs of each specific practice. However, there are some general guidelines applicable to any practice, based on the patient population, the physician's work habits, and the available facilities.

Patient population   The practice must consider its patient population and the location of the practice when choosing a scheduling system. Are mothers home with children, or do most parents work the traditional five-day business week? Are evening and Saturday and even Sunday appointments essential for some patients?

The specific amount of time allotted to patients should be based on their particular needs. This can be determined by asking patients to supply the following information:

- Purpose of the visit
- Age of the patient (Older patients often require more time than young adults.)
- Need to see both the physician and another staff member, which affects time needed

Physician's work habits   A physician's work habits must be considered in setting an appointment schedule. Does the physician faithfully arrive in the office before patient appointments are scheduled to begin? Does the physician like to see one patient after another and then complete the records and other paperwork at the end of the day, or does the physician need time between each patient visit to complete the documentation required.

The other responsibilities of the physicians must also be factored into the schedule, such as dedicated time to receive and return telephone calls, to examine and dictate reports, to review and answer mail, and to complete other business items. Sometimes the only way some of these items are addressed is to include them in the physician's appointment schedule so time is set aside for the specific tasks.

Facilities The available facilities are yet another important consideration in setting the appointment schedule. Depending on the number of examination rooms or offices in a facility, only a certain number of patients can be scheduled during a time period. If only one room is used for minor surgery, an appropriate schedule would be set up so that two physicians would not be trying to use the same room at the same time. (For details on office design, see Chapter 6, "Medical Office Components.")

Time Management

To determine the best use of a physician's time, the office manager can monitor time management through an informal practice analysis, noting the arrival time, treatment or conference time, departure time, and procedure performed over the course of a month. A definite time pattern usually emerges for each procedure. The office manager can arrange a schedule that has some long and some short appointments. The schedule should be reviewed with the physician at the beginning of each day. The use of computer scheduling software should allow for the printing of a schedule that can be posted or distributed to the staff.

Depending on the type of practice and the physician's specialty, there may be a need for same-day service for acutely ill patients or emergencies. Some physicians prefer to have at least one or two appointment slots open each day to accommodate such emergencies. Family practitioners may leave as much as 25 percent of their time open for emergencies and urgent-care patients.

Wave scheduling The flexible system called *wave scheduling* is a time schedule that books two or three people for the same time. Wave scheduling is based on the law of averages. If the average time per appointment is 20 minutes, three patients are scheduled for each hour and are seen in the order of their arrival; if one person arrives late, it will not disrupt the entire schedule.

A variation of wave scheduling books two patients to come on the hour and a third on the half hour, or it schedules all three patients to arrive at given intervals during the first half of the hour, with none scheduled to arrive during the second half. In any case, practices should avoid double booking, or scheduling two people for the same 20-minute slot. It is unlikely that both will be seen by the physician in a timely manner.

Grouping procedures Some physicians practice time management by scheduling groups of procedures together, such as an internist keeping the mornings for physical exams, or a pediatrician holding well-baby hours, which prevents sick children and infants from coming in contact with "well" children in the waiting or exam rooms.

Appointment Reminders

Appointments may be made with patients in person while the patient is in the office, over the telephone, and through a third party, such as a referring-physician's office. Several methods of reminders can be used to ensure the patient will remember to arrive on the correct date and time for the appointment. Many practices use small cards that are given to patients to remind them of appointments. Other offices send postcards to patients a week before the appointment as a reminder of the scheduled date and time. Still other offices make it a practice to call the patient's home or office one to two days before the appointment to remind the patient of the upcoming visit. The goal is to eliminate as many no-shows as possible that could occur when the patient simply forgets the appointment date or time, and to allow rescheduling of patients who find they cannot keep their appointments.

Failed appointments   Patients fail to arrive for scheduled appointments for a variety of reasons. They may simply forget, or another family or personal emergency may arise. It is important to determine the reason for failed appointments and reschedule patients if practical. This may involve a telephone call to the patient the same day or the day following the failed appointment. Patients who cannot be reached by telephone may be sent a letter or postcard asking them to call and reschedule the visit. Patients who are known to be acutely ill, as well as the elderly or disabled, may require more aggressive follow-up to make sure they are not in acute medical danger.

Whenever a patient fails to keep an appointment, a notation should be made in the patient's health record as well as in the appointment book or scheduling software. The notation should include the reason for the failed appointment, if known, and the action taken by the office to contact the patient and reschedule the visit. This would serve the practice as evidence of good-faith efforts to contact a patient if allegations are made at a later date that care was not available to the patient.

Patient Registration Information

Another process to collect health information occurs with patient registration, the capture of demographic and insurance information about the patient. A patient coming in for a first visit completes a patient information form, which is intended to gather basic information about the patient. The patient may be asked to complete the form or may be interviewed by the office staff. (See Figure 9.1 for a sample form.) The basic information obtained from each patient includes the following:

- Full name
- Date of birth
- Gender
- Home address and telephone number
- Names of parents if patient is a minor
- Occupation, employer, business address and telephone number
- Social Security number

Fig. 9.1 New Patient Registration Form

PATIENT REGISTRATION

Welcome to our office. We are committed to providing the best, most comprehensive care possible. We encourage you to ask questions. Please assist us by providing the following information. All information is confidential and is released only with your consent. Please fill in the blanks below the line.

Patient Name	Today's Date	Date of Birth	Sex	Age
Parent if Patient Is a Minor				
Patient's Social Security Number	California Driver's License No.			
Home Address	City	State	ZIP	
Mailing Address if Different	City	State	ZIP	
Home Telephone	Work Telephone			
Occupation	Employer's Name			
Employer's Address	City	State	ZIP	
Spouse Name	Employer			
Other Physician's Name				
Whom May We Thank for Referring You to Our Practice?				
NOTIFY IN CASE OF EMERGENCY				
Name	Relationship			
Address	City	State	ZIP	
Home Telephone	Work Telephone			
Nearest Relative (not living with you)				
Home Telephone	Work Telephone			
FINANCIAL INFORMATION: PERSON RESPONSIBLE FOR FEES				
Name	Telephone			
Address	City	State	ZIP	
Insurance Company	Claim Address			
Subscriber's Name	Subscriber's Date of Birth	Subscriber's Social Security No.		
Insurance ID No.				
Secondary Insurance	Claim Address			
Subscriber's Name	Subscriber's Date of Birth	Subscriber's Social Security No.		
Were You Injured on the Job? YES NO	Have You Informed Your Employer? YES NO			
Date of Original Injury				
Worker's Compensation Carrier Name	Address			

(Reprinted by permission, © 1995 Professional Management and Marketing)

- Name of spouse if married
- Name of referring physician or source of referral
- Name and address of person responsible for payment
- Method of payment
- Health insurance information

Insurance Forms

Insurance cards and Medicare or Medicaid cards should be photocopied (including both the front and back sides) to assure the collection of accurate information. Sometimes patients bring insurance forms to the office that must be completed for payment purposes.

Patients may be asked to sign several consent forms, such as an assignment of benefits, which authorizes the insurance company to pay the physician directly for all services rendered (see Figure 9.2 for a sample form). Patients should be asked to sign an authorization to release information to allow their confidential diagnoses and procedures and/or the codes be sent to the insurance company for processing of the claim. Patients may also be asked to sign a statement of financial responsibility to acknowledge their responsibility in paying for the services rendered regardless of their insurance coverage.

Information obtained from the patient is entered into the office computer system and also included as hard copy in the patient's health record.

For every subsequent visit to the office, the patient should be asked to verify the information is still correct. Photocopies of insurance cards should be made when the patient has a new insurance plan. Regardless of any change of insurance companies, it is wise to photocopy patients' insurance cards periodically as many employers frequently change deductibles, co-payments, and coverage.

Health Records Information—Format

Health records are compiled according to various formats, which describe the organization of the forms and the information within the health record. There are three types of formats: source-oriented, problem-oriented, and integrated.

Source-Oriented Health Record

The source-oriented health record is organized in sections according to the type or source of patient care rendered. There may be sections for history, physical exam, progress notes, problem list, laboratory reports, radiology reports, other miscellaneous tests and therapies, correspondence with other physicians, and other patient demographic or insurance information. Within each section the forms are arranged according to date. Usually the record

Fig. 9.2   Insurance Authorization Form

LIFETIME INSURANCE AUTHORIZATION

Provider name_____

I authorize the release of any medical information necessary to process claims.

I also authorize payments under my insurance programs to be made directly to the above provider for any services furnished to me.

This authorization also permits the release of information by HCFA (its intermediaries or carriers) on any UNASSIGNED Medicare claims to the above.

I further permit copies of this authorization to be used in place of the original.

_____

Patient Signature (or responsible party)

_____

Patient Name (or responsible party)   please print

_____

Date

(Reprinted by permission, © 1995 Professional Management and Marketing)

is arranged in reverse chronological order so the most recent information is at the front and the oldest information at the back of each section.

Advantages and disadvantages   The major advantage to the source-oriented format is that it organizes reports from each source together, thus making it easy to determine the assessment, treatments, and observations provided. Critics of the source-oriented record state it is not possible to quickly determine all of the patient's problems and treatments being provided at a given time, since the data from the various sections are not organized according to the problems of the patient or integrated in time sequence.

Problem-Oriented Medical Record

The problem-oriented medical record, commonly referred to as POMR, provides a systematic method of documentation to reflect logical thinking on the part of the physician directing the care of the patient. The physician defines and follows each clinical problem individually and organizes the problems for solution. The POMR has four basic parts: (1) database, (2) problem list, (3) treatment plan, and (4) progress notes.

Database   The database is a minimum set of data to be obtained on every patient, including chief complaint, present illness, patient profile (the patient's typical day) and related social data, past history and review of systems, physical examination of defined content, and baseline laboratory data.

Problem list   The problem list is contained on a form placed in the front of the record. The "problems" are anything that require management or diagnostic work-up, including medical, social, economic, and demographic problems, past and present. The list should state the problems at the level of the physician's understanding of a particular problem. Thus, the problem list may contain a statement of a symptom, an abnormal finding, a physiological finding, or a specific diagnosis. Conditions suspected or to be ruled out are not listed as problems but are noted in the treatment plan. Additions or changes are made to the list as new problems are identified and active problems resolved. Problems are not erased; they are marked "dropped" or "resolved" and the date of the change recorded. Problems are titled and numbered and serve as a table of contents to the record. (See Figure 9.3 for a sample problem list.)

Treatment plans   The plans describe what will be done to learn more about the patient's condition, treat the condition, and educate the patient about the condition. Specific plans for each problem are delineated and fall into three categories: (1) more information for diagnosis and management, (2) therapy, and (3) patient education. The plans are numbered to correspond with the problem they address.

Progress notes   Progress notes are the follow-up for each problem. Each note is preceded by the number and title of the appropriate problem and may consist of any or all of the following elements:

- Subjective (symptoms)
- Objective (measurable, observable findings)
- Assessment (interpretation or impression of current condition)
- Plan (statements that describe treatment)

The acronym for this process is SOAP, and the writing of progress notes in the POMR format is referred to as "soaping." (For an example of a SOAP record, see Figure 11.2 on page 297.) The emphasis is on unresolved problems. In addition to the narrative notes to describe the patient's progress,

Fig. 9.3   Problem List

MEDICAL PROBLEMS SUMMARY SHEET

Patient Name:

Medical Problems	Surgeries/ Injuries

Health Care Maintenance	Family History
Physical	Mother
Pap	Father
Mammo	ASVD
FOBT	HTN
Slg	DM
PSA	CA
Tetanus	Tobacco
Pneumovax	EtoH
TB	Allergies

(Reprinted by permission, © 1995 Professional Management and Marketing)

flowcharts may be used in situations in which there are several factors being monitored or when the patient's condition is changing rapidly.

Advantages and disadvantages   Proponents of the POMR identify many advantages to this format: the physician is required to consider all the patient's problems in total context; the record clearly indicates the goals and methods of the physician in treating the patient; medical education is facilitated by the documentation of logical thought processes of the physician; and the quality assurance process is easier because the data is organized. The major disadvantage of POMR is that the format usually requires additional training and commitment of the medical and professional staffs. However, many allied health professionals use the SOAP form of progress notes.

Integrated Health Records

In the integrated format, all forms in the health record are organized in strict chronological order. The key element is that forms from various sources are intermingled. Thus a record of a patient may have the history and physical followed by progress notes, then an X-ray report, additional progress notes, a consultation report, and so on. The forms for each episode of care are organized in separate sections of the record.

Advantages and disadvantages   The advantage of the integrated format is that all information on a particular episode of care is together, thus providing a clear picture of the patient's illness and response to treatment. The disadvantage is that it is difficult to compare similar information—for example, fasting blood sugar levels—over time because all reports of one type are not together in the record.

Integrated Progress Notes

There may be varying degrees of integration of information. The most common variation allows for integrated progress notes, with all providers recording on the same forms, in sequence. All other reports are maintained in source-oriented fashion.

Advantages and disadvantages   Advantages to using integrated progress notes are that a patient's progress can be determined quickly, because the current notes of all disciplines are grouped together. The number of specialized forms is reduced, thus the bulk of the record is reduced. The concept of teamwork among health care professionals is encouraged.

A disadvantage of integrated progress notes in a manual health record is that only one individual can document at a time. In addition, it may be difficult to identify the profession or specialty of the individual making a particular entry unless notes are always followed by the title of the recorder.

The decision regarding the format of the health record is usually made by the physicians in consultation with the other health care providers in the practice.

Health Records Information—Content

The content of the health record depends on the specialty of the physician and the type of health care delivered in the physician office. However, several broad categories of clinical data are collected on most ambulatory patients.

Medical History

The medical history is data the physician uses to establish a tentative provisional diagnosis on which to base the treatment of the patient. In the event that a reliable history cannot be elicited from the patient, the history must be obtained from the person best able to relate the facts. It is helpful to record the source of the history, such as the patient, parent, adult child, or friend. The history of a patient should be captured completely at the patient's first visit and updated at each subsequent visit to the physician's office. (See Figures 9.4 and 9.5 for sample forms.)

To promote uniformity and completeness, the physician should adopt a standard outline for the history, which may be printed on a history form. In a computerized system, the components of the history appear on the display screen for the physician to use. Positive (the presence of a symptom) and negative data should be recorded. The data should reflect what the patient states. The physician's point of view may be expressed in the physical examination and subsequent notes. (For examples of medical histories, see Chapter 11, "Medical Transcription and Correspondence.") The following information is suggested content for the history:

1. Chief complaint—nature and duration of the symptoms that caused the patient to seek medical attention, as stated in the patient's own words
2. Present illness—detailed chronological description of the development of the patient's illness from the appearance of the first symptom to the present time
3. Past medical history—summary of childhood and adult illnesses or medical treatment, such as infectious diseases, pregnancies, allergies and drug sensitivities, accidents, operations, hospitalizations, and current medications
4. Psychosocial or personal history—marital status; dietary, sleeping, and exercise patterns; use of coffee, alcohol, other drugs, and tobacco; occupation; environment; daily routine, religious beliefs; and outlook on life
5. Family history—diseases among relatives in which heredity or contact may play a role, such as allergies; infectious diseases; mental, metabolic, endocrine, cardiovascular, or renal diseases; or neoplasms; as well as the health of immediate relatives, ages at death, and causes of death
6. Review of systems—a systematic inventory to reveal subjective symptoms that the patient either forgot to describe or seemed relatively unimportant

Physical Examination

The physical examination provides baseline data about the patient that will assist the physician in determining a diagnosis. The exam should include all

Fig. 9.4   Medical History

HEALTH HISTORY SHEET

Welcome to our practice! To provide you with the best, most comprehensive care possible, we request that you provide the following information. All information is held strictly confidential and is released only with your written permission.

Last Name: First:			Age: Sex:		Doctor Notes *please do not write in this area*
Presenting Problem or Proposed Surgery:					

Have you or any blood relative had:					
	Yes	No	Who	Year	
Allergies, asthma, hay fever					
Anemia					
Alcoholism					
Arthritis					
Bleeding problems					
Birth defects					
Cancer					
Emphysema					
Epilepsy or seizures					
Heart trouble					
Mental illness					
Migraine headaches					
Rheumatic fever					
Stroke					
Suicide					
Thyroid disease/goiter					
Tuberculosis					
Ulcers					
Venereal disease					
Osteoporosis					
Glaucoma					
Gallstones					

Have you ever been turned down for military, job, insurance? ❑ Yes ❑ No

Names of Other Present MDs Last Visit		Childhood Immunizations	Year
		Tetanus	
		"Childhood" Diphtheria	
		"Childhood" Polio	
		Pneumovax	
		Flu Shot	
		Last TB Test	
		TB: ❑ Positive ❑ Negative	

ALLERGIES: Please list type and reaction   ❑NONE

Name of Drug/Item	Reaction	Name of Drug/Item	Reaction

(Reprinted by permission, © 1995 Professional Management and Marketing)

Fig. 9.4 *(continued)*

HEALTH HISTORY SHEET

Patient Name:

MEDICATIONS Have you EVER TAKEN:	Yes	No	Year	How Long?	Brand/Descr/Dose
Blood pressure pills					
Cortisone/steroids					
Diet pills					
Diabetes pills					
Thyroid pills					
Tranquilizers					
Water pills					
Are you NOW taking:					
Antacids					
Aspirin					
Antibiotics					
Birth control pills					
Blood thinner pills					
Laxatives					
Pain pills					
Sleeping pills					
Vitamins					
OTHER *Please list*					

Doctor Notes
please do not write in this area

OB/GYN HISTORY	Date or no. if requested	Yes	No
Date of last menstrual period:			
Are your menses regular?			
No. of days between periods			
No. of days periods last			
Spotting between periods?			
Do you do self breast exams monthly?			
Are you pregnant?			
No. of pregnancies			
Date of last pregnancy			
No. of live births			
No. of abortions or miscarriages			
Date of last Pap smear			
Was it normal?			
Have you ever had an abnormal Pap?			
Are you currently using contraception?			
Type of contraception			
Types of contraceptives used in past			
Did your mother take DES during her pregnancy?			
Have you ever had a mammogram? If yes, date			

SURGICAL HISTORY: Name of Operation	Date	Complications

Have you ever had bleeding problems? ❏ Yes ❏ No
Have you ever had a blood transfusion? ❏ Yes ❏ No Date: _____

MAJOR ILLNESS OR INJURY: list any illness or injury requiring
hospitalization, prolonged care, or use of medication. Include approx. date.

Fig. 9.4   *(continued)*

HEALTH HISTORY SHEET

Patient Name:

PERSONAL HABITS/RISK FACTORS	Yes	No		Doctor Notes *please do not write in this area*
Do you smoke or chew tobacco?			No. packs/day:	
Have you ever smoked in the past?			Date started:	
			Date stopped:	
Do you eat 3 meals/day?				
Do you eat snacks regularly?				
Do you have an eating problem?				
Any diet preferences/restrictions?				
Type				
Dietary habits			Frequency or No.:	
❑ Low fat				
No. servings/day vegetables/fruits				
No. servings/day grains				
No. times/week you eat red meat				
No. servings/day dairy				
No. caffeine drinks/day				
Alcoholic drinks			No./day: No./week:	
type: ❑ wine ❑ beer ❑ hard liquor				
Ever had a drinking problem?				
Ever had a drug problem?				
Ever used intravenous drugs?			Date last used:	
Do you use seat belts?				
No. hours sleep daily				
Highest grade level achieved				
Do you know how to swim?				
Do you exercise regularly?				
What do you do?				
How often?			Duration:	
What do you do to relieve stress?				
Any pets?				
Any hobbies?				
Occupation:				
Do you like your job?				
Is your job a risk to your health?				
If yes *(in any way)*, please explain				

SOCIAL HISTORY	Do you have children?	
Are You: ❑ Married ❑ Divorced ❑ Single ❑ Widowed ❑ Living with "signif. other"	❑ Yes ❑ No If yes, please list No. and age(s):	*If there are any special concerns you would like to discuss with the doctor, please continue on the reverse of this sheet. Thank you for providing us with this important information.*

SEXUAL HISTORY	Yes	No		
Are you sexually active?			Sexual partners in past year:	
Is sex satisfactory?			No. men	
History of chlamydia?			No. women	
Gonorrhea?			No. both	
Venereal warts?			AIDS, cont'd	
Are you concerned about AIDS?			Would you like to have a test? ❑ Yes ❑ No	

Fig. 9.5   Medical History Update

PATIENT HEALTH HISTORY UPDATE

Patient Health History Update

DATE _____

NAME _____

CURRENT ADDRESS _____

CURRENT PHONE NO. Home_____ Work _____

Any changes in insurance coverage?   ❑ yes ❑ no   ❑ N/A

Since your last checkup with us, have you:

1. Had any major surgery? If so, what?
   ❑ No
   ❑ Yes, please list _____

2. Had any heart problems diagnosed? If so, what?
   ❑ No
   ❑ Yes, please list _____

3. Any change in your medications?
   ❑ No
   ❑ Yes, please list _____

4. Contracted or been exposed to hepatitis?
   ❑ No
   ❑ Yes, please list type _____

5. Contracted or been exposed to HIV (AIDS virus)?
   ❑ No
   ❑ Yes

6. If female, are you pregnant?
   ❑ No
   ❑ Yes

7. Any other health problems we should know about?
   ❑ No
   ❑ Yes, please list _____

(Reprinted by permission, © 1995 Professional Management and Marketing)

body systems. The degree of detail depends on the age and gender of the patient, the patient's symptoms, other findings, and laboratory data.

The diagnosis portion of the physical exam may be a statement of a provisional or tentative diagnosis. The physician records the impression based on subjective statements of the patient in the history and objective findings of the physical examination. The physician may have several diagnoses that are considered possible for the patient. The stating of several different diagnoses is referred to as the "differential" diagnosis.

A complete physical exam may be performed at the time of the initial visit of the patient to the physician. Physicals may be repeated annually. In the interim, physicians may elect to perform system-focused physicals based on the limited complaints of the patient at the time of subsequent visits.

Physician Orders

Physician orders are written requests for services to be provided by nursing or allied health staff. The orders should specify the what, when, and how a particular request should be carried out. All physician orders should be dated and signed. When directed to another staff member, that staff member should acknowledge the processing of the order. For example, a nurse or medical assistant may initial the order page to indicate the order has been received. Some physicians communicate "orders" to nurses and allied health staff orally. Without the written documentation, it is often difficult to later ascertain exactly what was requested and what was performed for a patient if a dispute arose.

Progress Notes

Each patient's visit to a physician's office must include a progress note that describes in detail the services rendered during the visit. Reports on the patient's progress are continually being added to the health record. Each progress note must include the date preceding any notations and the signature or authentication of the individual making the entry. If a service is being provided by a nurse, medical assistant, or other allied health personnel, a progress note must be written by that individual describing the services rendered to the patient.

Every instruction, prescription, or telephone call for advice should be entered with the correct date. This includes all contacts with the patient, whether in person or not.

Laboratory Reports

Today laboratory reports are frequently computer-generated summaries of tests performed and results determined. Each report must contain the name of the patient, the ordering physician, a date of service, and the name of the responsible staff member performing the test. If outside reference laboratories are used, the name of the laboratory must be clearly identified on the report. If laboratory personnel in the physician's office perform tests, reports must be generated and included in the patient's record as well. Lab summary sheets with an appropriate section for recording each specific test are often used.

Lab reports are typically filed in a specially marked section within the health record. The ordering or responsible physician should review the findings before the report is filed in the patient's record. A good practice is for the physician to initial and date the report to indicate the review has been performed. Some offices use the lab report as a reminder to call the patient with test results before filing the report in the record. Any call to the patient and subsequent instructions for care should be documented in the progress notes or on the lab report itself.

Radiology Reports

Radiology or X-ray reports are usually typed reports of the findings and diagnoses identified by the radiologist who reviews the X-ray films. X-ray reports should always be prepared, even if the X rays are interpreted by a physician other than a radiologist. A routine should be established to call the patient with test results before filing the report in the record. Any call to the patient and subsequent instructions for care should be documented in the progress notes or on the radiology report itself.

Other Diagnostic Procedures

Physician office personnel may perform a variety of diagnostic procedures, including electrocardiograms, electromyographic studies, audiology tests, and visual studies. Regardless of the type of test performed, a report of the procedure and the findings must be documented. Each test must include the name of the patient, the date of service, the ordering physician, the objective test findings, any interpretations or impressions based on the results and any recommendations for follow-up or further study. Other reports are typically filed in a specially marked section within the health record.

Medication Sheet

The medication sheet provides documentation of the medicines given orally, topically, or by injection, inhalation, or infusion. The date, time, name of the drug, dose, and route by which it was given are documented after the drug has been administered. Intentional omission of medication is also documented in the record and the reasons noted. The signature of the nurse administering the drug or its nonadministration must be included.

Printed immunization forms may be used for children's and adolescents' records, to provide a complete summary of immunizations received and to serve as a reminder of immunizations due at a later date. Copies of immunization forms are typically given to parents. Again, the date, time, name of the vaccine or drug, dose, and route by which it was given are documented after the medication has been administered. The signature of the nurse administering the immunization must be included. (For an immunization schedule, see Appendix B.)

A medication list may be used to summarize all medications currently being taken by a patient or medications administered in the past. Such a list includes the medication and dosage, the date started, and the date discontinued. A special listing alerts the physician to the medications that the patient is currently taking, including those medications ordered and monitored by other physicians. Maintaining a special medication list also facilitates prescription renewals.

Consent Forms

Documentary evidence of the informed-consent process is provided by consent forms, which are legal documents permitting the physician to render a specified type of treatment, perform a specific procedure, or release confidential medical information to a specific individual or agency. Evidence of informed consent must also include the benefits and risks of proposed and alternative procedures and the patient acknowledgement of such benefits and risks. Consent forms must be completed with great care and must be signed by the patient or by a responsible representative of the patient, such as a parent or guardian. All consent forms should be filed in one section of the health record.

Consultation Reports

Consultation reports contain an opinion about a patient's condition by a physician other than the primary care physician. This opinion is based on a review of the patient's health record or history, an examination of the patient, and possibly a conference with the primary care physician.

When a patient is sent to a consulting physician for an examination and opinion, the consulting physician completes a consultation report and files it in the patient's record within the consultant's office. A copy of the consultation report, often with an accompanying letter, is sent to the primary care physician. This report must be filed within the patient's health record in the primary care physician's office. The ordering or responsible physician should review the consultant's report before filing it in the patient's record. A good practice is for the physician to initial and date the report to indicate the review has been performed. Follow-up with the patient may be documented in a separate progress note or in the progress note of the patient's subsequent visit to the physician's office. (For examples of a consultation and other reports, see Chapter 11, "Medical Transcription and Correspondence.")

Making Corrections to Health Records

Error correction is a particularly important aspect of documentation. It is also very important for legal purposes (see Chapter 2, "Health Law"). Alterations can easily raise questions of authenticity and negligence. When it is necessary to correct an error (such as when the health care provider has mistakenly written in the wrong patient's health record), the health care provider should be advised to draw a single line through each line of the error, add a note explaining the error (such as "entry made in wrong patient's record"), date and sign the note, and then make the correct entry in chronological order, indicating which entry it is replacing. If there is any doubt about the subsequent admissibility of the entry, it is a good practice to have a professional colleague witness the correction process.

Erasing or obliterating an entry is forbidden and must *not* be attempted. Also, entries must not be squeezed in between existing documentation; instead, corrections should be written in the next entry space.

Errors in documentation can occur as honest mistakes. The correction of these erroneous entries should be made simply and honestly to indicate the error was not intentional and the correction has been made with diligence and care.

Documentation Guidelines for Health Records

The following guidelines provide standards for careful and complete documentation.

1. Develop a separate health record for each individual to whom care is provided.
2. Record each visit precisely and thoroughly.
3. Document or dictate each encounter at the time the service is rendered.
4. On each page of the record, note the patient's name and identifying information such as health record number or date of birth.
5. Record the date and time, and sign each entry
6. Write all record entries legibly, or dictate them. Record all written entries in black or blue permanent ink.
7. Document all patient and family encounters, including those by telephone.
8. Identify progress notes by the physician specialty, or by the nursing or allied health professional responsible in a group practice.
9. Note the extent of any counseling or coordination of patient care during the encounter with the patient or family.
10. Use a limited number of abbreviations and only those that are standard.
11. Be as specific as possible when a diagnosis is known; specify *acute* to distinguish from *chronic* conditions.
12. When a diagnosis is unknown, support rule-out, suspected, or probable diagnoses with the patient's description of symptoms or complaints.
13. Avoid nonspecific or vague language (such as "doing well" or "activity as tolerated"). If such phrases must be used, support them with objective, precise documentation about the patient's condition.
14. Include drawings and relevant notes as necessary.
15. Avoid preprinted, prescribed, or fill-in-the-blank narratives. Documentation should be individualized for each patient.
16. Document so that each record entry stands alone and enables other

health care professionals to carry out or continue patient care in the absence of the primary care physician.

Releasing Health Information

Confidentiality

One of the most important responsibilities of a health care provider is to safeguard the confidentiality of health records. Confidentiality is the underpinning of the legal aspects of health records. It is the reference point for security measures that affect medical data and is the underlying reason for most of the state and federal legislation regarding health records.

Confidentiality and *privacy* are terms often used interchangeably in reference to medical data. Although not precisely synonymous, they are quite similar when applied to medical information. Reduced to a simple definition, *privacy* is the right to be left alone. Medical confidentiality can be viewed as a special case of the right to privacy. Simply defined, *confidentiality* means keeping a secret. This implies that two people are involved and precludes sharing with a third. Confidentiality becomes an issue, however, only when the third person is involved, that is, only when there is a need to share the secret. Therefore, *medical confidentiality* is concerned with the restrictive use of information obtained from and about a patient.

Federal regulations   Carrying out the responsibility to protect the medical confidentiality of patient information requires a knowledge of the laws and regulations affecting disclosure of information, including the conditions under which it can be disclosed without the patient's consent and the circumstances in which patient consent is required. At the present, the only federal regulations concerning confidentiality of health information addresses drug-abuse treatment and alcohol-abuse treatment and prevention.

State regulations   However, many state laws exist concerning privacy and confidentiality of medical information. In particular, states often have detailed laws regarding the privileged status of the records of psychiatric, mentally retarded, and developmentally disabled patients as well as information pertaining to HIV status. Health care providers must be knowledgeable about their specific state laws concerning all medical information.

A valuable resource is each state's health information management association, many of which publish a state-specific guidebook that addresses the requirements for the proper patient consent and release of information in each state. The American Health Information Management Association in Chicago (312-787-2672) can be contacted to provide the name and address of each state's association.

Consent to Release Information

Because the information in the health record belongs to the patient, the patient may authorize the health care provider to release it to a third party. Consents to release information from the health record must always be in writing and should be an informed consent. *Informed consent* means that the patient is aware, in a general way, what information will be released and the use that will be made of the information.

A consent or authorization to release information must be obtained when the information is requested by other doctors and institutions, insurance companies, attorneys, government agencies not entitled to access by law, and the media. No consent form is usually necessary for releasing medical information to a health care facility to which the physician has arranged admission for a patient or for follow-up care, or to an institution for the maintenance of its cancer or other disease registry. However, some medical conditions may require specific consent forms, as detailed under state regulations.

Written authorization   The written authorization to release information should contain at least the following data:

1. Name of physician or practice that is to release the information
2. Name of the individual or institution that is to receive the information
3. Patient's full name, address, and date of birth
4. Purpose or need for the information
5. Extent or nature of the information to be released, with inclusive dates of treatment
6. Specific date, event, or condition upon which the authorization will expire, unless revoked earlier
7. Statement that authorization can be revoked but not retroactive to the release of information made in good faith
8. Date the consent is signed (Note: the date of signature must be later than the date of care for which the information is to be released—that is, a patient cannot consent to release information about care before the care is rendered, as the patient would be "uninformed" as to the nature of information that could be released.)
9. Signature of the patient or legal representative of the patient

The signed consent to release information may be given by (1) the patient, (2) a legally qualified representative of the patient (such as a parent or guardian), (3) an executor or administrator of an estate, or (4) an agency designated by the court as a guardian. A parent cannot sign for an adult child (usually over age 18); nor can a spouse for the husband or wife.

Policies and Procedures

A physician's office should have detailed policies and procedures regarding the release of information to cover all possible situations. The policies and procedures must be approved by the physicians in the practice and the practice attorney.

Upon receipt of a written authorization for medical information, the signature on the authorization form should be compared to a signature of the patient contained in the health record. The information released should be strictly limited to that which is required to fulfill the purpose of the authorization. The authorization form should be retained as part of the patient's health record. The individual who released the information should make a notation on the authorization form following the release showing what information was released and the date released, and then sign the entry. (See Figure 9.6 for a sample release form.)

Methods of Releasing Information

There are basically four methods of releasing properly authorized information from health records: (1) direct access, (2) abstracting information, (3) oral release, or (4) photocopying all or portions of the record.

Direct access   Direct access may be by the patient or by the authorized representative. Individual medical practices may have specific guidelines that apply before allowing access. In general, care should be taken that the person directly reviewing the record does not alter the contents or remove any part of the record. An office staff member should sit with the reviewer to ensure that neither of these occur and to assist the reviewer with locating desired information.

Abstracting information   Abstracting information from a patient's health record should be delegated to an individual properly trained, so that only essential information (as stipulated on the authorization) is abstracted onto the requesting form or insurance claim report.

Oral release   An oral release should be limited to those circumstances when other methods of release cannot be used, such as in an emergency situation. The identity of the caller should be verified by returning the call. Only the information required to satisfy the emergency should be released orally. Some physicians prefer to handle an oral release of information personally. A record should be made of the oral release. (See Figure 9.7 for a sample oral release form.)

Photocopying   Photocopying all or a portion of the record in response to a legitimate request is the method used most often. Care must be taken not to release more information than is covered by the patient's authorization. The record must be carefully reviewed to assure that highly sensitive data is not inadvertently disclosed.

Fax Transmission

Fax transmission is a system of sending and receiving copies of information instantly over telephone lines. Faxes have become everyday methods of communication.

Fig. 9.6   Patient Release of Information

AUTHORIZATION FOR DISCLOSURE OF HEALTH INFORMATION

(1) I hereby authorize _____ to disclose the following information from the health records of:
                                [name of provider]

Patient Name: _____   Date of Birth   _____

Address: _____   Telephone   _____

                _____   Patient Number   _____

covering the period(s) of healthcare:

From (date) _____ to (date) _____

From (date) _____ to (date) _____

(2) Information to be disclosed:
- ☐   Complete health record(s)   ☐   Discharge Summary
- ☐   History & Physical Examination   ☐   Consultation Reports
- ☐   Progress Notes   ☐   Laboratory Tests
- ☐   X-Ray Reports   ☐   Other (please specify) _____

I understand that this will include information relating to (check if applicable):
- ☐   Acquired Immunodeficiency Syndrome (AIDS) or infection with HIV (Human Immunodeficiency Virus)
- ☐   psychiatric care
- ☐   treatment for alcohol and/or drug abuse.

(3) This information is to be disclosed to _____ for the purpose
    of _____.

(4) I understand this authorization may be revoked in writing at any time, except to the extent that action has been taken in reliance on this authorization. Unless otherwise revoked, this authorization will expire on the following date, event, or condition: _____.

(5) The facility, its employees, officers, and physicians are hereby released from any legal responsibility or liability for disclosure of the above information to the extent indicated and authorized herein.

Signed: _____
                    (Patient)   (Date)

        _____
        or (Legal Representative)   (Relationship to Patient)   (Date)

(Reprinted by permission of American Health Information Management Association)

Fig. 9.7 Verbal Release of Information

RECORD OF VERBAL DISCLOSURE OF HEALTH INFORMATION

Patient Name _____ Date of Birth _____

Patient Number _____

Date of Disclosure _____

Information Disclosed to: _____

Reason for Disclosure: _____

Specific Information Disclosed:

_____
Signature of Individual Making Disclosure   Date

(Reprinted by permission of American Health Information Management Association)

From a legal standpoint, protecting the patient's confidentiality in the fax process is critical. Fax transmissions of medical information should be avoided when other methods of communication are available, such as mail or delivery services. Documents containing information on highly personal matters such as sexually transmitted diseases, drug or alcohol treatment, or HIV status should never be faxed. Fax machines should be located in secure or restricted-access areas.

Confidentiality   If it is absolutely essential to convey confidential medical information via fax, several steps should be taken. To ensure protection, a cover sheet should be used for all transmissions (see Figure 9.8). It should contain the name of the recipient, name of the sender, date, total number of pages, fax and telephone numbers of the sender in case of transmittal problems, and a statement that the fax is personal, privileged, and confidential information intended for the named recipient only.

Coded mailboxes   A good practice is to make arrangements with the recipient for a scheduled time for transmission, or to send the fax to a coded mailbox. Coded mailboxes require the sender to enter a code indicating the individual the fax is addressed to; the recipient then must enter the same code number to activate the printer.

Another practice to assure receipt of the confidential information is to request the authorized recipient to sign and return a receipt form that may be printed on the bottom of the fax cover sheet.

Faxes have become an important communication tool. However, the protection of the patient's privacy and the confidentiality of the patient's medical information cannot be sacrificed to the convenience of the rapid, sometimes impersonal communication that fax machines have created.

Patient Access to Health Records

In slightly more than half the states, no patient-access statutes or regulations exist. In those states with statutes guaranteeing patients access to their health records, the content of the laws varies. The majority, however, allow for inspection of health records with language such as "upon written request," "upon demand," or "within a reasonable period of time."

Health care providers must be knowledgeable about the statutes within their states concerning patient access. In states without a law addressing this issue, physicians must determine their own internal policies and procedures. The American Health Information Management Association (AHIMA) asserts that unless prohibited by state law, the patient or the patient's legal representative should have access to health information. In the case of psychiatric records, the patient's physician should be contacted prior to disclosure.

The patient or the patient's representative should be allowed to view the record or to obtain copies of the record upon written request. As with any authorized release of information, the physician's practice may charge a sufficient fee to cover the cost of the photocopies made.

Fig. 9.8   Fax Cover Sheet

FACSIMILE COVER LETTER

[sending facility name]
[address]
[city, state, zip code]
[telephone number]
[facsimile number]

DATE:_____   TIME: _____   NO. OF PAGES _____

TO: _____
       (name of authorized receiver)

       _____
       (name and address of authorized receiver's facility)

TELEPHONE:_____ FAX:_____
            (of receiver)   (of receiver)

FROM: _____
       (name of sender)

TELEPHONE:_____ FAX:_____
            (of sender)   (of sender)

*****CONFIDENTIALITY NOTICE*****

The documents accompanying this telecopy transmission contain confidential information, belonging to the sender, that is legally privileged. This information is intended only for the use of the individual or entity named above. The authorized recipient of this information is prohibited from disclosing this information to any other party and is required to destroy the information after its stated need has been fulfilled.

If you are not the intended recipient, you are hereby notified that any disclosure, copying, distribution, or action taken in reliance on the contents of these documents is strictly prohibited. If you have received this telecopy in error, please notify the sender immediately to arrange for return of these documents.

COMMENTS:

(Reprinted by permission of American Health Information Management Association)

If the patient or the patient's representative disputes any information within the record, AHIMA recommends first discussing the dispute with the practitioner who made the entry. If the practitioner agrees that the entry contains an error, the practitioner should make the correcting entry in the record by amending the first entry and adding the correct information. If the practitioner does not agree that the entry is in error, the patient should be allowed to write a statement concerning the disputed information and the statement should be added to the health record.

Using Health Information for Insurance Billing

Many forms of health insurance coverage are currently in effect in the United States. Health insurance is available through group policies, individual policies, and subscription to prepaid plans. Many people are covered by government plans. All insurance companies may be referred to as *third-party payers*. Indeed the insurance company is the third party in the relationship between the physician, the patient, and the insurance company.

For payment purposes, third-party payers need health information about the patient for whom the visit or encounter was necessary, such as the reason the patient was seen, evaluated, examined, or treated. This information is illustrated in the chief complaint, the diagnosis, and the assessment and impression of the physician.

The insurance company needs to know what was done during the encounter. For example, was a history, physical, review of diagnostic data, assessment, review of management options, or risk assessment performed? Was a plan made? Was surgery performed, and if so, by what surgical procedures?

The minimum information required by third-party payers includes the following:

1. Type of service or procedures
2. Reason for service or procedure, expressed in ICD-9-CM diagnosis codes
3. Date performed
4. Place of service
5. Name or identification number of health care provider

Diagnosis Codes

Coding is the process by which a number or other symbol is substituted for a more extensive item of information, such as a description of a disease entity or diagnosis. Medical services and surgical procedures can also be coded by converting the narrative text description of the service into a number or other symbol. The International Classification of Diseases, 9th revision, Clinical Modification (ICD-9-CM) is a two-part classification system in current use for coding or converting patient diagnoses, symptoms, or complaints into a standardized numerical system for communication.

Numerical diagnostic and procedural coding was developed for a number of reasons: (1) to track disease processes, (2) to classify medical problems, (3) for medical research, and (4) to evaluate health care utilization. The two-part classification system of ICD-9-CM allows for the coding of both diagnoses and procedures. Its codes are predominantly numeric and vary from three to five digits in length. ICD-9-CM is updated annually by the federal government, with changes effective October 1st. The system is governed by rules for code selection and guidelines for reporting the codes.

Procedure Codes

CPT-4 Current Procedural Terminology, 4th edition (CPT-4) is a comprehensive listing of medical terms and codes for the uniform designation of diagnostic and therapeutic procedures. Its purpose is to provide standard terminology and coding for consistency and comparability in reporting claims for third-party reimbursement. CPT-4 is limited to procedure and service codes; the codes are strictly five-digit numeric.

CPT-4 is used by physicians for coding all services and procedures for reimbursement; it has highly detailed procedural descriptions. Modifiers can be added to CPT-4 codes to distinguish special circumstances associated with the services provided. Modifiers are suffixes to codes that show a variation to a standard procedure. For example, a physician may use a particular modifier if unexpected discoveries during surgery required action beyond the customary procedures. A modifier also may be used when multiple procedures are performed. Physicians or coding specialists should not hesitate to use modifiers when warranted because they can affect reimbursement.

CPT-4 is governed by a system of rules for code selection and guidelines for reporting the codes; it is updated annually by the American Medical Association, with changes effective January 1st.

HCPCS A second procedural coding system is the Health Care Financing Administration Common Procedural Coding System (HCPCS). HCPCS, based on the current edition of the CPT-4 system, is a five-digit alphanumeric coding system used primarily by Medicare and some Medicaid plans. There are three levels of codes assigned and maintained by the Medicare carriers: Level I includes approximately 98 percent of all Medicare Part B procedural codes and uses only CPT-4 codes; Level II codes are assigned by the Health Care Financing Administration (HCFA) for physician and nonphysician services not contained in the CPT system; Level III codes are assigned by each local fiscal intermediary, and represent services not included in the CPT system and not common to all carriers.

Resource-Based Relative Value Scale (RBRVS)

The RBRVS is not a coding system but a payment system. In use since 1992, the RBRVS is an outcome of Medicare's physician payment reform. It changed the fee-for-service system that was based on the customary, prevailing, and reasonable (CPR) charges formerly used by Medicare to pay physicians.

The RBRVS determines payment by measuring three factors: physician work, charge-based professional liability expenses, and charge-based overhead. Physician work includes the amount of time and effort the physician spends on a particular service or procedure; it is expressed in terms of the CPT-4 procedure codes. The professional-liability and overhead factors are computed by HCFA. The fee schedule provides uniform payments that are adjusted to include different practice costs across the United States.

Since the reporting of physician services through the use of CPT-4 codes drives much of the RBRVS reimbursement system, great care must be taken to correctly assign the most appropriate CPT-4 code to describe the services rendered by the physician.

Documentation and Coding

Documentation is linked to reimbursement through the standard nomenclature in the coding systems noted above. Coding systems and nomenclature are the standards for reporting the services rendered to a patient.

The documentation in the health record must be matched with the terms in the coding systems to code and report diagnoses and services for billing purposes. When documentation, for whatever reason, does not readily correspond to the uniform language, accuracy of coding and reporting will be more difficult to achieve. Payment may be affected as well. Payers, upon record review, must verify that the coded service or procedure and the record documentation agree.

Confidentiality of Codes

In addition to the release of information in a patient's health record discussed earlier, the use of ICD-9-CM or CPT-4 coding systems to release medical information to third-party payers also requires the authorization of the patient. Patients or their legal representatives must be asked to sign a release-of-information form before confidential patient information is submitted in the form of ICD-9-CM or CPT-4 codes.

The HCFA Health Insurance Claim Form (HCFA-1500) has been designed to meet the needs of most basic health care insurers, and is used for Medicare and Medicaid claims by physicians and suppliers. Item 12 on the HCFA-1500 form requires the patient's or authorized person's signature to release medical or other information necessary to process the claim. (For a copy of the HCFA-1500 form, see Figure 9.9.)

Some commercial insurance companies provide their own forms. These forms also contain an entry for the patient's or authorized person's signature to release medical information. Physician offices or their billing services must obtain the patient's or authorized person's consent to release medical information as part of the claims processing. A copy of the consent must be maintained by the medical practice.

Fig. 9.9 HCFA-1500 Insurance Form

Managing Health Information

Managing health information requires systems that allow for the appropriate storage and retrieval, retention, and disposal of health records according to laws, regulations, and professional practice.

Storage and Retrieval

Two major concerns determine how health information and health records are stored. One concern is ease of access. Records should be stored in such a manner that allows them to be easily retrieved. In fact, many state laws and regulations require that health care facilities and providers maintain health records in this way.

Security

The security of health information is another concern. The loss of information contained in health records could have catastrophic consequences. The records must be protected against loss, damage, destruction, or unauthorized access or release. To adequately protect health information, the health care provider must consider personnel security, physical security, and system security.

Personnel security The most effective way to ensure the security of health records is to make certain that qualified individuals are responsible for safeguarding health information. A careful screening of employees who have access to confidential records is essential. Security consciousness must be promoted during new-staff orientation as well as regularly reminding all staff of their responsibility for the records. All staff members should sign a confidentiality agreement verifying that they understand the policies and procedures concerning record disclosure, security, and retention (see Figure 9.10 for a sample form). Staff members must understand that consequences exist if policies and procedures are not followed.

Computer security Computer security, with appropriate access and passwords, is also crucial. There must be a system to recover keys and badges and delete computer access codes when personnel are no longer employed by the practice. (For details on computer security, see Chapter 5, "The Computer in the Medical Office.")

Physical security Protection of records against various forms of destruction is essential. Records should be stored in a fireproof or fire-resistant storage facility with a sprinkler system.

The physical environment of the storage area must be considered: a temperature of approximately 70 degrees and humidity between 50 and 60 percent are considered safe for most paper and filmed documents. Higher temperature and humidity cause deterioration of paper and other storage media.

Fig. 9.10   Employee Confidentiality Agreement

EMPLOYEE/STUDENT/VOLUNTEER NON-DISCLOSURE AGREEMENT

[Name of health care facility] has a legal and ethical responsibility to safeguard the privacy of all patients and protect the confidentiality of their health information. In the course of my employment/assignment at *[name of health care facility]*, I may come into possession of confidential patient information, even though I may not be directly involved in providing patient services.

I understand that such information must be maintained in the strictest confidence. As a condition of my employment/assignment, I hereby agree that, unless directed by my supervisor, I will not at any time during or after my employment/assignment with *[name of health care facility]* disclose any patient information to any person whatsoever or permit any person whatsoever to examine or make copies of any patient reports or other documents prepared by me, coming into my possession, or under my control, or use patient information, other than as necessary in the course of my employment/assignment.

When patient information must be discussed with other health care practitioners in the course of my work, I will use discretion to assure that such conversations cannot be overheard by others who are not involved in the patient's care.

I understand that violation of this agreement may result in corrective action, up to and including discharge.

_____

Signature of Employee/Student/Volunteer

_____

Date

(Reprinted by permission of American Health Information Management Association)

Confidential records should be stored in a secure area that is kept locked unless a staff member is present. Storage cabinets or rooms that contain records should be locked overnight or when the facility is closed, especially if contracted services, such as cleaning and maintenance, have access to the area when staff members are not present.

System security System security is related to both personnel and physical security. Having a security-conscious staff and good physical security will not prevent loss, damage, destruction, or unauthorized disclosure of records if there is not also a good system to control access to and disclosure of the records. This involves a requisition and charge-out system for health records. Procedures must be followed to properly release records to authorized individuals. Close monitoring of the reproduction or photocopying of records is essential to prevent unauthorized disclosure of confidential information. Finally, proper destruction of records is the final step in ensuring confidentiality.

Filing Systems

Managing health information requires appropriate filing systems that ensure ease of access and security.

Alphabetical Filing

Alphabetical filing by name is the most commonly used system for filing health records in medical offices, particularly in small practices. Alphabetical filing follows the sequence of letters in the alphabet and the sequence of letters in patients' names. In alphabetical files, the needed information can be retrieved by direct reference without the use of a separate index.

However, errors in alphabetizing and misspelled names can often cause retrieval problems. Another disadvantage is that alphabetical filing units are difficult to plan for in terms of expansion; as more space is needed for different sections of the alphabet, folders must be moved from drawer to drawer or shelf to shelf.

Phonetic classification Phonetic classification systems have been developed to overcome the difficulties associated with misspelled names in alphabetical filing. Phonetic classification systems are based on a numerical code that represents consonant sounds. Vowel sounds are ignored. Each name is reduced to one letter and three digits. For example, in a phonetic file, the names *John Smith* and *Jon Smythe* would be filed together.

The main advantages of phonetic filing are (1) similar sounding names are grouped together; (2) silent letters and double consonants are disregarded, thus reducing retrieval time; and (3) duplicate entries are avoided because names that may have been spelled incorrectly or that contain typographical errors still can be filed correctly.

The disadvantage of the phonetic filing system is that special training is needed before it can be used by staff members. Also, filing errors can occur when more than one person is responsible for coding, filing, and retrieving from a phonetic file.

Numerical Filing

With a numerical filing system, each new patient is assigned a sequential number. Although numbers are easier for some people to remember than names, the maintenance of numerical files is time-consuming because additional filing procedures are required. For example, a separate alphabetical index file must be consulted to locate the record of a specified patient.

Nevertheless, the advantages of the numerical filing system are that (1) orderly expansion is possible, thus eliminating the shifting of files, (2) the number of misfiles is reduced, and (3) speedy retrieval is possible because it is unnecessary to search through several files labeled with the same name in order to find the right patient's record. Numerical filing requires more training, but once the system is mastered, fewer errors occur than with alphabetical filing.

The three basic methods of numerical filing are (1) the straight numerical, (2) the middle digit, and (3) the terminal digit.

Straight numerical method   In straight numerical filing, consecutively numbered folders are filed in exact numerical order. Anyone who can count can become proficient in filing with the straight numerical method. However, errors can occur in large files because all digits of the record number must be considered at one time, thus increasing the inadvertent transposition of numbers.

Middle digit and terminal digit methods   In middle digit and terminal digit filing, the number of a given folder is divided into three groups of two digits for filing. In middle digit filing, for example, folder 12-34-56 is filed first by 34, then by 12, and finally by 56.

In terminal digit filing, the records are filed backward in groups. Numbers are read in groups of two from right to left instead of from left to right. For example, folder 12-34-56 is filed first by 56, then by 34, and finally by 12. The sequence of numbers in each method is as follows:

Middle Digit Files	Terminal Digit Files
12-34-56	12-34-56
12-34-57	13-34-56
. . . . . .	. . . . . .
12-34-99	99-34-56
13-34-00	00-35-56
. . . . .	. . . . .
13-34-99	99-35-56
14-34-00	00-36-56
. . . . .	. . . . .
99-34-99	99-99-56
00-35-00	00-00-57

Advantages and disadvantages   Middle digit and terminal digit filing can eliminate traffic jams in the files, because each file section contains recently assigned numbers; new folders do not become backed up at the end of the files as occurs with straight numerical filing. Responsibility for a specific file section also may be assigned to one staff member, thus promoting greater accuracy. Sorting the records before filing is facilitated because two digits are sorted at a time.

The chief disadvantage of these two methods is the need to give special training to the staff filing the records. Although most employees are able to learn terminal digit filing rapidly, middle digit filing is difficult for some people to learn. The filer must read the middle of the number first and then move to the far left and finally to the right, which some people find illogical.

The terminal digit system is considered the most effective numerical method of filing for organizing, storing, and retrieving health records. This method offers a virtually perfect distribution of folders throughout the file. It also greatly increases filing speed and retrieval because the filer works with only two numbers at a time.

Social Security numbers Some practices use the last four digits of each patient's Social Security number to file health records.

Alphabetical index for numerical files If a numerical filing system is used, an alphabetical index entry must be created for each patient folder. The entry can be a manual card or list, or a computer-generated index. The alphabetical index should include the patient's name, address, birth date, and health record number. Additional information such as visit dates and billing information may be included. The alphabetical index is used to locate a health record given the patient's name. It may also make it unnecessary to pull a patient's record to handle some requests for information.

Number-access register for numerical files With numerical files, adequate controls must be established to ensure that a patient's number can be located and that two patients are not given the same number. A number-access register is a paper log or a computer-generated listing of all numbers assigned to patients in order of their occurrence. Only three entries are required: a list of numbers in numerical order, the name of the person to whom each number has been issued, and the date of issue.

A number-access register is different from an alphabetical index. When only a patient's name is known, the alphabetical index is used to locate the patient's record number. If only the health record number is known, the number-access register is used to identify the patient assigned to that number.

Filing Rules

For the sake of accuracy, written filing rules should be prepared and new staff members thoroughly instructed in file maintenance procedures. While individual offices may have their own procedures, some appropriate rules for arranging alphabetical files include the following:

1. Alphabetize the names of individuals by surname, then given name, then middle name or initial.

> Jones, M. Arthur
> Jones, Mary Ann

2. Arrange all health record folders in alphabetical order letter by letter to the end of the surname, then by given names and initials.

   > Morison, John A.
   > Morison, John Thomas
   > Morrison, John Andrew

3. Treat hyphenated or compound names as one word.

   > Fitz-Smith, Patrick
   > Foster Brown, Joan

4. During alphabetizing, disregard titles such as *Dr., Mrs.,* or *Senator.* However, these designations may be used to provide additional identifying information.

   > Peters, Susan (Dr.)
   > Smith, Walter (Senator)

5. Disregard religious titles (such as *Reverend* and *Sister*) in filing. File the material according to the patients' last names.

   > Raphael, Mary (Sister)
   > Smith, John (Reverend)

6. Alphabetize abbreviated prefixes such as *St.* according to the complete spelling *Saint.*

   > St. Peter, Joanne
   > Saint-Simon, Paul

7. Disregard designation such as *Jr., Sr.,* or *2d* in filing.

   > Smith, John T. (Sr.)
   > Smith, John Thomas (Jr.)

8. Consider the legal signature of a married woman's name in filing. Her husband's name may be cross-referenced if desired.

   > Jones, Mary Ann (Mrs. John)

9. File "nothing" before "something" if initials are used for a given name.

   > Peters, J.
   > Peters, J.G.
   > Peters, John

10. Arrange surnames having the prefixes *de, La,* and *Mac* just as they are spelled.

    > MacDougal, John
    > Mbasdeken, Joan
    > McDover, Mary

11. File as written those surnames in which it is impossible to determine the given name or middle name.

  Chin Sing Hop
  Hope Big Feather
  Osak Wong

Filing Equipment

Some considerations in selecting filing equipment depend on the following: (1) available office space, (2) building structural systems, (3) cost of equipment, (4) total number of records, (5) time needed to retrieve records, and (6) fire protection. Two common types of filing methods use drawers or open shelves.

Vertical drawer files Full-suspension drawer files should roll smoothly and close securely. Adequate floor space should be planned to enable the drawer to be opened completely. One disadvantage of the vertical drawer file is that only one person at a time can access the files. In addition, file retrieval is slower because the drawer must be opened and closed each time a file is accessed.

Open shelf files Shelf files can accommodate more patient records per square foot of floor space than can vertical drawer files. Records in open shelf units are filed sideways, and file retrieval is faster because several staff members can work at the same time. While an open shelf system is the most cost-effective, it does not protect the confidentiality of the records. However, open shelf files can be placed in a room that can be locked, an alternative that allows for record security.

Lateral files Lateral files use more wall space than do vertical files, but they do not need as much floor space. The records are filed sideways as in the open shelf system. Some lateral files have pull-out drawers, similar to vertical files; others have retractable doors.

A variation of open shelf files is a movable system that offers a great volume of storage in a small space. The files are mounted on tracks in the floor, and the units slide to allow access to the needed record. These mobile files may be moved manually or they may be electrically powered. One disadvantage, depending on the physical layout of the system, is that not all records are available at the same time. The system is also more expensive than other systems.

Filing equipment should be standardized in a practice. If shelf filing is going to be used for the storage of records, then only shelves should be used. It is not efficient to mix active records in file cabinets and shelf units because the design of vertical and lateral filing supplies differ.

Estimating Storage Needs

A fairly accurate estimate of the amount of record storage space that will be needed in a given practice can be established first by measuring the number of records that can be filed per filing inch and then by multiplying that figure by the number of new records initiated each year. About three to four records can be filed per inch, but the situation can vary according to the type of practice. For instance, a family practitioner with a stable patient population may have thicker records than those of a specialist with a referral practice.

To estimate the number of records that will be initiated by a physician in a year, count the new patients for a month and multiple this number by 12. Divide the number of records initiated per year by the number of records filed per inch to obtain an estimate of the number of inches of filing space required per year. Filing space should be considered in terms of estimated practice growth over 10 years.

Filing Supplies

The management of paper-based records systems requires several types of filing supplies.

Shelf guides   To expedite the filing and retrieving of records, each file drawer or shelf should be equipped with dividers and guides. One guide for every 50 records is usually adequate unless the records are very thick. Shelf guides may be used in both alphabetical and numerical files.

Since durability and visibility are important considerations, shelf guides should be of quality pressboard or sturdy plastic. The tab on each guide should project far enough beyond the record folders to ensure complete visibility. The shelf guides are intended to reduce the area of search and serve as supports for the files. With straight numerical files, the guides are added constantly, but with terminal digit and alphabetical files, the guides are usually permanent.

Outguides   An outguide is a heavy guide or pocket that is filed in place of a record that has been temporarily removed from the file. The outguide should be a bright color for easy identification, to facilitate accurate refiling. Several colors may be used, each to correspond with a temporary location for the file. The outguide may include a plastic pocket for inserting a requisition form that indicates the location of the file, the date it was removed, and the date it should be returned to the permanent file. The plastic pocket is useful for holding loose reports that may be sent to the file while the folder and record have been removed. When the folder is returned to the file, the loose reports are then filed in the folder. Outguides must be audited on a periodic basis, preferably weekly, to determine which records are due to be returned to the file and to follow up with the requesters.

Folders   Most records are filed in tabbed folders. Four types of folders are commonly used:

1. Manila folders are the most common and least expensive; they are available with wax or Mylar coating for extra durability and come in multiple colors.

2. Kraft folders are heavier and darker in color than manila; they are durable and do not soil easily, but are more expensive than manila folders. Kraft folders are especially useful if they are subjected to much wear and tear.
3. Pressboard folders are made out of expensive heavy-duty material, which is more suitable for shelf guides than folders.
4. Vinyl or plastic folders are durable and available in a variety of colors. Since the texture is smooth, the folders can be slippery and do not stack well on a desk or table.

The most commonly used folder is a general-purpose manila folder that may be expanded to three-quarters of an inch. Folders are available with a reinforced tab, which will lengthen the life of the folder. Folders kept in drawers have tabs at the top. Folders kept on shelves have tabs at the side.

Some folders can be used to separate papers in one record into categories, such as history, progress notes, or lab reports. Another type of folder, with a vertical pocket that folds down for easy access to contents, may be used for bulky records or correspondence. Folders with fasteners to hold papers offer security and help to organize the information contained within the folder.

Labels Labels can be used to identify each shelf, drawer, shelf guide, and folder. The label should indicate the alphabetical, numerical, or chronologic range of the material filed in that space. The label on the folder identifies the content of that folder only. This may be the name of the patient or, for nonpatient records, the subject matter within the folder. Labels may also indicate the physician's name or the health record number. Year labels are also useful on a folder to indicate the last visit of a patient to the practice. This is useful when older records are removed from an active file area and relocated into a storage area.

Filing Procedures

Filing of all materials involves several procedures that ensure records are protected and secured in the appropriate area.

Maintenance and repair Maintenance and repair of paper files involves removing paper clips or loose staples and securing the papers into the folder either with fasteners or prongs. Damaged and torn paper should be mended to prevent further destruction. Half or quarter sheets of paper should be attached to a full sheet to prevent their loss within a large file.

Sorting The next step is to sort the papers in filing sequence. Folders being returned to a numerical or alphabetical file should be placed in sequential order to facilitate faster filing. For example, loose pages that need to be added to the record, consultation reports for outside physicians, and reports should be sorted into the numerical or alphabetical sequence of the files. A basic rule of filing is to sort and file all loose reports within 24–48 hours of receipt. Health record files should be returned to the permanent file the same day that the record is returned from the provider.

Color-coding   A system of color-coded folders is desirable in large file units or in situations when more than one person has regular access to the files. There are many color-coding systems available that provide immediate visual recognition of filing errors. Filing errors are reduced by using color-coded folders, and the time needed to find misfiles is minimized.

Color-coding may be used with either numerical or alphabetical filing systems. The simplest system requires colored folders. Most commonly, the record number is color-coded. Ten colors indicate the numerals 0 through 9. In straight numerical files, the third digit from the right is coded since it is where the most filing errors occur. In alphabetical files, colored folders can also be assigned to certain letters of the alphabet; the second letter of each patient's last name is color-coded, since the first letter is rarely misfiled.

Extensive color-coding systems necessitate the purchase of preprinted folders. Companies that sell health record folders offer assistance in the selection of the most appropriate color-coding method for the particular practice.

Preventing Misfiles

Careful training of personnel, color-coding of folders, and well-organized files reduce the incidence of misfiled records in both alphabetical and numerical filing systems. However, occasional misfiles are inevitable. To conduct a search for a misfiled record, consider the following:

1. Think of alternate ways that the patient's name might have been spelled.
2. Search for transposed letters due to typographical errors.
3. Check the folders just before and after the one that is needed; it may have been put into another folder rather than between two folders.
4. Look for transposition of the last digits of the number or the hundred and thousand digits.
5. Look for misfiles that may have been caused by unclear numbers; for example, look for a missing *3* under *5* or *8,* and a missing *1* under *7,* and vice versa.
6. Check for a missing number in the hundred group just preceding or following it; for example, look for *288* in the *188* and the *388* sequences.
7. Look next to the folders of patients seen on the same day as that of the one whose record is lost.

Health Records Retention

Patients' health records are preserved for several reasons: (1) to fulfill statutory and regulatory requirements, (2) to secure continuity of patient care, (3) to serve as evidence in possible future litigation, and (4) to fulfill research and educational needs.

Practical experience sometimes causes a practitioner to keep records longer than legally required. Even when a law provides for such a period of time, other considerations may require records be retained for longer period of time. Practical concerns, like the availability of resources such as space and funding, will also affect the decision of how long to retain records.

Statutory and Regulatory Requirements

All levels of government have the authority to require that health records be retained. A statute, an executive order, or an agency regulation may lawfully require records to be kept for a specified length of time. The government's power to require records and reports in the area of health services is necessary to ensure the public welfare. The government, whether acting through the courts or through an administrative agency such as a health department, has the power to enforce sanctions for failure to maintain required records. Such sanctions may include fines, contempt citations, or default judgments. Often a federal, state, or local law will define how long records are to be retained.

Continuity of Patient Care

An effort must be made to decide whether or not a particular record is likely to be of future medical, economic, or social benefit to the patient. Experience demonstrates that a health record documenting a prolonged period of care will be needed in the future to help provide the patient with appropriate care or to establish the presence or absence of disability. However, records documenting care for minor, self-limiting problems are less likely to be of great future benefit to the patient or the physician.

Potential Evidence in Future Litigation

Regardless of whether a regulation specifies how long to retain a record, the statutes of limitations within state law must be considered. Statutes of limitations usually run from the date of the incident, such as the malpractice, or from the date the plaintiff learns of or reasonably should have learned of the incident, whichever is later. Thus, at a minimum, you should retain records for the period of the statute of limitations. And, because the statute may not begin to run until the prospective plaintiff learns of the causal relation between the injury and the treatment received, records should be kept for a longer period than required by the statute of limitations. Also, if the patient was a minor or under some other legal disability, such as insanity, records must be kept until the patient reaches the age of majority or becomes competent, plus an additional period of the statute of limitations.

Even if a law or regulation specifies how long a record must be kept, good risk management may dictate keeping it for the period of the statute of limitations plus an additional period to cover the situation where the statute does not begin to run until the plaintiff learns of the alleged malpractice.

Most states have different statutes of limitations for different lawsuits. Because statutes of limitations are so complex, the practice attorney must be consulted to make certain which statute of limitations governs any specific situation.

Research and Education Needs

The physician's involvement with basic medical or continuing medical education and research will also affect the retention of health records. Physicians actively involved in teaching have greater use for past health records to demonstrate outcomes based on medical care. An active research program promotes a longer retention period so that physicians and others have access to medical data over long periods of time. Past treatment protocols that today are resurfacing as cancer-causing or disease-producing attest to the research potential of office records in identifying and documenting long-term sequelae of accepted treatment protocols.

Medical office records are becoming more important in medical education today. The growing emphasis on the education of physicians for primary care translates to more medical education being conducted in the physician office. Office records are actively used to teach students documentation guidelines and to study the course of a patient's illness over time.

Retention Schedules

Unless longer periods of time are required by state law or regulation, the American Health Information Management Association (AHIMA) recommends that patient health information be retained for adults for 10 years after the most recent encounter. Records of minors should be kept until the age of majority plus the period of the statute of limitations.

The American Hospital Association (AHA) recommends a similar 10-year retention period but also recommends that basic information such as dates of treatment, names of responsible physicians, diagnoses, operative reports, pathology reports, and discharge summaries be kept permanently. AHA recommends that records for minors and persons under mental disability be kept until the age of majority or until competence is established plus the established statute of limitations as prescribed by law. Another AHA recommendation is to retain complete health records for longer periods when requested in writing by the attending or consulting physician of the patient, by the patient or someone acting legally in the patient's behalf, or by legal counsel for a party having an interest affected by the patient's health records.

The federal government requires that health records for patients whose care has been financed by government programs should be maintained for a minimum of five years to protect the physician from fraud charges.

While few statutory or regulatory requirements apply to health records maintained by medical offices, the medical practice act of the state where a specific practice is located should be reviewed to determine if it imposes any requirements pertaining to record retention. In the absence of specific regulations, medical offices should follow general requirements that are written for all health care providers and institutions.

A retention schedule should specify the following for each type of document being evaluated: (1) its active life—the period during which the record is readily accessible in its original form, (2) its inactive life—the period during which the record is retained but may be transferred to storage or microfilm, and (3) its destruction—the point when further retention is not justified by usage or law.

Active, Inactive, and Closed Files

Medical practices often file patient records according to three classifications:

1. Active files—for patients currently receiving treatment
2. Inactive files—for patients not seen by the physician in the past year or longer
3. Closed files—for patients who have died, moved away, or otherwise ended their relationship with the physician

In some practices, it may be more efficient to maintain only two sets of files: active and inactive. The active files contain records of all patients who have consulted the physician within a five-year period. All other records are then considered inactive.

Records for patients who are currently hospitalized may be kept in a special section for quick reference, then placed in a regular active file when the patient is discharged from the hospital.

The use of a date stamp on the outside of the folder or a color-coded year bar on the folder helps to facilitate the transfer of records by date from the active files to the inactive files.

Record Storage

Inactive records may be placed into storage. If closed file cabinets are not available, sturdy file storage boxes with lift-off lids or drawers are good options for long-term storage. Covered boxes protect the paper records from dust and moisture and prevent decay. Each box should be clearly labeled so that needed records can be retrieved rapidly. The boxes can be kept in the office if cool, dry, humidity-controlled space is available. Otherwise, the boxes can be stored commercially. When it is necessary to store records outside the practice, a list of the contents of each box should be kept in the office. A firm specializing in record storage should be used, if possible, because this type of firm can assure confidentiality and can promptly produce requested records.

Microfilming

Microfilm saves space by reducing the original document to a very small size on film. Because microfilm is self-reproducible, microfilming also reduces paper handling, as a microfilm copy can be easily made while the original master remains in the file.

Health records are usually filmed on 16-mm film at a reduction ratio of

24:1 (the original document is reduced to an image $\frac{1}{24}$ its original size). Microfilm lasts for many years, and the cost of microfilming is approximately equal to that of storing a record in an active filing area for 10 years. However, some states require the original record to be retained, even if a microfilm copy exists.

The admission and acceptance of microfilmed records as primary evidence is legal throughout the United States, regardless of whether a state has a law to that effect or not. The application of microfilming to the health care industry for patient, departmental, and corporate storage of records has become a common practice.

Formats   Medical records can be microfilmed in a variety of formats. With *roll film,* documents are filmed sequentially in alphabetical or numerical order on a 100-foot roll of film. This is the least expensive form of microfilming. *Microfiche* is a single sheet of film with a number of images exposed on the sheet; one microfiche is produced for each patient. *Jacket* format uses roll film converted to flat film by cutting the roll and inserting each patient's record into a separate jacket. The microfiche and jacket formats are more expensive than roll film.

Advantages and disadvantages   The advantages of microfilming health records are that (1) record storage space requirements are reduced by 90–98 percent depending on the microfilming format used, (2) retrieval time spent going to secondary storage areas is eliminated, (3) protection against record loss or misfiling is provided with roll film, and (4) record content alterations are eliminated.

The disadvantages of microfilming are that (1) a special viewer is required to read the microfilm and print paper copies of the film and (2) there is an additional cost of record preparation, filming, and storage.

Health Records Disposition

Health records may be destroyed in one of two situations: pursuant to the established records retention schedule, or on a one-time basis. The latter is often necessary to eliminate very old records that the retention schedule does not cover. Because courts are suspicious of any record destruction that is not part of a records retention schedule or plan, the one-time destruction of health records must be conducted properly.

One-time destruction   When conducting a one-time destruction of a group of records, rather than destroying records pursuant to the retention schedule, the records must be reviewed to make certain all are to be destroyed. An excellent technique is to send out notices to interested parties, such as physicians within the practice, former physician partners, legal counsel, and the liability insurance carrier, announcing the planned destruction of records.

The parties should be given a date by which to respond if they object to the destruction plan. Otherwise, the notice would state the destruction will occur on a particular date.

If records are on computer media, a hard copy should be reviewed prior to the destruction. If the decision is made to destroy the information, both the hard-copy printout and the electronic media (tape, disk, etc.) are destroyed.

Any one-time destruction of records should not include any records that are to be retained according to the established retention schedule. Likewise, records of minors or others under mental disability, records that someone has requested to be retained, and records involved with litigation or government investigation or audit should not be destroyed.

Destruction methods   State or federal statutes or regulations will normally prescribe how records may be destroyed. Allowable destruction methods are usually shredding or burning. However, some states allow paper recycling and even disposal in landfills. Often, the controlling law will require that the health care provider create an abstract of any pertinent data in the record prior to its destruction.

A commercial document-destruction company may be used for the process. In the contract with the firm, it should be set forth how the records will be destroyed, how confidentiality will be protected, including indemnification from loss due to unauthorized disclosure, and how documentary proof of destruction will be given to the practice.

Proof of destruction   Regardless of whether records are destroyed on site or by a commercial firm, the practice must be certain that the records are completely destroyed and that dated certificates of destruction of the records are kept permanently. These certificates may be used in court or before a government agency to show how records were destroyed in the regular course of business. It is very important to be able to demonstrate that any record destruction is pursuant to the normal retention schedule or as a one-time carefully planned event.

Disposition of Records During Practice Mergers or Closings

Some states have statutory or regulatory guidelines regarding the handling of information when a practice closes or merges with another practice. In the absence of statutory guidance, medical societies and professional associations may provide opinions and advice. It is absolutely essential that the practice's legal counsel be involved in the management of information during mergers or closings.

Practice merger   The American Health Information Management Association (AHIMA) recommends that when two or more facilities are involved in a merger or acquisition, patient records should be consolidated and linked with a master patient index. A records retention policy should be developed and implemented to meet the needs of patients and other legitimate users and to assure compliance with legal, regulatory, and accreditation requirements.

Practice closing When a medical practice is being closed, AHIMA recommends that the provider begin planning for proper disposition of patient health records. The primary objective is to protect the confidentiality of the information contained in the records. The second objective is to assure future access by patients, future health care providers, and other legitimate users.

To assure accurate information for continuing care, all health information must be completed before the records are archived. This includes transcription of all dictated reports and interpretation of any diagnostic tests.

Before records are transferred to an archive or another provider, patients should be notified, if possible, and given the opportunity to obtain copies of their records. Patient notification is required in some states, including Maryland, New Jersey, Pennsylvania, and Utah. Letters may be sent to former patients, or announcements may be repeated in local newspapers and professional journals to notify patients and their physicians about the upcoming dissolution of the practice. Patients should be given a reasonable amount of time (at least one month) to request copies of their records.

Practice sale If a medical practice is sold to another health care provider, patient records may be considered assets and included in the sale of the property. As part of the agreement, the provider should retain the right to access the records and obtain copies, if needed, from the new owners. In addition, if the new owner considers a sale to a third party, the original provider should retain the right to reclaim the patient records.

If the medical practice is sold to a non–health care entity, the patient records should not be included in the assets available for purchase. The provider then must make arrangements to transfer the records either to an archive or to another provider who agrees to accept responsibility for maintaining them.

If a medical practice dissolves without a sale, arrangements should be made with another health care provider where patients may seek future care, unless otherwise required by state law. That provider should agree to maintain the records, permit access by authorized persons, and destroy the records when applicable time periods have expired. Prior to transferring the records, a written agreement outlining the terms and obligations should be executed. The original provider is responsible for assuring the records are stored safely for an appropriate length of time.

Transfer to archive If transfer to another provider is not feasible, records may be archived with a reputable commercial-storage form. Specific provisions should be negotiated and included in the written agreement with the firm. Such provisions include but are not limited to the following:

1. Agreement to keep all information confidential, disclosing only to authorized representatives of the provider or upon written authorization of the patient or the patient's legal representative

2. Prohibition to sell, share, discuss, assign, transfer, or otherwise disclose confidential information with any other individuals or business entities
3. Agreement to protect information against theft, loss, unauthorized destruction, or other unauthorized access
4. Return or destruction of information at the end of the mutually agreed-upon retention period
5. Assurance that provider, patients, and other legitimate users will have access to the information

During the required retention period, the original provider may need access to the records for the provider's own business reasons.

Computer Use in Health Information Management

Numerous computer software applications are available to assist with the management of health information in a physician's office. Most medical offices now use a computer to perform administrative procedures that were previously performed manually.

Medical management software programs consist of a number of systems or areas of specialization. Examples of systems included in the medical management programs are patient registration, appointment scheduling, posting transactions, patient billing, insurance billing, and reports.

Specialized Medical-Office Systems

Typical systems that manage health information for the medical office are described in the following paragraphs.

Patient registration system The patient registration system is designed to create a registration record for each patient in the practice, and it includes demographic and insurance information. The system is used to review and update information on existing registration records during subsequent patient visits. Information entered into the patient registration system is used for preparing clinical records, posting transactions, and processing patient statements and insurance claims.

Appointment system The appointment system handles all procedures related to appointment scheduling, such as making an appointment, canceling an appointment, finding an appointment slot, printing an appointment log, and printing a patient reminder card. This system replaces the handwritten appointment book for patient scheduling.

Posting transactions system When a patient has been seen by the physician, office staff must post the charges of the office visit and any payments made by the patient. This system allows the staff to enter charges for all the services and procedures performed for a patient. It permits posting of payments made by the patient or the third-party payer. In most programs, the system creates a hard copy for the patient of the superbill, patient statement, or insurance claim.

Patient billing system   The function of a patient billing system is to prepare bills and print billing statements. When patient charges and payments are posted, this information is stored in the computer and is available when needed by the patient billing system. This system is responsible for searching the medical practice database to obtain the information necessary to generate bills for patients with outstanding balances.

Insurance billing system   The function of an insurance billing system is to prepare and generate insurance claims. As procedure and diagnosis codes are entered into the computer during the posting of transactions, they are stored in the medical practice database. From the information stored in the database, the computer is able to generate a standard insurance claim form.

Reports system   The function of the reports system is to generate a variety of reports for the medical practice. The reports are designed to allow the physician to review and analyze many business and practice activities.

Business Applications to Health Information Management

Specific systems or areas of specialization included in medical management programs rely on four important applications that are built into medical software programs and which form the foundation on which the programs work. These applications are word processing, spreadsheets, communications, and database management.

Word processing   Word processing involves the use of the computer to enter, edit, file, and format text. A medical management program uses the word-processing application to produce mailing lists, letters, medical histories, and other reports. Examples of commercially available word processing programs include WordPerfect and Microsoft Word.

Spreadsheets   A spreadsheet is an electronic ledger designed to perform repetitive calculations quickly. Spreadsheets are used to produce financial reports and to analyze and process statistics. Medical management programs rely on spreadsheets to generate financial reports for the office such as the daily report and the accounts receivable report. In addition, spreadsheets are used in the medical office for practice analysis, such as printouts of the revenue generated by each physician in the practice, a list of procedures performed during a specified period of time, and total revenue generated by each procedure. By analyzing practice statistics, a physician can identify specific areas needing improvement. Commercially available spreadsheets include Lotus 1-2-3, Quattro Pro, and Excel.

Communications The communications application provides the means for one computer to "talk" to another over telephone lines. Electronic communication between computers greatly reduces the time it takes to send information. Medical management programs rely on this application for the electronic submission of insurance claims. In addition, some offices use the communications application to send letters and messages electronically.

Database management Database management allows the user to store large amounts of data that can be easily retrieved and manipulated. Medical management programs rely heavily on a database to perform the majority of the administrative procedures in the medical office. The database for a medical practice consists of patient records, patient transactions, diagnosis codes, procedure codes, insurance carriers, and other information.

The advantages of using a computer to perform database management are numerous. Once information is stored in the computer, it becomes easier for office staff members to retrieve and share the data. Data entered into a database is easier to keep track of, eliminating the need to locate various notes, folders, memos, and so on. Finally, the computer helps to eliminate the redundancy of maintaining the same information in different types of records stored in different ways, and it provides a system of safeguard to guarantee both data integrity and security.

The most significant aspect of a database is that the computer can cross-reference all of the information stored in its database. For example, information can be obtained from a patient registration record and combined with transaction and insurance carrier information for the batch processing of insurance claims. A database also provides the ability to add new information, to modify existing information, and to delete unneeded information. Numerous database programs are available on the market; commonly used products are dBASE, Paradox, and Access.

Each medical management program has specific capabilities that refer to both the systems included in the program and the tasks performed by those systems. Most medical offices use programs that are commercially available through local or regional computer software vendors. (For more details on computer use, see Chapter 5, "The Computer in the Medical Office.")

Chapter 10

Financial Management

Introduction   256
Physician Fees   257
Billing and Collection   263
Banking   273
Internal Financial Controls   277
Budgeting   279
Taxes for Medical Practices   280
Insurance for Medical Practices   281
Retirement Plans   284
Conclusion   286

Introduction

The Importance of Financial Management

While patient care is the heart and soul of a medical practice, sound financial management is also essential. In an era of rising overhead and diminishing reimbursement, practice managers must be exceptionally efficient at setting fees, collecting from patients and third-party payers, and managing other tasks related to the practice's financial well-being, such as budgeting, banking, paying taxes and insurance, and establishing retirement plans. Fees set too low or too high may result in lost revenue. Improperly timed billing causes uneven cash flow. Too passive (or too aggressive) efforts to collect also let money slip away.

Without good financial management, it is difficult for practices to remain open for the primary task of providing patient care. It also is harder for practices to compete in a changing environment where hospitals, health systems, managed care companies, and others are acquiring medical practices and integrating them into networks. The most successful practices, and those most likely to flourish within an integrated health system, are practices whose managers can adjust to new financial challenges and provide sound financial management.

The Financial Counselor

To assist in the day-to-day financial management, every practice should invest an employee with the responsibility of ensuring financial stability. Often called a financial counselor, this staff member performs tasks such as preregistration and collecting payment at the time of the patient visit. Qualifications for the job of financial counselor include financial and billing background, computer literacy, and a knowledge of local insurance plans.

A large practice may have a full-time financial counselor. Smaller practices may find it more practical to add these responsibilities to the job description of another staff member, such as the individual who does coding and charge entry. Responsibilities of the financial counselor include:

- Preregistering new patients
- Verifying insurance
- Accepting payments
- Providing receipts
- Making follow-up appointments
- Checking on patient satisfaction at the end of the visit
- Developing budget plans for patients
- Preparing financial summaries for the physicians

Another function of the financial counselor or other financial staff member would be to develop and maintain a system for keeping track of the requirements and guidelines of each managed care and insurance plan the practice accepts. One method uses a binder with sections for information on each plan, separated by dividers. Another method uses a sheet on which comparable information for each plan is listed in rows or columns; for example, one row might list the amount of co-payment for each plan, and another might list whether a second opinion is required before performing certain services (see Figure 10.1 for a sample sheet).

In all practices, the financial counselor will assist the other staff members in the efficient financial management of the medical office.

Physician Fees

Until a few years ago, most physicians derived all their practice revenue from fees charged for services. Whether the patient paid directly or the bill was covered by insurance, fees were the main source of cash. Physicians had few restrictions on what they could charge. The situation is changing, however, for patients in government programs such as Medicare and for those with private insurance.

Capitated medicine is the most significant factor altering the financial picture of physician practices. With capitation, physicians are paid a set fee each month per patient enrolled in a managed care plan. Physicians also may receive small administrative fees to cover paperwork or management responsibilities. From these monthly fees, physicians are expected to provide all necessary care for a particular patient population.

Capitation is designed to reward physicians for efficiency and appropriate

Fig. 10.1   Managed Care Tracking Sheet

Managed Care Participation

Managed Care Carriers	Type	Co-payment	Referral	Phone

Practice Does Not Have Contracts With:

Notes:

use of services, tests, and procedures. There is no incentive to perform a test or procedure that might not be medically necessary because extra services will not generate additional revenue. Under capitation, the fee for a procedure is largely irrelevant because it is not the basis for reimbursement.

Many details about how capitation should be put into effect in primary care and specialty practices must still be resolved. Until the health care system is largely or completely capitated, fee-for-service revenue will continue to be important in medical practices.

Every practice should develop a fee schedule that is in line with prevailing standards. If the fees are too low, the practice is not generating revenue to which it is entitled. If the fees are too high, the physician must write off the unpaid amount. A series of steps called a fee analysis can show a practice how its fee schedule compares to the standard used by health insurance plans or by government programs such as Medicare or Medicaid.

Fee Analysis

To conduct a fee analysis, obtain a guidebook to the relative value system. Several books are readily available, such as *Relative Values for Physicians* or *Physician Fee Analyzer*. These guides list units of value and the CPT-4 code for every medical procedure. Because of regional and local differences in medical practices, some books provide values only for a particular state, such as California or Florida. Others list median values based on nationwide data. The values are derived through extensive research and surveys of physicians.

Comparison   The values are used to perform a *gross conversion*, which is a calculation used to compare fees. Using a fee guide, the physician and practice manager should select 20 to 30 procedures most often performed in their practice, list the average reimbursement for each procedure from three major insurance carriers, and perform a series of calculations that result in a recommended fee for each medical procedure. (See Figure 10.2 for a sample worksheet.)

Fig. 10.2   Gross Conversion Factor Worksheet

Procedure Code	Your Base Fee ($)	Relative Value Units	Revenue Streams			Calculated Fee	Recommended Fee
			Carrier	Carrier	Carrier		
1							
2							
3							
4							
5							
6							
7							
8							
9							
10							
11							
12							
13							
14							
15							
16							
17							
18							
19							
20							

Fig. 10.2 *(continued)*

Procedure Code	Your Base Fee ($)	Relative Value Units	Revenue Streams Medicare Carrier	BC/BS Carrier	Healthwise Carrier	Calculated Analysis Fee	Result
72040	40.00	3.0	27.58	34.90	40.00	39.27	45.00
72050	60.00	4.8	40.14	0.00	60.00	62.83	65.00
72070	40.00	3.3	29.01	37.48	40.00	43.20	45.00
72100	40.00	3.3	29.58	41.50	0.00	43.20	45.00
72110	40.00	4.5	32.50	44.00	40.00	58.91	50.00
72114	80.00	5.4	50.77	57.00	56.00	70.69	0.00
72170	30.00	3.0	22.97	28.00	30.00	39.27	35.00
72220	40.00	3.0	24.61	0.00	30.00	39.27	0.00
73010	40.00	2.7	20.92	35.00	38.00	35.34	0.00
73020	30.00	2.2	20.92	26.10	30.00	28.80	35.00
73030	40.00	2.7	24.92	22.88	40.00	35.34	45.00
73060	35.00	2.8	24.61	26.62	35.00	36.65	40.00
73070	40.00	2.6	22.35	24.10	40.00	34.03	45.00
73100	30.00	2.5	21.80	23.50	30.00	32.73	35.00
73110	40.00	2.7	23.54	38.50	40.00	35.34	45.00
73120	30.00	2.2	21.80	31.80	30.00	28.80	35.00
73510	40.00	3.0	26.41	28.00	40.00	39.27	45.00
73550	40.00	2.8	24.61	28.02	40.00	36.65	45.00
73560	30.00	2.5	22.97	24.75	30.00	32.73	35.00
73562	45.00	2.8	25.20	45.00	45.00	36.65	50.00
73565	30.00	4.5	22.42	0.00	30.00	58.91	35.00
73600	40.00	2.3	21.80	23.50	39.20	30.11	45.00
73610	50.00	2.8	23.54	41.00	42.00	36.65	0.00
73630	40.00	2.7	23.54	40.00	40.00	35.34	45.00
73650	30.00	2.3	21.23	24.87	30.00	30.11	35.00
	1,000.00	76.4					

GCF = 13.09

Conversion factor *Relative Values for Physicians,* the guide most widely used by insurance carriers, practices, and consultants, outlines these steps for reaching the conversion factor:

1. Select the basic procedures.
2. List the relative value for each and total the values.
3. List the fee for each procedure and total the fees.
4. Divide total fees by total relative values to reach the gross conversion factor.
5. Develop a gross conversion factor for all relevant sections of a practice, such as surgery, medicine, radiology, and non-CPT-4 codes required by the Health Care Financing Administration.
6. Multiply the gross conversion factor by any relative value within the appropriate section to reach a suggested fee for the procedure.

Results Results of the fee analysis may reveal that a physician has been charging significantly less for many procedures than the accepted standard. If so, rates should be adjusted upward to the maximum allowable level. However, if a practice's fees are higher than the standard, it may be necessary to reduce them. A practice that persists in charging higher-than-average fees will have artificially high write-offs that in turn may cause budget problems. It is usually better to set fees close to the norm in the local area.

To supplement the formal fee analysis, physicians or practice managers may want to compare fees with colleagues in the same specialty. However, no attempt should be made to form an alliance or group that agrees to charge the same rates for certain procedures. Doing so would violate regulations designed to prevent price-fixing.

Often, physicians are surprised by the results of a formal fee analysis or an informal comparison among peers. Many physicians are unaware of terms such as *relative values* and have never analyzed their fee structure. As a result, their fees are likely to be significantly below current standards. It is far less common for a practice to discover that its fees are much higher than customary levels. Once fees have been brought in line, they should be reanalyzed every year.

Resource-Based Relative Value Scale

Fees for treating Medicare patients are set by a system known as the Resource-Based Relative Value Scale (RBRVS), introduced as a Medicare payment reform plan in 1992. Under this system, payment for treatment of Medicare patients is based on uniform procedural coding, with each procedure having a code and a set fee. Before RBRVS, physicians were paid 80 percent of the prevailing charge in their area for a procedure. Every physician participating in the Medicare program was assigned a different prevailing charge, based on individual billing history and averages in their geographic area.

RBRVS was introduced to bring more uniformity and fairness to the payment system. All participating physicians are reimbursed according to the same set of prevailing charges, with geographical adjustments. Physicians receive 80 percent of the allowable charge per procedure.

Medicare patients   Physicians may choose not to participate in Medicare yet still see Medicare patients. Fees for these patients must follow a list of maximum allowable charges set by Medicare. After a patient visit, a claim is filed based on the appropriate CPT-4 code and its maximum allowable charge. The check for payment is sent to the patient, who is then supposed to pay the physician.

Physicians might see nonparticipation as a way of avoiding Medicare red tape. However, the disadvantage to nonparticipation is lack of control over revenue flow. Elderly patients may be confused about the payment process or forget to make payments to their physician. If physicians choose not to participate in Medicare, they should begin appropriate collection methods to ensure that they receive payments from Medicare patients. A practice might offer to help Medicare patients with paperwork or train special counselors to work with them on payment plans.

Reimbursement under Managed Care

As noted earlier, the fee-for-service system is no longer the only method by which physicians are paid. As managed care becomes more widespread, more physicians will receive reimbursement under some form of capitation. The most common forms of compensation at this time are modified fee-for-service compensation, primary care capitation, and overall or global physician capitation.

Modified fee-for-service compensation   Under this system, physicians are paid on a unit-of-service basis, typically with one of several modifications. In the first modification, a portion of each payment is withheld and placed in a reserve fund until the end of the year. This portion, usually 10 to 25 percent, is withheld to provide protection against overutilization of health services. At the end of the year, the physician may receive all, some, or none of the withheld amount. Disbursement is likely to be based on the utilization records of both the physician and the health care system as a whole.

The second form of modification requires the physician to submit bills directly to the system and accept the system payments as full payments, except for applicable co-payments. To protect patients enrolled in managed care plans, most states require physician contracts to contain a provision stating that they will "look solely to the system for payment." As a result, physicians can bill patients only for co-payments or deductibles, regardless of the amount of payment they receive from the system.

The third modification involves risk-sharing agreements between the contracting physician and the system. Physicians may receive additional payments if hospital utilization is lower than expected. If utilization is higher, they may lose a portion of their withheld fees.

Primary care capitation   In this form of compensation, each primary care physician receives a set amount each month for each member enrolled in the managed care plan who has chosen that physician as his or her primary care doctor. A portion of the capitation payment may be withheld and placed in a reserve fund.

Specialists are compensated differently, usually under the modified fee-for-service method. However, primary care physicians may be allowed to join a risk-sharing arrangement in which they may gain or lose a portion of the funds withheld for both specialty and hospital services.

Overall or global physician compensation   Under this method of compensation, each primary care physician is credited with a monthly, capitated amount for each enrollee who has chosen him or her as a primary care physician. The physician receives a portion of the capitation at the beginning of each month. The remainder is held in a reserve fund to pay for specialty services the physician's patients may require from other physicians. At the end of the year, the physician receives any money remaining in the reserve fund. If there is a deficit, it is either carried forward or paid by the physician. (For details about managed care models, see Chapter 4, "Managed Care.")

Billing and Collection

The most critical business function for a medical practice is billing and collection. Revenue from patients and third-party payers covers physician and employee salaries, rent, supplies, fees for maintaining and leasing equipment, and other practice expenses. Establishing an effective system for managing accounts receivable is a top priority.

Cycle of Reimbursement

The management of accounts receivable requires a series of interrelated steps, called a *cycle of reimbursement.* The cycle starts with patient registration and culminates in collection, with many steps often dependent on having obtained accurate information at registration. (See Figure 10.3 for an illustration of the reimbursement cycle.)

Patient registration   Proper billing and collection procedures begin before the patient arrives at the office. When a new patient calls for an appointment, the receptionist should explain the practice's payment policy and ask the patient if he or she has the time to provide registration information over the

Fig. 10.3   Cycle of Reimbursement

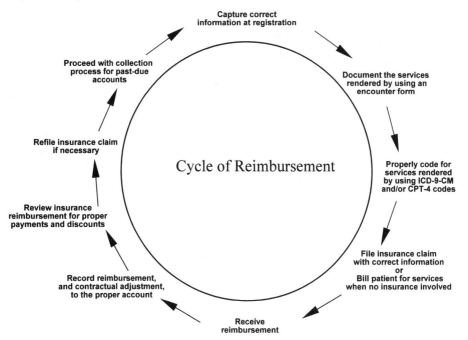

Capture correct
information at registration

Proceed with collection
process for past-due
accounts

Document the services
rendered by using an
encounter form

Refile insurance claim
if necessary

Cycle of Reimbursement

Properly code for
services rendered
by using ICD-9-CM
and/or CPT-4 codes

Review insurance
reimbursement for proper
payments and discounts

File insurance claim
with correct information
or
Bill patient for services
when no insurance involved

Record reimbursement,
and contractual adjustment,
to the proper account

Receive
reimbursement

telephone. If the patient is willing, the receptionist or financial counselor should obtain enough information to complete the registration form. The financial counselor should then contact the insurer to verify coverage and check on the guidelines in that plan, such as the need for second opinions and list of services covered.

Upon arrival, new patients who were not preregistered should complete a patient information form (see Chapter 9, Figure 9.1, for a sample form). Ask current patients if any information has changed, such as a new address, new employer, or new insurance carrier. Registration is also the time to ask for a patient's Medicare or insurance card. Make a photocopy of a new or updated card to place in the patient's file.

Documentation of services   The second step in the cycle of reimbursement is determining which services are provided to the patient during the visit. A patient encounter form identifies the services provided in the practice setting and the charge.

Encounter form   An encounter form should be designed around the needs of each individual practice. Standard information should include evaluation and management codes, also known as E&M codes. Other than that, the services listed and other information depend on the nature of the practice and its most frequently performed procedures. Leave space to write information about services not covered under the standard categories. (See Figure 10.4 for a sample form.)

The encounter forms should be numbered and used in sequence. This helps with record keeping since a missing number suggests a discrepancy that should be checked. A missing encounter form may simply have been misplaced, or it may be a warning sign of employee theft. Encounter forms should be "balanced back" to the computer or manual bookkeeping system.

Because they contain the information on which the practice's revenue will be based, encounter forms pass through many hands within the practice. After the doctor completes the form, an employee skilled in coding should verify the accuracy of the diagnosis and procedure codes and ensure that they follow insurance guidelines. Next, the encounter forms should be routed to the data entry department to make sure demographic information is accurate and for entry of charges.

Out-of-office journal   An out-of-office journal is used to record charges for services provided out of the office, at sites such as nursing homes, jails, outpatient settings, or emergency rooms. The out-of-office journal should be compact so that it can be carried in a physician's pocket. If a new journal is used every day, a simple card or single-fold brochure may be adequate to contain one day's records. Completed out-of-office journals are given to the staff member responsible for charge entry. After the information is transferred, journals are filed with other financial records for that day.

For surgeons or hospital-based physicians, a transcribed medical records

Fig. 10.4 Encounter Form

W 0200001

☐ New
☐ Established

Family Medical Center
2500 West Haven Avenue
Middle Island, NY 10035
(516) 555-1212 • (516) 555-1234 FAX

☐ Melanie Jones, M.D.
☐ Brett Asher, M.D.
☐ John Mason, R.N.
☐ _____

✓ OFFICE VISIT NEW	CODE	FEE	✓ INJECTIONS (CONT D.)	CODE	FEE	✓ X-RAYS (CONT D.)	CODE	FEE	✓ SURG. PROC. CONT	CODE	FEE
FOCUSED	99201		EPINEPHRINE	J0170		TOES	73660		2.6CM-7.5CM	12002*	
EXPANDED	99202		CELESTONE, UP TO 3MG	J0702		CLAVICLE	73000		7.6CM-12.5CM	12004*	
DETAILED	99203		AMPICLN., UP TO 500 MG	J0290		HIPS UNILATERAL-2 VIEWS	73510		✓ PROCEDURES	CODE	FEE
COMP. & MODERATE	99204		PENICLN. PROC. 600,000U	J0530		FACIAL NOSE	70150		ANOSCOPY	46600	
COMP. & HIGH	99205		PENICLN. BENZ. 600,000U	J0580		NASAL BONES	70160		EKG	93000	
W/SURG. PROCEDURE	99205*		KETZAL (ANCEF)	J0690		PELVIS	72170		ENDOMETRIAL BX	58100	
✓ OFFICE VISIT ESTAB	CODE	FEE	ROCEPHIN 250 MG.	J0696		SPINE, CERVICAL	72050		NEBULIZER TX.	94664	
MINIMAL	99211		ZINACEF, 750 MG.	J0697		SPINE, LUMBAR, AP & LAT.	72100		PODOPHYLIN FEMALE	57061	
FOCUSED	99212		COMPAZINE 10 MG.	J0780		SPINE-THOR., AP & LAT.	72070		PODOPHYLIN MALE	54050*	
EXPANDED	99213		ACTH 40U	J0800		SPINE-THOR., COMPL.	72074		SPIROMETRY	94010	
DETAILED & MODERATE	99214		ESTROGEN 5 MG.	J1000		✓ SURGICAL PROC	CODE	FEE	SPIROMETRY PRE/POST	94060	
COMP. & HIGH	99215		DEPOMEDROL, 20 MG.	J1020		CAUT. 1ST LES. NON FAC.	17100		TRIGGER POINT INJ.	20550	
✓ PREVENTATIVE MED.	CODE	FEE	DEPO TESTADIOL	J1060		BURN 1ST DEG. INIT. TX	16000		3 SPLINT APPLICATION		
NEW PATIENT			TESTOSTERONE 100 MG.	J1070		BURN DSG. & DEBRID.	16020*				
LESS THAN 1 YR.	99381		DECADRON 4 MG.	J1100		CAUTERY WARTS	17110*		CAST APPLICATION		
1-4 YRS.	99382		TORADOL 15 MG.	J1885		CERUMEN REMOVAL	69210				
5-11 YRS.	99383		LASIX	J1940		COMPLEX REMOVAL	10121		SUPPLIES	99070	
12-17 YRS.	99384		LINCOCIN	J2010		CONJ. FB REMOV.	65205*		✓ LABORATORY	CODE	FEE
18-39 YRS.	99385		DEMEROL	J2175		CONJ. FB REMOV. EMBED.	65210*		VENIPUNCTURE	G0001	
40-64 YRS.	99386		TERRAMYCIN, UP TO 50 MG	J2460		CORNEAL FB REMOVAL	65220*		HANDLING/COLLECT.	99000	
65 YRS. AND UP	99387		PHENERGAN	J2550		CORNEAL FB/SLIT LAMP	65222*		AMYLASE	82150	
ESTABLISHED			SOLUMEDROL 125 MG.	J2930		EXCISION SKIN TAGS	11200*		ANEMIA PROFILE		
LESS THAN 1 YR.	99391		VISTARIL 25 MG.	J3410		EYELID FB REMOVAL	67938		ARTHRITIS PROFILE	80072	
1-4 YRS.	99392		VITAMIN B-12	J3420		FB REMOVAL SKIN	10120*		CBC WITH DIFF.	85025	
5-11 YRS.	99393		IMITREX 6 MG.	J3490		I & D ABSCESS	10060*		CK ISOENZYMES	82550	
12-17 YRS.	99394		STADOL	J3490		I & D PILONIDAL CYST	10080*		C&S. ROUTINE	87070	
18-39 YRS.	99395		NUBAIN	J3490		NAIL EXCISION	11750		C&S. URINE	87086	
40-64 YRS.	99396		✓ X RAYS	CODE	FEE	EXCISION FACIAL LESION			CULT., CHLAMYDIA & GC		
65 YRS. AND UP	99397		WATER'S VIEW	70210		<1CM	11441		DRUG SCREEN-MULTIPLE	80100	
✓ IMMUNIZATIONS	CODE	FEE	SKULL-4 VIEW	70260		<2CM	11442		HEMOGLOBIN	83030	
DPT	90701		COCCYX/SACRUM	72220		<3CM	11443		HEPATITIS A, B, C	80059	
DT	90702		SPINE 1 VIEW	72020		<4CM	11444		HIV	86689	
TD	90718		1 VIEW OF ABDOMEN	74000		EXCIS. NCK-SCLP-HND-FT.			IRON PACKAGE		
ORAL POLIO	90712		FLAT/UPRIGHT	74020		<1CM	11421		KOH PREP	87210	
MMR	90707		PELVIS	72170		<2CM	11422		LIPASE	83690	
MEASLES	90705		CHEST 2 VIEW	71020		<3CM	11423		PAP & PSA		
HIB VACCINE	90737		RIBS UNILATERAL	71101		<4CM	11424		RPR	86592	
HEPATITIS B	90731		SHOULDER	73030		>4CM	11426		SED RATE	85651	
INFLUENZA	90724		HUMERUS	73060		EXCIS. TRUNK-ARM-LEG			SERUM HCG	84703	
PNEUMOCOCCOL	90732		ELBOW 3 VIEW	73080		<1CM	11401		SMA 25	80019	
IMMUNE GLOBULIN	90741		FOREARM	73090		<2CM	11402		STREP SCREEN	86588	
TB TINE	86585		WRIST	73110		<3CM	11403		TSH	84443	
PPD	86580		HAND	73130		<4CM	11404		THYROID PROFILE, COMP.	80092	
RUBELLA	90706		FINGERS	73140		>4CM	11406		URINALYSIS	81000	
✓ INJECTIONS	CODE	FEE	FEMUR	73550		LACERATION REPAIR FACIAL			URINE, HCG	81025	
ALLERGY INJ.	95115		KNEE	73560		2.5CM OR <	12011*		VIP 7	80007	
INFUSION 1 HR.	90780		TIBIA/FIBULA	73590		2.6CM-5CM	12013*		WET PREP.	88160	
ADDED HRS.	90781		ANKLE	73610		5.1CM-7.5CM	12014				
IV INJECTION	90784		FOOT	73630		TRUNK & EXTREMITIES					
TETANUS TOXOID	90703		OS CALCIS	73650		.5CM OR <	12001*				

DR.'S. SIGNATURE

RETURN

_____DAYS _____WKS. _____MOS.

NEXT APPOINTMENT:

_____ DAY _____ MO. _____ TIME

DIAGNOSIS:

PREVIOUS BALANCE	$
TODAY'S CHARGES	$
PAYMENT	$
BALANCE	$

___ CASH   ___ CHECK #   ___ CHARGE

report provides the information necessary to document delivery of patient services.

Coding   The third step in the reimbursement cycle is coding. Both a diagnosis code (ICD-9-CM code) and a procedure code (CPT-4 code) must be assigned for each service.

Third-party carriers use these codes to decide how much to reimburse the physician for each service provided. It is essential to use the most current codes and to select the codes that best describe the services provided. (For details on codes, see Chapter 9, "Health Information Management.")

When assigning a code, the physician should choose the one most accurately describing the level of service provided. Using codes that are too low will result in lower reimbursement; inappropriately high codes may trigger an audit or review of the practice's financial records.

Insurance claims   The next step in the cycle of reimbursement is to prepare an insurance form for billing the third-party carrier (such as an insurance company, managed care organization, or Medicare) or to prepare a billing statement if the patient does not have insurance. If a patient is insured, it is customary to bill the insurance company first, then bill the patient for the remainder of the balance. Patients enrolled in a managed care plan typically pay a fixed co-payment at the time of the visit, while the practice bills the insurance company for the remainder. The practice absorbs the cost of services that are not reimbursed.

Reimbursement   The next phase of the cycle focuses on the reimbursement itself. When payment is received from the patient or the insurance company, the money is deposited in the bank. The payment is posted to the patient's account, and a contractual adjustment is made, if the physician participates in an HMO, Medicare, or Medicaid.

When posting payment from an insurance company, check to see if it is within the expected range of reimbursement. If it is lower, ask the insurance company to review the claim and consider an adjustment. Every carrier has a procedure to follow for reviewing claims with problems. Follow the guidelines from the pertinent carrier when a claim has been rejected or paid at a lower than expected rate. It is not advisable to send a duplicate claim. A coding specialist within the practice should also check to see if the claim was coded correctly.

Collection   The final step in the cycle of reimbursement is collection. Every practice should have a policy on internal collection efforts. Specify how many statements are to be mailed and at what interval, how many telephone calls will be made, and when—or if—accounts will be given to a collection agency.

Managing Collection

Depending on the size of the practice, one or more employees should be trained to work in collections. This may be a role for the financial counselor, if that position is staffed. Physicians should rarely become involved in billing matters. Instead, a trained staff member should meet with patients to work out payment arrangements.

The best policy is to collect from patients before they leave. The financial counselor or other designated employee should be responsible for the end of the patient visit. The employee should ask the patient if everything is satisfactory, make another appointment if needed, and ask how the patient wants to pay the bill or make a co-payment. If the patient needs to discuss payment concerns, set up a private consultation away from other patients and employees.

Be reasonable with collection efforts. Increasing aggressiveness yields higher returns, but rudeness and harassment are unacceptable. Most patients want to pay their bills. To do so, they will need to know what is expected of them and be offered a reasonable plan for meeting their obligation.

While the goal should be to collect the full payment, the practice must consider each patient's ability to pay, the size of the debt, and the cost of pursuing collection of overdue amounts. Review each overdue account and obtain approval from a physician or the practice manager before assigning it to the collection agency. There may be times when a practice chooses not to pursue payment of an overdue account, perhaps because a patient is terminally ill or there are other personal circumstances justifying an adjustment.

Schedule   The collections procedure should follow a schedule. Third-party payers often take a considerable amount of time to pay claims. For private payers, a practice may want to wait as long as 150 days before turning accounts over to a collection agency; 90 to 120 days is a more typical waiting period. During that time, the practice should send at least three statements or letters and make at least three telephone calls requesting payment. (See Figure 10.5 for samples of letters requesting payment.)

Goals   Each practice should have goals or targets for its accounts receivable and collection. A good benchmark for accounts receivable is to receive payment on most accounts within 90 to 120 days. A bad-debt ceiling of about 5 percent is reasonable. However, a practice may have a higher average percentage of bad debt because of its patient mix or other characteristics. Generally, a net collection rate of 95 percent or more is the sign of a well-run practice.

If an outside collection agency is used, it should submit a monthly report showing how much money was received on each account. The report should also state the amount the physician owes for collection services. Collection firms usually charge a percentage of the amount they bring in, generally 20 to 50 percent.

The practice manager should monitor results of collection efforts from the staff and from outside collection firms, if used. Collection ratios should be reviewed quarterly and adjustments made if the rate of return seems too low. A change to a different outside collection firm may improve cash flow.

Fig. 10.5   Series of Collection Letters

Family Medical Center
2500 West Haven Avenue
Middle Island, NY 10035

October 3, 19--

John B. Patient
112 Oak Avenue
Pleasant Ridge, NY 10038

Dear Mr. Patient:

We did not receive your payment last month, and assume that you may have overlooked the unpaid balance on your account.

Unfortunately, the account is now past due; however, immediate payment will bring it back to current status.

Please contact me by telephone about your intentions; perhaps we can place you on a budget plan if finances are a concern.

Sincerely,

Joan Smith
Business Manager

Collection telephone calls   Letters, memos, and other requests for payment are not always effective. Collection telephone calls are another way of reaching patients to remind them of overdue accounts. However, collection calls must follow a certain protocol. Every state has laws regulating debt collection. Typically, these laws outline matters such as the hours during which collection calls can be made and the places to which calls may be made. Some states prohibit collection calls to workplaces. The practice manager and employee responsible for collection efforts should be familiar with local debt collection guidelines.

Before beginning a series of collection calls, gather patient charts and account information. Have a pen or pencil and paper for taking notes during the conversation. Because these calls deal with confidential, sensitive informa-

Fig. 10.5 *(continued)*

Family Medical Center
2500 West Haven Avenue
Middle Island, NY 10035

November 3, 19--

John B. Patient
112 Oak Avenue
Pleasant Ridge, NY 10038

Dear Mr. Patient:

There has been no response to our previous correspondence; therefore, I must assume that an unusual situation is preventing you from making payment on your account.

I would like to remind you that our office will extend credit terms to patients with a financial need. We also accept payment by Visa, MasterCard, and American Express.

In order to protect your credit, you must contact us to make credit arrangements or mail payment immediately to delay further action against your account.

Sincerely,

Joan Smith
Business Manager

---

tion, make them from a location in the office where they cannot be overheard by other patients.

Call the patient's home first. Give information only to the patient. Do not provide details to family members, coworkers, or anyone else who may answer the telephone. Since many patients will be away from home during the day, try again in the evening or call at work if this is allowed. If a coworker answers the telephone, keep the reason for the call confidential. Saying that the call is from "Dr. Smith's office" is sufficient. Patients may prefer not to discuss the bill at work. Respect the patient's wishes and arrange another time and place to call.

Always be specific about the reason for the call, and ask for payment. Listen carefully to what the patient says and look for solutions that will enable

Fig. 10.5 *(continued)*

Family Medical Center
2500 West Haven Avenue
Middle Island, NY 10035

December 3, 19--

John B. Patient
112 Oak Avenue
Pleasant Ridge, NY 10038

Dear Mr. Patient:

We regret that you have not responded to our previous requests for payment. We provided service to you in good faith and expected that your account would be paid in a timely manner. However, since you have not fulfilled your obligation, we must now submit your account to a collection agency.

We will hold your account for 30 days before taking action. Should you wish to clear your balance, please call immediately.

Sincerely,

Joan Smith
Business Manager

---

the patient to pay. The result of the call should be a mutually agreeable plan that covers the amount of payment, the time and method by which payment will be made, and who will make the payment (the patient, an insurer, another party). Patients may become angry or defensive during a collection call. Try to remain calm and cheerful, and always treat patients fairly but firmly. (For details on using the telephone and a sample script asking for payment, see Chapter 8, "Human Relations in the Medical Office.")

More than one call may be needed to resolve the issue. Set up a tickler or reminder system to keep track of calls and payments. Follow the practice policy for ending collection efforts. If an account has been given to a collection firm after several months of internal efforts, give the agency about three months to secure payment. If payment is not received by this time, about six months since the charges were incurred, it is unlikely that the bill will ever be paid. Close the account and write off the charge as bad debt.

Managing Accounts Receivable

Accounts receivable are a practice's primary source of cash. Despite this fact, too few practices manage accounts receivable effectively. This may be due to a lack of management training. However, practices must meet the challenge of improving results of accounts receivable if they want to remain viable.

A good starting point for managing accounts receivable is a plan that includes specific goals and targets for collections. The plan should address these questions:

- How effective (in measurable terms) is your practice today?
- How effective do you want to be?
- When do you want to reach your goals?
- How do you plan to monitor results

It is essential to monitor results and make changes accordingly, and to establish internal controls and a clearly defined reporting structure. When these steps have been accomplished, the manager can monitor activity daily, twice a month, or monthly. After the plan has been in effect long enough for collections to run smoothly, the frequency of formal review and monitoring can be reduced, perhaps to quarterly. Compare the actual effectiveness of collection efforts to the goal. Review results of each financial class or source of revenue (for example, self-pay, Medicare, Medicaid, commercial insurance, HMO, workers' compensation) as well as the total.

The practice manager should set realistic targets for accounts receivable activity. These targets will vary from practice to practice, but here are some suggested goals:

- Gross days in accounts receivable: 60 to 65
- Bad-debt percentage: 5 percent
- Net collection percentage: 95 percent

Billing cycle   The key to steady cash flow is billing regularly. Bill daily, not weekly or monthly. Billing daily ensures a constant flow of cash to the practice from patients and third-party payers. To manage this flow of bills, establish a plan for a monthly billing cycle. There are several options for the cycle.

The bills can be sorted by financial class. For example, private-pay bills could be sent the first week of the month, Medicare bills (the portion for which the patient is responsible) could be sent the second week, and other bills would be sent the third week. The largest of these categories could be subdivided and spread over two weeks to maintain the monthly cycle.

Another approach is to sort bills alphabetically. Divide the alphabet into four segments and mail one segment per week. Similarly, bills can be sorted and mailed by zip code.

Insurance claims also should be filed promptly, preferably daily. As with patient bills, a steady flow of claims sent to insurance companies produces a steady flow of payments in return.

Several office functions must be performed smoothly to ensure effective management of accounts receivable. These include data entry, receipt processing, and patient services.

Data entry The goal of effective data entry is to see that patient charges and demographic information are entered into the computer system regularly. Another goal is to see that the optimal charge codes and diagnosis codes are used for each patient visit so that the maximum allowable reimbursement is received. Finally, an effective data entry system is one in which the level of backlog is reasonable for the practice setting.

Receipt processing Deposit checks and cash daily. Only payments that arrive in late afternoon should be held at the practice until the next day. A backlog is permissible for posting receipts and adjustments, but it should be no more than 24 hours. Correct posting of receipts is also important in preparing management reports based on accurate information.

When receipt processing is handled properly, totals from different sources will add up correctly. The deposit ticket total will match the batch total generated by the computer system, and the manual batch totals for the adjustments will agree with system batch totals. A *batch* is a term covering all of the charges for patient visits in a single day.

Other components of receipt processing include billing secondary insurance if the primary carrier has processed its total portion, reclassifying accounts into the appropriate financial class when necessary, and recognizing and posting appropriate contractual allowances.

Patient services Several steps are important to efficient management of patient services in accounts receivable management.

- File insurance claims regularly, preferably daily.
- Use electronic filing as much as possible. When necessary, edit claim forms manually or electronically to make sure that all the required information is provided.
- Post approved adjustments for professional courtesy and similar items promptly.
- Conduct collection activity according to a schedule and avoid backlog.

Every practice can improve its accounts receivable by developing, monitoring, and adjusting a plan. However, the improvements may have a cost. To achieve the best results, the practice may need to invest in new computer software or hardware, outside services (such as billing and collection firms or consultants), additional employees, or training courses. Balance the required investment against an estimate of how much additional revenue and productivity could be gained through the improvements.

Outside Services

Billing and collection are becoming increasingly complex because of changing requirements for reimbursement in government and private insurance programs. A practice may have dozens of managed care contracts and arrangements with other payers, all of whom have different requirements for filing claims.

Handling this function well can be difficult and time-consuming. It may be more sensible, even in small practices, to use outside services for as many business functions as possible. Besides billing and collection, practices may want to send out functions such as payroll, administration of retirement plans, and transcription. Outsourcing may save money and allow more efficient use of employee time.

Billing and collection are a popular practice function to outsource for several reasons. First, practices usually need sophisticated computer hardware and software to manage this function. Hardware and software rapidly become obsolete. Practices may find that it is not feasible to replace their computer systems every few years. Also, at least one employee will be required who is skilled in medical billing and familiar with the computer equipment. If this person is ill or on vacation, or leaves, it may be difficult to find someone who can assume the responsibility, and revenue may quickly drop.

Outsourcing may be more practical than retaining the function in-house if vendors offer competitive rates, regularly upgrade their equipment, and continually train their staff.

The main reason physicians choose to keep billing and other business functions in-house is the feeling of control. They see the staff on a daily basis and can check on their work at any time. If a practice has the resources to hire and train the staff and maintain the necessary equipment, maintaining business functions in-house may be an appropriate choice.

If billing and collection are kept within the practice, use an off-the-shelf computer software package designed for this purpose. Unless the practice is large enough to have its own staff of programmers or to contract with programmers, it is unwise to develop a custom financial management program. Some useful software packages are G.P.M.S., Medic Software, Promed, and Medical Manager.

Banking

Although their main focus is on patient relationships, physicians also should become well acquainted with banking and bankers. Banking transactions such as deposits take place daily, and practices also may look to banks for services such as loans for practice expansion or major equipment purchases.

Location and Services

Because banking transactions occur frequently, the first rule for selecting a bank is to look for one close to the office. A bank with many branches is ideal for a large practice with multiple sites.

Besides a convenient location, a good choice for a bank is a facility whose staff is knowledgeable and friendly. It is also important to choose a facility offering the services the practice will need, besides such basics as checking accounts. For example, the bank should offer safe-deposit boxes and lockbox service and have a notary public on its staff.

Lockbox service   The term *lockbox service* has come to have two meanings. In one sense, it is similar to a safe-deposit box, a place where valuable practice records can be placed for safekeeping. Although most practices would think of the lockbox as a storage site for seldom-used documents such as a lease or contracts, the lockbox also can be a storage site for computer backup copies of items such as accounts receivable. New paper copies or computer disks should be placed in the box monthly, as a backup in case of fire or natural disaster.

The other meaning of lockbox service is a system of making bank deposits. The practice rents a post office box to which all payments are mailed. Through an arrangement with the bank, a bank employee picks up the payments, records and deposits them, and sends a list of those payments to the practice daily.

Relationships with Bankers

After a bank has been chosen, the physician (or a designated physician from a group) should develop relationships with bank officials. This personal acquaintance can be very helpful if the practice later needs to establish a line of credit or resolve other problems, such as checks returned because of insufficient funds.

Getting acquainted is simple. The physician should call the bank and set up an appointment with an appropriate officer. In a small bank, the president or chief executive officer may be highly accessible. In larger facilities, the physician may meet with a vice president or other officer who oversees business accounts.

During the visit, ask for information about the bank's services and products, particularly those that might be relevant to the medical practice's current and future needs. Also tell the banker about the practice and its plans for growth. Invite the banker to visit the practice, preferably at an arranged time so that the physician can spend a few minutes with the banker.

Getting acquainted with the bank and the banker is highly recommended for new physicians, but established physicians can take these steps as well. In either case, it is better to have established a relationship before asking for a loan.

Checking Accounts

Banks offer a variety of checking accounts for business and personal needs. Differences among a bank's business accounts may include the minimum level of funds required to be in the account at any time, the amount of monthly service charges, the number of checks and other transactions that can take place in a month without incurring additional charges, and the type of checks available. The physician or practice manager should study the options and choose the account that seems best suited to the needs of the practice.

Each individual authorized to write checks needs to complete a signature card for the bank's records. In banking terminology, the depositor is called the *drawer*, and the company or individual to whom the check is made out is the *payee*.

Deposit slips   A deposit slip must accompany funds being deposited. The slip lists the amount and types of funds (currency, coins, checks) being deposited. When the money is deposited, the bank teller will issue a deposit receipt verifying the total amount deposited. Save deposit slips and file them in the daily activity folder.

Checkbooks   The most common style of checkbook for a medical practice is one with three checks to a page. Prenumbered stubs are attached by perforation to the prenumbered checks. The date, amount, payee, and reason for the disbursement should be written on the stub when the check itself is written. The stubs provide a permanent record of payments.

Many new computer software packages integrate check writing with a bookkeeping function.

Writing checks   Checks may be typed, printed, or written in ink. The signature should be written or printed in facsimile. If a mistake is made, write *VOID* on the check and the stub, and prepare another check.

Overdrafts   Occasionally, a check inadvertently will be written for a sum higher than the amount on deposit. As a customer service, the bank may honor the check and ask the account owner to deposit sufficient funds. The bank also has the option to refuse to honor overdrawn checks; a service fee may be charged. A dishonored check may be returned to the depositor with a notice indicating the reason for its return. The term *NSF* (not sufficient funds) is usually stamped on the notice. A good relationship with the bank may allow the practice to avoid the embarrassment and cost of returned checks.

Stop payment   If a check is lost or stolen or contains an error, the practice should immediately request the bank to stop payment. Make the request by telephone, then follow it up in writing. A stop payment order means that the check cannot be cashed. However, an order cannot be issued if a check has been cleared.

Check endorsements   Before a check can be deposited or cashed, the payee must endorse it on the reverse side. Some checks are printed with lines indicating where the endorsement should be written. There are several types of endorsements. A blank endorsement is the signature only of the person to whom the check is made out. Private individuals often sign checks this way, but it is not recommended for medical practices. If a check has a blank endorsement, the bearer can cash it or negotiate it further.

A full endorsement contains the name of the company or person to whom the check is being given, followed by the payee's signature. Only the new payee can negotiate the check further. A restrictive endorsement indicates the condition of endorsement and limits the check's negotiability. The phrase *for deposit only* is often used as a restrictive endorsement, meaning that the check must be deposited in the payee's bank account and cannot be negotiated again.

Bank Statements and Bank Reconciliations

Depositors receive monthly statements from their banks that show the previous month's beginning balance, deposits made, and checks paid during that month, other charges or additions, and the ending balance. The statement and the practice's financial records may show different ending balances. This is because certain transactions will not have been entered into the records of both parties by the end of the month. For example, checks the practice has written and subtracted from its balance may not have been cashed and therefore have not been deducted from the bank's current account balance. The practice accountant, bookkeeper, or other employee responsible for the financial records should reconcile each monthly bank statement and show the reasons for the disparity between ending balances.

Canceled checks   These are checks that have been paid by the bank and are returned to the practice in the envelope containing the bank statement. However, a bank may offer a checking account option in which canceled checks are not returned. Be aware of this option when selecting an account.

Outstanding checks   A check is considered outstanding if it has not cleared the bank by the end of the previous month.

Deposits-in-transit   A deposit is termed in transit or late if it is entered in the practice records but does not reach the bank by the last day of the previous month, in time to be listed on the bank statement.

Service charges   Banks may charge depositors for services such as the collection of notes and stop payments. Most banks also charge a fee each month for the basic checking service; some accounts have a fixed charge each month, while others charge per check written or other transactions. The bank can provide a list of the type and amount of its service charges.

Bank memos   Deductions and additions indicated on bank statements are sometimes explained in debit and credit memos sent along with the statement to the bank customer.

Internal Financial Controls

Well-run medical practices have effective internal control systems for charges, claims, and reimbursement. The foundation for effective internal controls is having accurate job descriptions and lists of responsibility. When it is clear who is to be doing what, there is less chance of things slipping through the cracks. However, medical practice employees should be "cross-trained" to fill in for other staff members as needed. Cross-training and occasional rotation of responsibilities also are precautions against one employee developing too much control over financial matters and being in a position to steal from the practice.

Division of Responsibility

Divide responsibility for financial management among several staff members. No single employee should have complete authority. This is a security measure against employee embezzlement. One person could easily devise a way to siphon funds, but it is less likely that a staff member could enlist a coworker in the scheme.

Internal Monitoring

Most physicians and practice managers assume their employees are honest, and usually they are right. However, medicine is not immune from its share of dishonest workers, and embezzlement is more common than most people think. Medical practices can be easy targets for unscrupulous employees because physicians rarely want to be involved in the financial workings of the practice. With little oversight from the top, an employee may seize the opportunity to steal. With tighter security, the same employee would probably not try anything.

However, a few people take jobs in medical practices with the intent to steal. Often, they are accomplished at embezzlement and can easily conceal their actions from physicians and other employees. Periodic outside audits are a good idea and often can detect sophisticated employee theft schemes.

While physicians do not need to take on the role of accountants to prevent employee theft, they should show interest in their practice's financial standing. Simple spot-checks that physicians or managers can perform include comparing the day sheets with the appointment book to make sure every patient who was seen has an entry on the day sheet. Also verify that payments received equal the amount deposited.

Physicians may want to review a daily summary of charges, payments, and adjustments. If they review the report daily, while their memory is fresh, they can remember seeing particular patients and are more likely to notice if there is no record of payment. They can also readily remember authorizing any professional courtesy discounts, charity write-offs, or patient refunds. If they question any item, they should be able to easily obtain the source documents for verification. Physicians should also review monthly and quarterly financial reports, looking for unusual short-term or long-term variations.

Another internal control measure that can help prevent losses is to compare reports from the practice's collection agency with office records. This review could turn up evidence that an employee has been writing off accounts as bad debt and keeping money secured by the collection agency.

Check-Writing Procedures

Accounts payable also should be managed wisely. Certain employees should be authorized to write checks for practice expenses, but only a physician should sign them. In a group practice, one physician should have primary responsibility for signing checks, but a few others should also have signing privileges so that payments are not delayed in the absence of the primary contact. Only checks with attached invoices should be signed.

Before signing checks to unfamiliar vendors, the physician or practice manager should check on the company. An unscrupulous employee may have prepared a phony invoice and slipped it in with legitimate bills. It is easy to have fake invoices made at any print shop; a quick telephone call to the number on an invoice will usually reveal whether a business is legitimate.

Physicians should also verify any patient refund checks before signing them. Make sure there actually is a patient, or that the request is genuine.

Accounts Receivable Verification

As part of its internal control program, the staff should verify the accuracy of accounts receivable each month. Compare the total amount of the individual accounts with the accounts receivable balance recorded on the day sheets and the general ledger at the end of the month. Any errors should be traced to their source. It is also advisable to retain an accounting firm to review the practice's records, including accounts receivable, at least once a year.

Internal Control of Claims

A practice also needs a system to ensure that claims are properly managed. After claims are generated, they should be reviewed and balanced with the daily charge report or edit report. An *edit report* is a report generated by a computer when errors are found in a claim. An error message usually occurs because the claim has not been filled out according to the payer's specifications. Clean claims (those with no errors) should be sent to their respective third-party payers daily, and those with errors should be corrected and submitted as soon as possible. Prepare a daily activity folder with encounter forms, deposit slips, balance reports, computer printouts, and any other items pertinent to the day's work.

Internal Control of Reimbursement

Cash and checks flowing into a practice can tempt even the most honest employees. As a safeguard against theft, practices should either use a lockbox at a bank for deposit of checks or divide responsibility for opening mail and making deposits between different employees.

If payments arrive directly at the practice, the recommended procedure to follow is to total all monies received and retain the adding machine or computer printout. A second employee processes the money, totals it, and compares the tape with the first one. Explanation of benefit forms should be processed for correct payment, and adjustments should be accounted for. Any claims that were denied or not paid as expected should be reviewed so that follow-up steps can be taken.

After checks have been deposited, compare the total of the deposit with the tape or printout of checks received. When checks have been returned from the bank, they should be photocopied, attached to a copy of the deposit slip, and filed in the daily activity folder.

Budgeting

Budget preparation is an important function in a physician practice. Both revenue and expenses must be estimated as accurately as possible to develop a realistic budget. For solo and small partnership practices, use of cash accounting principles can be a sound approach to budget planning. Large group practices that use accrual-based accounting still must prepare a cash-flow budget.

In budgeting, revenue projections are made first. The revenue projection is based on how the physician (or each individual physician in a group practice) expects to practice. Factors to estimate include the following:

- Number of days a week the physician will work
- Number of weeks worked per year
- Number of patients per day the physician expects to see
- Anticipated hospital admissions
- Anticipated procedure volume
- Estimated cash collections

After revenue projections are completed, a detailed profile of practice expenses must be developed. Expenses can be divided into two broad categories: operating expenses and physician-related expenses. Major items classified as operating expenses include:

- Staff salaries and benefits
- Clinical expenses
- Office rent, furniture, and equipment
- Office supplies and services
- Legal and accounting services

The physician-related expenses include fees to physician consultants, malpractice premiums, and benefits such as dues, memberships, travel, and automobile allowance.

Physician salaries are a critical factor in budget planning. A physician's salary is defined as the anticipated W-2 income before taxes. Physician compensation should be budgeted and paid in some manner that reasonably reflects actual revenue generation or cash collections.

When physician salaries and the estimated total annual expenses are subtracted from anticipated revenue, the resulting balance is the net profit or loss. If budget projections indicate a net loss for the year or other planning period, steps should be taken to reduce expenses, generate additional revenue, or both.

Taxes for Medical Practices

The legal structure of a practice defines the way in which certain financial matters are managed. Practices may be set up as a sole proprietorship, a partnership, or a corporation. State regulations set the requirements for these entities. Since regulations vary from state to state, a health law specialist should be retained to help set up a practice.

All practices need to obtain a federal identification number, also known as an FIN or EIN (employee identification number). An application for an FIN can be obtained from a certified public accountant or the Internal Revenue Service (IRS). Once completed, the form should be filed with the IRS.

The FIN or EIN is required on forms the practice must complete for state unemployment taxes, Social Security withholding, and other taxes applicable to employers. Incorporated physician practices are also liable for state income taxes (where applicable) and federal income taxes.

A tax identification number is required for financial transactions with third-party payers such as insurance companies and governmental programs such as Medicare and Medicaid.

Another number to obtain is the provider number. Every payer (Medicare, Medicaid, Blue Cross/Blue Shield, and others) assigns its own number. A knowledgeable accountant can steer new providers through the process of obtaining all the necessary forms, filing applications, and setting up bank accounts.

State and Federal Taxes

Employers, including medical practices, must withhold a variety of taxes from their employees' gross salaries or wages as the money is earned. The withheld funds are sent periodically to the city, state, and federal governments. The amount withheld for federal taxes is determined by using wage bracket tables published by the IRS. Local experts are the best source of information on municipal and state tax regulations.

FICA (Social Security Withholding)

FICA (Federal Insurance Contributions Act) is the term used to describe payroll deductions withheld for Social Security. FICA deductions support programs for the elderly, the disabled, and survivors of wage earners; they also support the Medicare program. To determine the amount of the FICA deduction, use FICA tables supplied by the government and multiply gross pay by the current FICA rate.

Each year, Congress sets a tax rate and the maximum amount of gross pay from which FICA taxes are deducted. The law requires employers to match the taxes deducted from their employees' pay. Both the employee deductions and the equal amount from the employer must be sent to the government.

Federal Unemployment Tax

This tax supports unemployment insurance programs. In most states, only employers are required to pay this tax; the government defines an employer as anyone who has paid wages of $1,500 or more in any quarter of the previous calendar year or has had one or more employees during each of 20 calendar weeks. It is not necessary for employees to have worked full time or for the work period to have been 20 consecutive weeks. Unemployment taxes are filed by using Form 940, the Federal Unemployment Tax Return. The return and tax payment are due by January 31 of the year following the taxable year.

State Unemployment Tax

As at the federal level, state unemployment taxes fund unemployment benefits. Most states apply this tax only to employers. Tax rates vary by state; the tax is usually paid quarterly.

State Disability Insurance

In many states, employers must withhold a disability or sickness tax from their employees' gross pay. The tax rate and applicable wage level are set by each state. Funds from this tax support benefit payments to employees who cannot work because of disability.

Insurance for Medical Practices

Medical practices require several forms of insurance coverage. Some are unique to the medical profession, while others are standard for any business setting. Ideally, practices should select an insurance broker who can arrange all forms of coverage, including malpractice insurance.

When practices join integrated health care delivery systems, as is occurring more frequently, the larger organization typically assumes responsibility for all forms of medical practice insurance except malpractice. Physicians are usually responsible for their own malpractice coverage, even if much or all of the management responsibility for their practice has been transferred to another entity. However, if a practice is owned by another organization and the physician is an employee, the larger organization generally assumes responsibility for the malpractice insurance premiums as a standard practice expense.

General Insurance

General liability is an umbrella term that can include coverage for both internal and external features of the medical practice. Building liability or occupancy liability insurance is a more specific form of coverage that is necessary if the physician owns the building in which the practice is housed. If the practice occupies leased space, the landlord is responsible for providing this coverage. However, the physician (or lessee) is responsible for the internal contents, such as medical equipment.

The general or building liability policy covers the external features of the practice, such as the roof, and damage from vandalism or natural causes. It also covers the internal contents, such as medical and office equipment and furniture or damage to the interior. The liability coverage also would cover incidents such as a fall in the parking lot or an injury inside the office, unrelated to the reason for the patient's visit.

Workers' Compensation

Workers' compensation insurance provides compensation for disability or death that results from work-related accidental injury or disease. It is a mandatory employment benefit in all 50 states; however, the provisions vary from state to state. Workers' compensation is not the same as group insurance that practices may purchase to cover illnesses or accidents affecting employees and their dependents.

Employers pay premiums for workers' compensation, either directly or through their insurance company. Actual payments to an injured party are made by the insurance carrier through the state's workers' compensation program. Compensation is paid regardless of fault.

Under workers' compensation, employees are entitled to receive reasonable medical care to cure or relieve the effects of work-related injuries and diseases. They are also entitled to weekly benefits as long as the disability and wage loss persist. The amount of the weekly compensation depends on the date and type of injury.

Payment of workers' compensation benefits can cease under several sets of circumstances. For example, compensation will end when the employee returns to work at his or her regular job or a different job. Payments will also cease if the employee dies from causes unrelated to the original injury or disease. If death results form the work-related injury or disease, benefits must be paid to the employee's dependents for a specified period of time. A third way in which workers' compensation benefits can end is when the case is resolved by a settlement in an agreement approved by an administrative law judge.

Professional Liability Insurance

Every physician and certain health care professionals need to obtain professional liability insurance to pay for the cost of defending a malpractice case. Proof of liability coverage is a requirement to practice in most hospitals. Malpractice is defined as the negligence or carelessness of a professional.

Four elements must be proved in a malpractice case:

- A duty to provide care existed; there is a physician-patient relationship.
- The physician was derelict in that duty and failed to adhere to the standard of care.
- The patient must have suffered damage or injuries.
- The harm suffered by the patient was directly caused by the physician's breach of duty to that patient.

There is a time limit within which people can initiate a malpractice lawsuit. The statute of limitations varies widely from state to state; although state statutes rarely change, the information for your state should be verified periodically. (For details on malpractice liability, see Chapter 2, "Health Law.")

Employee Insurance

A practice may wish to offer employees group health insurance, life insurance, and disability insurance. Group health insurance provides coverage for illnesses and injuries affecting staff members and any family members also enrolled in the plan. In addition to the standard health insurance, practices may offer supplementary insurance to cover dental care or vision care. Life insurance provides benefits to the survivors of the insured individual. Disability insurance provides income for individuals who are injured off the job and unable to continue working. (For details on employee insurance, see Chapter 7, "Personnel Policies.")

COBRA (Consolidated Omnibus Budget Reconciliation Act) COBRA is a law that requires employers to offer continuation of group health coverage to employees who have left their jobs or have had their hours reduced so that they are no longer eligible for health coverage under their employer's group health plan. Continuing coverage must be offered for at least 18 months. Employers must also offer continuing coverage to dependent spouses and children if they lose group health coverage because of the employee's death or divorce, or because a minor child has reached the maximum age limit under the health plan.

COBRA applies to all employers who employed 20 or more people during the previous calendar year and who maintain a group health benefit plan. However, some states have adopted COBRA rules that apply to employers with fewer than 20 employees; this may include small medical practices. Eligible employers who fail to comply with COBRA cannot take the federal tax deduction normally allowed for the expenses of group health plans.

Family and Medical Leave Act (FMLA)   While FMLA may not be insurance in the strictest definition of the word, medical practices may be obligated to comply with its requirements. FMLA entitles eligible employees to take up to 12 weeks of unpaid, job-protected leave in a 12-month period for specified family and medical reasons, such as caring for children or elderly parents.

To be eligible for FMLA leave, an individual must work at a site where the employer employs at least 50 people within a 75-mile radius. A worksite can be a single location or a group of bordering locations. Other eligibility requirements include having worked for the employer at least 12 months and for at least 1,250 hours during the 12-month period immediately before the leave begins.

Insurance Management in the Practice

Oversight of insurance programs in a medical practice can be handled in several ways.

- The practice manager or administrator of a solo or small practice may assume responsibility in addition to other roles.
- A large practice may hire a benefits administrator whose only responsibility is insurance-related issues.
- Insurance management may be administered by an outside professional human resources company.
- If the practice is owned by a hospital or health care system, responsibility may be shifted to the benefits administration department of the larger organization.

Because insurance is a complex and constantly changing subject, practices must be sure that they remain well-informed of current requirements. Seminars are one way for practice managers to stay abreast of insurance requirements and regulations.

Retirement Plans

Retirement plans for physicians and employees should be part of the financial management program in a medical practice. Retirement plans have many advantages, for the practice and for employees. Employers gain substantial tax deductions, while both physicians and employees can accumulate retirement funds. In addition, a retirement plan can be a valuable benefit for recruiting and retaining practice employees.

Most retirement plans are complex and highly regulated by governmental agencies such as the IRS and the Department of Labor. Because of their complexity, a professional tax or financial adviser should design and set up these plans.

Simplified Employee Pension Plan (SEP)

As its name implies, this is a relatively easy plan to administer. The basic premise is that the employer contributes directly to Individual Retirement Accounts (IRAs) for each employee participating in the retirement plan. The allowable annual contribution is higher than for other IRAs: currently 15 percent of compensation up to $22,500. In addition, the annual contribution can vary from year to year. The practice can deduct all contributions to the IRAs.

Salary Reduction Simplified Employee Pension Plan (SARSEP)

SARSEP is funded by employees rather than by the employer, as in a SEP plan. Contributions allow employees to save for retirement and reduce their taxes. Salary reductions are limited to 15 percent of compensation, but the limit increases with the cost of living. The physician employer may supplement employees' contributions. Combined, contributions must not exceed 15 percent of compensation up to $22,500.

Guidelines for SARSEPs limit their availability to companies with fewer than 25 eligible employees, and 50 percent of those employees must participate. These plans also must meet nondiscrimination guidelines that guarantee a favorable balance between pretax contributions made by highly compensated employees and those who earn significantly less.

Profit Sharing Plan

The name of this plan is misleading, It does not have to be linked to profits. A medical practice that lacks a current or accumulated profit may participate. The premise of this plan is similar to that of the SEP, in which the employer makes contributions to employees' retirement accounts. The limit for contributions is the same, 15 percent of total employee compensation up to $22,500. However, profit sharing plans have more restrictions than the simplified pension plans. In their favor, though, is flexibility. Contributions may vary from year to year.

Money Purchase Pension Plan

This plan requires an annual mandatory contribution at a fixed percentage of compensation, up to 25 percent or $30,000 per person. This form of plan may work well in practices that have consistent earnings. It allows rapid accumulation of retirement funds.

Combined Profit Sharing and Money Purchase Pension Plans

To gain maximum contributions for highly compensated physicians or employees (in excess of $150,000 annual compensation) some practices may choose to combine two types of plans. A 10 percent money purchase plan could be combined with a profit sharing plan, which would allow a deduction of up to 25 percent or $30,000, whichever is less. If the practice were unable to make that high a contribution in a given year, it would be required to contribute only the 10 percent from the money purchase plan. Contributions from the profit sharing plan are discretionary.

401(k)

The 401(k) is a very popular retirement plan, named after the IRS regulation paragraph that created it. A 401(k) is an extension of a profit sharing plan that allows for pre-tax salary deferrals of up to $9,240 per year by each employee. This is combined with profit sharing from the practice but still cannot exceed $22,500, as required by law.

The 403(b) is the same as a 401(k) except that is it designed for use by nonprofit entities.

Keogh Plan

A Keogh Plan is a very popular option similar to a profit sharing plan for solo practitioners.

Conclusion

The importance of financial management in physician practices has grown in recent years and shows no signs of diminishing. Practices must have proper systems in place for accounts receivable, claims, accounts payable, and internal controls so that they can produce reports that track the practice's financial health. A financial status report is the foundation for making critical decisions that enable the practice to stay in business. For additional information about practice management, one of the best sources of information is the Medical Group Management Association (MGMA), based in Englewood, Colorado.

Chapter 11

Medical Transcription and Correspondence

The Transcriptionist in the Medical Office   287
Dictation/Transcription Equipment and Reference
  Material   290
Transcription in Practice   292
Medical Correspondence   302
Proofreading and Editing   305

The Transcriptionist in the Medical Office

Those charged with the recording and transcribing of medical documents are called *medical transcriptionists* or medical language specialists. The medical transcriptionist does all the physician's transcription for medical records. This person must have strong skills in typing and transcribing, as well as a broad knowledge of medical terminology. The medical transcriptionist also prepares reports and correspondence to other physicians involved in the patient's care. The work performed by medical transcriptionists is extremely important since the material they are transcribing is a critical part of the patient's medical record, documenting what the physician did and creating the history for future treatment for the patient.

Medical transcription requires personnel with one or more of the following attributes: detail-oriented, a "word person" rather than a "number person"; able to sit for long periods, concentrating and tuning out distractions; someone who loves the medical field and the interesting path to diagnosis but does not need to participate in patient care. These are the employees who make excellent, successful medical transcriptionists.

The normal route of progress from dictation to transcription is as follows: the physician dictates a report and delivers it on audiocassette to the transcription section of the medical office; the transcriptionist receives the dictated tape, transcribes it, prints it out if necessary, then sends it back to the physician for review and signature. The dictation is usually done via recording devices that are increasingly sophisticated, although some physicians prefer to handwrite their medical records. In addition, there are transcriptionists who choose to do their work on typewriters rather than computers. These are personal choices, and can be accomplished without sacrificing accuracy or legality.

Reference books are the tools of the trade for medical transcriptionists, who are constantly looking for the newest and most comprehensive medical reference material. In the medical office, the transcriptionist is the ideal staff member to be charged with keeping the office reference material up to date. (For a list of references, see Appendix B.)

American Association for Medical Transcription (AAMT)

The professional association for medical transcriptionists is the AAMT, based in Modesto, California. The AAMT publishes a bimonthly journal, and holds annual meetings and regional symposia. Various state associations and local chapters also exist, offering information on networking and job opportunities.

The AAMT certification board administers a two-part examination for those transcriptionists who wish to be certified. The first part contains written questions on medical terminology, grammar, punctuation, pharmacology, and disease processes. The second part consists of a number of dictated medical reports that the candidate transcribes within a given time period. Those who pass both parts earn the title Certified Medical Transcriptionist, and they must maintain that certification through continuing education credits, 10 per year in a three-year cycle for a total of 30 every three years. For more information, call AAMT at (800) 982-2182.

Production Standards

Various production standards are used to determine the salary and/or fees for medical transcriptionists. Whether your medical office has an in-house transcriptionist who earns a salary or uses an outside transcription service that charges a fee, production standards play a big part in how the salary or fee is structured. Production norms for one medical office cannot be applied to another medical office because of variables; these include the following:

- Type of practice
- Number of dictating physicians in an office for whom English is a second language
- Type of keyboarding and transcribing equipment
- Duties assigned to MTs other than transcription
- Availability of current reference material
- Method of measuring production—by the hour, page, line, keystroke, or byte

For additional information, contact several medical offices, hospital medical records departments, and transcription services in your area to determine the production standards in your particular locale.

Transcriptionist's Workstation

Even if the transcriptionist cannot control major office-design decisions, the desk and the space immediately adjacent to it—the workstation—can be organized for maximum efficiency. To set up the most effective workstation, sit in your chair and face the work surface. Stretch your arms straight out about six inches above the surface; then swing your arms carefully out to each side, making a wide arc, and look to see what areas of the desk your arms cover. This is the surface on which you should have all of the articles with which you frequently work—and only those articles. The far corners beyond this work area should be clean and free from clutter and may house a personal item or two. Choose a nonglare work surface, which will be easier on the eyes than glass or shiny plastic.

If your telephone is not installed where it is handy, request permission to have it moved. Essential reference books and material should be readily available on your desktop or on a shelf within your work area.

Work organizer Have a work organizer on the desk to hold documents. This may be a set of closely spaced shelves, a multilevel desk tray, or a vertical sorting rack. Separate areas are needed for dictation that is ready to be transcribed, for completed transcription that is ready for signature and/or delivery, for pending items, for projects in process, and so on.

Keep your area and equipment neat and clean. Alcohol wipes are useful for cleaning headsets, telephones, and keyboards. Keep food and drink away from the computer. Store loose papers at day's end inside the desk or otherwise out of sight.

The contents of desk drawers should also be organized. There are many types of organizers that fit into both large and small drawers to keep small, loose items orderly.

For maximum comfort and convenience, you should be able to sit at your workstation and reach your telephone, audiocassettes, computer disks, CD-ROMs, and printer while still having an accessible flat surface on which to keep open a manual or other reference book.

Accessories Important accessories for each workstation include wrist supports or wrist rests; these attach to the computer keyboard and enable you to rest your wrists during prolonged periods of keyboarding. Footrests are good to support your legs and improve circulation. A transcriptionist's foot pedal might sit on top of a footrest, as long as it does not interfere with leg room. Other accessories useful at your workstation are a copyholder, computer keyboard cover and cable cover.

Lighting In most offices, the pattern of ceiling lights is generally a symmetrical grid for the entire office space and may have no relation to where individual desks and workstations are placed. Make sure your workstation is adequately lit and that there is no glare reflected on your computer screen. The glare guards available in office supply stores do a good job of reducing the glare on the computer screen.

Noise can be a big problem for medical transcriptionists. Without doors to close, the sound of several computer printers can be distracting. If you are sensitive to noise, there are various enclosures on the market for printers. Laser printers are relatively quiet and ideally suited to the open environment.

Ergonomics   As office operations have become increasingly automated, concern for the effects of this automation has produced the discipline of ergonomics, the study of the effects of the physical design of equipment on the physical and emotional well-being of its users. Specialists in ergonomics have studied the effects of all the various office technologies and accessories, examining everything from the color of a computer screen to the shape of a chair. As a medical transcriptionist, you can profit from the considerable body of knowledge that exists when selecting or recommending products for your office.

It has been shown that computer monitors are better placed below eye level and tilted away from the face. By looking down at the computer monitor, headaches, eye strain, and fatigue are reduced, according to an ergonomic study. (For details on computer use, see Chapter 5, "The Computer in the Medical Office.")

Dictation/Transcription Equipment and Reference Material

Those in a medical office who dictate and those who transcribe use specific equipment, including various types of dictation units, transcribing equipment, typewriters, word processors, computers, and printers, in addition to the usual office machines such as photocopiers, fax machines, modems, and telephones.

Dictation Equipment

Dictation equipment must be evaluated from the usefulness to both the person recording and the transcriptionist. With any dictation equipment, the quality of sound and convenience of the machine are important. High-quality dictating units allow the recorder to fast-forward, rewind, correct dictation, mark the end of documents, and indicate priority work. The volume is adjustable and most models can record at two speeds. (Speech recorded at the slower speed does not have the quality of that recorded at the faster speed, but a tape recorded at slow speed can hold about twice as much dictation.)

In some cases a single unit can serve multiple purposes: when a microphone is attached to it, it becomes a dictating unit; when a foot pedal is attached, it becomes a transcriber. In other cases these units are separate. In any case the transcriber should include such features as earphones, on/off foot controls, rewind ability, an indexing system to indicate the length of the documents, controls for dictation corrections and insertions, and adjustments for speed, volume, and tone.

Desktop dictation machines   A desktop dictation machine is more durable than portable models, and usually comes with more features that can enhance the quality of the dictated material and in general facilitate a smooth dictation-to-transcription process.

Portable dictation units   Most physicians use handheld, portable dictation units. These are about the size of a deck of cards and fit easily into a pocket or briefcase. They are also, unfortunately, relatively easily lost or damaged. In general portables require more service than desktop models.

Central dictation systems   In an office with many physicians and other health care personnel, the volume of dictation may indicate the need for a dictation system with a central recorder and several extension microphones. Some central dictation systems use endless-loop recorders; others use a group of cassettes. Central systems can receive input by private or public telephone from local or long-distance sources. A machine with an endless-loop system can also accept dictation at the same time the transcriptionist transcribes from it. However, even though dictation and transcription can occur simultaneously, usually only one person may dictate at a time.

New digital equipment, which records on computer disks rather than tape, enables the transcriptionist to type during dictation, calculate the length of each document, and preview changes before beginning transcription. The sound quality of digital recording is a distinct advantage, since it results in improved accuracy, thus speeding transcription.

Such equipment is now combined with voice mail, which not only allows physicians to call in and dictate but also permits patients to leave messages. Such messages can be accessed from outside the office and can then be transcribed to be later reviewed by the physician and placed in the patient's file. This equipment allows two listeners or recorders to access the equipment at the same time.

Transcription Equipment

Transcriber   Medical transcribers are machines in which an audiocassette tape is placed after dictation. The sound of the dictation is easily controlled by changing the volume, tone, and speed. The transcriber is essential to the medical transcriptionist, as it allows the transcriptionist to receive dictation, to decipher and encode it, and to turn the spoken words into written material. The transcriber is the device that makes it possible to transform voice recordings into transcripts.

The transcriber consists of a base, where the audiocassette is inserted, headphones, and a foot pedal. The transcriber usually has separate controls for speed, tone, and volume, allowing the user to adjust the sound to suit personal needs. There are also play, stop, rewind, and fast-forward buttons on the base control board. These controls are useful when previewing or scanning tapes before they are transcribed.

The foot pedal, however, is the control primarily used for playing and rewinding the audiocassette. The transcriptionist will listen to an "earful" or just a few words more than can be transcribed, then continue to keyboard as the foot comes off the pedal briefly, finally pressing the foot pedal to continue hearing the dictated report. After a little practice, this becomes a very smooth motion, allowing for fast and accurate transcription.

Audiocassette tapes   Medical transcribers use various sizes of audiocassette tapes, from standard to microcassette and minicassette tapes—some machines can take a combination of tape sizes. The new digital transcription systems do not use tapes at all; transcriptionists access each report by simply dialing in a code number. As described above, these are convenient to use for off-site dictation and/or transcription.

Reference Material

Medical transcriptionists recognize the importance of maintaining a library of reference material. Keeping current is an ongoing and expensive effort; however, current editions and up-to-date reference materials are critical to the accuracy of medical transcription. There are professional journals and newsletters available by subscription for medical transcriptionists, which allows the medical transcriptionist to keep abreast of new words, drugs, and changes in the field of medical transcription. (For a list of references, see Appendix B; for a list of medical abbreviations, see Appendix C.)

Some considerations for maintaining a library of reference materials include building a basic library before branching out to the specialty and subspecialty areas, unless you happen to work in one of these areas. A basic library would include current editions of the following:

- Medical dictionary (unabridged)
- English dictionary (one unabridged for the office, and a desk edition for each workstation)
- Style guide for English grammar and punctuation
- Style guide for technical and scientific writing
- Drug book with information on spelling, dosage, and usage
- Laboratory tests and values information
- Medical abbreviations book, frequently updated with new abbreviations and new meanings ascribed to old abbreviations

Transcription in Practice

Health Records

In all medical settings, the health information gathered for each patient includes demographic information and specific reports that deal with a patient's examination and experience within the health care setting. These reports may include the following: history and physical examination, radiology report, laboratory reports, consultation, operative report, pathology report, discharge summary (or, if required, death summary), autopsy report, and others.

The health records most widely dictated and transcribed are the history and physical exam (H&P), consultation report, operative report, and discharge summary. These records are called the *basic four,* and are shown in sample form on the following pages. (For details on the organization and maintenance of health records, see Chapter 9, "Health Information Management.")

Each patient seen in a physician's office or admitted to a hospital has a history and physical examination and a discharge summary as part of the permanent health record. If the patient has surgery, an operative report will be part of that record as well. In addition, for medical or surgical patients, a consultation is often the fourth part of the basic four reports that make up the medical record. These reports are considered legal documents that are subject to subpoena. They contain information that is arranged according to guidelines developed by AHIMA and/or AMA. (Samples of the basic four reports and others in this chapter are taken from different regions of the United States and represent a variety of medical conditions.)

History and Physical Examination (H&P)

The primary purpose of the history and physical examination is to assist the physician in establishing a diagnosis on which to base the care and treatment of the patient. Elements of the H&P using a general format are arranged as follows:

> Patient Name:
> Age/Sex:
> Chief Complaint:
> History of Present Illness:
> Past Medical/Surgical History:
> Current Medications:
> Allergies:
> Habits/Exercise:
> Family/Social History:
> Review of Systems:
>   HEENT & Neck
>   Cardiovascular
>   Pulmonary
>   Gastrointestinal
>   Genitourinary
>   Musculoskeletal
>   Neurologic
> Physical Examination:
>   Vital Signs (blood pressure, pulse, respiration, temperature)
>   General Condition

HEENT & Neck
Skin
Heart/Lungs
Abdomen
Pelvic/Rectal
Extremities
Neurologic
Assessment:
Plan/Recommendations/Treatment:

Signature of health care professional
Initials of originator and transcriber
Date dictated:
Date transcribed:

An H&P using the general format

The sample H&P shown in Figure 11.1 follows the general format outlined above; it includes those elements that apply to a particular patient.

Follow-up Notes in SOAP Format

The SOAP (*s*ubjective, *o*bjective, *a*ssessment, *p*lan) format was created to provide a concise summary of chart notes in the patient's health record. It helps physicians and other health care providers locate information about a patient quickly. An example of notes written in the SOAP format is shown in Figure 11.2.

Consultation Report

Consultation reports are commonly written to physicians who have referred patients to other specialists. One example of such is shown in Figure 11.3.

Operative Report

This is a report of the surgeon's findings during the course of an operation and of the procedures used. The surgeon generally includes the following items in the report:

- Preoperative diagnosis—made before the operation and based on clinical findings
- Postoperative diagnosis—based on findings at operation
- Name of operation or procedure
- Procedure—a detailed description of the techniques, equipment, and devices used
- Specimens—identification of any tissues or other specimens sent to the pathologist or to the laboratory.

The sample operative report in Figure 11.4 describes a surgical patient admitted by an orthopedic surgeon. This patient has a medical diagnosis of diabetes mellitus, but is in need of surgical attention.

Fig. 11.1   History and Physical Examination

Patient Name: J.R.O.
Age/Sex: 64-year-old male
Date Seen: 8-28-95

<u>Chief Complaint:</u>   This 64-year-old, married pediatric neurologist, born 2-19-31, has a known diagnosis of prostatic carcinoma and comes in for flexible sigmoidoscopy due to perianal discomfort.

<u>History of Present Illness:</u>   Patient with known localized prostate cancer completed a course of radiation therapy last year following a positive biopsy report after being observed for several years with a gradually rising prostatic-specific antigen level and negative interval biopsy specimens. Certainly there has been no evidence of metastatic disease, and he continues to exhibit excellent well-being with no constitutional symptoms or skeletal symptoms. He has experienced long-standing low-backaching discomfort and stiffness, severe enough several years ago to prompt an MRI that showed no major abnormalities. He has had recurrent back spasms and morning stiffness but no radicular pain or past radiculopathy. No recent change in these symptoms. Current well-being is good with a fine psychological outlook. No nocturia or other major voiding symptoms. Not apparently overburdened by his cancer diagnosis. Regular followup with Dr. P.C. Recent prostatic-specific antigen (PSA) equals 2.4.

<u>Past Medical/Surgical History:</u>   As above. No past history of urinary tract infection. Excision of basal cell carcinoma from nose in approximately 1985. Remote tonsillectomy and adenoidectomy.

<u>Current Medications:</u>   None. Has no known drug allergies.

<u>Habits/Exercise:</u>   Nonsmoker, social drinker, takes no illicit drugs. He follows a vigorous activity schedule, playing coed soccer and swimming on a regular basis without limiting cardiopulmonary symptoms.

<u>Family History:</u>   Father died at age 89, Alzheimer-type dementia, diagnosed with colon cancer at age 88. Mother died at age 88, breast cancer. One sister died of breast cancer. One brother alive with alcoholism. Two other sisters alive and well save one who may be hypertensive.

<u>Social History:</u>   Lives with his wife of >30 years. Two grown children plus two teenagers still at home. Pediatric neurologist at S.W. Hospital.

<u>Review of Systems:</u>   Endocrine, no known diabetes or thyroid disease. Respiratory, positive PPD after Peace Corps service, 1965. Apparently normal chest X-rays and no INH preventive therapy. No history of

Fig. 11.1 *(continued)*

asthma. No cardiovascular, GI, or GU tract symptoms. Hematopoietic, no history of anemia. Neurologic, no troublesome headaches. Musculo-skeletal, patient does experience intermittent bilateral aching discomfort in both shoulders with a bout of apparent bicipital tendinitis on the left several months ago, now improved.

Physical Examination: In general, a healthy-appearing male. Vital signs show a weight of 167 lb., BP 128/70, heart rate 60 and regular, respirations 22 and not labored, oral temperature 97.6 F. Skin shows no rash or suspicious lesions. No lymphadenopathy. HEENT are negative. Neck, thyroid not palpable, no bruits. Lungs are clear. Heart is regular rate and rhythm. Abdomen flat and nontender. Extremities show peripheral pulses 2+ and symmetric. No edema. Extremities are normal except for slight left bicipital groove tenderness. Full ROM of shoulders, although downward movement on abducted arms does provoke anterior discomfort, left more than right. Neurologic exam not performed. External genitalia are normal. Rectal exam shows slight diffuse prostate enlargement with no areas of hardness or nodularity. Stool guaiac negative for occult blood.

Flexible Sigmoidoscopy: Indication, mild perianal discomfort on screening exam. Informed consent obtained and discussed.

Procedure: Flexible sigmoidoscope gradually passed to 60 cm from anus. No mucosal abnormalities or lesions seen. Minimal edema of distal rectum but no erythema, friability, or other markers of inflammation.

Impression: Essentially normal rectosigmoid. No clear radiation proctitis.

Assessment:
1. Overall, generally healthy man of age 64.
2. Apparently localized prostate cancer with uncomplicated course of radiation therapy administered last summer. Recent normal PSA.
3. Recent hemoccult tests negative with two stool samples submitted today also negative. Recent screening laboratory studies WNL.

Plan: Continued follow-up with his primary care physician as scheduled.

L.E.F., M.D.
Internal Medicine
LEF:dt
D: 7-21-95
T: 7-27-95 at 2 p.m.

Fig. 11.2   Follow-up Notes in SOAP Format

Patient Name: V.A.R.
Date of birth: 9-7-62
Date of visit: 8-8-95

<u>Subjective:</u>   This 32-year-old, gravida 2, para 1, abortus 1 patient comes in for a Pap and pelvic. No new problems except malodorous urine for six months. Treated herself in June for vaginal yeast infection with good results. Has gained 10 lb. over the past six months due to lack of exercise and possible overeating. The right posterior arm and wrist have had intermittent swelling over the past nine months. She has consulted her orthopedic surgeon about this. Arthritis and back pain are under good control with Voltaren. Status post abdominal hysterectomy in 1994 due to fibroid uterus.

<u>Objective:</u>   Neck exam shows negative thyroid, no nodules or enlargement, no supraclavicular or axillary nodes. Lungs are clear. Heart, regular rate and rhythm without murmur or gallop. Abdomen is obese with no organomegaly, mass, or tenderness. No costovertebral angle or suprapubic tenderness. Pelvic exam, external genitalia are normal female. Speculum exam shows pink vaginal walls. Cervix is absent. Adnexa are nontender. Pap smear is taken at the vaginal cuff. Rectal exam is negative for pain, mass, or blood. Extremities, the right arm has slight soft tissue swelling, nontender, in the forearm. Wrists and upper extremities have full range of motion and intact strength. Deep tendon reflexes in upper extremities are +2/4 and symmetric.

<u>Assessment:</u>
   1. Postmenopausal syndrome.
   2. Dysuria.
   3. Obesity.
   4. Family history of diabetes mellitus and hypertension in a first-degree relative.

<u>Plan:</u>   Premarin 0.625 mg, No. 90 dispensed with refill for 1 year. Labs—urinalysis, lipid profile, glucose. Return to clinic for weight loss and exercise program. Blood pressure check in six months. Contact patient regarding lab results.

<u>C.W., D.O.</u>
CW:jg
D: 8-8-95
T: 8-9-95

Fig. 11.3 Consultation Report

Patient Name: T.W.
Age/Sex: 4-year-old male
Consultant: W.B., M.D., Plastic Surgeon
Attending Physician: D.C., M.D., Pediatrician
Date of Accident: 11-25-95
Reason for Consult: Evaluate extent of burn injuries.
Burning Agent: Fire in a fireplace.

   Thank you for asking me to see this 4-year-old, right-hand-dominant black child who appears in mild distress due to an upper extremity burn after having fallen into the family fireplace.

   Using the Lund-Browder chart, the severity of burn is first- and second-degree. The total body surface area burned includes right lower arm 3%, right hand 1%. The joints involved include the right elbow, right wrist, and right hand.

Treatment Plan:
   Splinting of right hand.
   Positioning: Elevation with splint on.
   Range of motion: Good mobility.
   Pressure therapy: Will follow for induration or pressure fracture.

Goals:
   1. Reduce risk of contractures of involved joints by positioning, splinting, and maintaining range of motion.
   2. Reduce scar tissue formation by using Jobst bandages, pressure therapy, and splinting.
   3. Obtain maximum mobility and strength of upper extremities.
   4. Maximize independence in activities of daily living.
   5. Provide education for patient and family regarding high-calorie, high-protein diet.

   I will follow the care of this child at the Burn Clinic in two weeks and will keep you posted on his progress. Referral to physical/occupational therapy remains a possibility to be determined at follow-up.

W.B., M.D.
Plastic Surgeon
WB:pai
D: 11-25-95
T: 11-26-95
cc: V.I., PT/OT

Fig. 11.4   Operative Report

Patient Name: A.R.
Age/Sex: 54-year-old female
Date of Surgery: 9-10-95
Surgeon: W.W., M.D.
Assistant: J.L.S., PA-C
Anesthesia: None.

Preoperative Diagnosis: Persistent cellulitis, left ankle.

Postoperative Diagnosis: Persistent cellulitis, left ankle.

Name of Procedure: Incision and drainage, left ankle.

Indications: Persistent left ankle cellulitis following open reduction, internal fixation in a diabetic patient.

Procedure: After informed consent was obtained, the patient was taken to the operating room and placed in the supine position. The patient's left lower extremity was prepped with Betadine and draped in the usual sterile fashion. Secondary to the patient's diabetic neuropathy, no anesthetic was used. Patient's skin was firmly pinched using a pair of Adson forceps, and she felt no pain. Several times during the operative procedure the patient was checked, and she had no sensation of pain during the entire procedure.

Using a No. 10 scalpel, the area overlying the infected tendon was opened and sharply debrided, exposing good granulation tissue along the inside portion of the tendon and along the edges of the incision. Approximately 50% of the tendon was left intact with the necrotic portion being removed. The tendon and the surrounding wound were thoroughly irrigated with >3000 cc of normal saline. The wound was then gently packed with Xeroform gauze and covered with sterile 4 × 4 gauze pads and Kerlix dressing. The patient tolerated the procedure well and was returned to her room for a 23-hour observation.

Estimated Blood Loss: <10 cc

I/O Fluids: Approximately 400 cc

Complications: None

Specimens: Wound culture sent to microbiology.

W.W., M.D.
WW:kly
D: 9-10-95
T: 9-10-95

Fig. 11.5 Discharge Summary

Patient Name: V.G.I.
Age/Sex: 65-year-old male
Date Initially Seen: 7-19-95
Referring Physician: L.G., M.D., Family Practice

Problem List: (1) Atherosclerotic coronary vascular disease, status post
bypass surgery in October 1994. (2) Essential hypertension. (3) Abnormal signal-averaged electrocardiogram without sustained ventricular
tachycardia postoperatively. (4) Hyperlipidemia, hypercholesterol-
emia, on simvastatin therapy as of April 1995. (5) Musculoskeletal
chest discomfort.

Medications: Zocor (simvastatin), 1 tablet p.o. b.i.d. Dyazide, 1 tablet p.o.
q.d. Enteric-coated aspirin, 1 tablet p.o. q.d. Multivitamins.

History: V.G.I states that he has been doing very well. He is currently
able to work in his garden. He states that after doing some physical
activity, particularly with the upper extremities, he has discomfort on
the external aspect of his rib cage on the left side. He states that this
is not similar angina. In addition, he says that his congestion improved
remarkably after his Dyazide therapy, which he is continuing at this
point.

Physical Examination: Vital signs show BP 120/82, temp 97 F, pulse 72,
respiratory rate 12, weight 201 lb. (Last weight was 207 lb., and dry
weight post surgery was 195 lb.) HEENT are unremarkable. Neck:
No bruits. Lungs are clear to auscultation and percussion but with an
increased anteroposterior diameter. Heart: Cardiac exam shows jugular
venous pulsation normal, single S1 and S2, no S3 or S4. Abdomen is
soft, nontender. Extremities show only trace edema on the left side.
Skin is warm and dry, tanned.

Assessment: The patient is doing very well at this time, and his congestion
has improved with mild Dyazide therapy. As far as I can tell, he has
normal left ventricular systolic function. However, I cannot rule out
that some of his failure symptoms may be secondary to left ventricular
diastolic dysfunction from concentric left ventricular hypertrophy as a
result of hypertension. Currently, hypertension is well controlled on
medication. The left-sided musculoskeletal chest discomfort seems
characteristic postoperatively.

Plan: We will have the patient return to see us in six months. In addition,
we will check a lipid panel, CPK panel, liver function tests, and SMA-
7 to rule out (1) hypokalemia from Dyazide, (2) to ascertain adequate
lipid-lowering effect from simvastatin, (3) and to detect simvastatin-

Fig. 11.5   *(continued)*

---

induced hepatic or muscular enzyme abnormalities, if present. We will send copies of the lab results to Dr. Godwin; patient's further treatment will be dependent on those results.

F.Z., M.D.
FZ:dh
DD: 7-20-95
DT: 7-21-95
cc: L.G., M.D.

Fig. 11.6   Cytology Report

Patient: A.L.
Age/Sex: 27-year-old female
Specimen Source: Combined cervical/vaginal smear
Date Collected: 7-25-95
Date Received: 7-26-95
No. of Slides: One
Last Menstrual Period: 7-15-95
Past History: On 7-25-95, endocervical curettings, nondiagnostic study (mucus only).

Ectocervical Biopsy: Mostly low-grade squamous intraepithelial lesion with a minute focus of high-grade squamous intraepithelial lesion (corresponding to CIN-2).

Statement of Adequacy: Satisfactory for interpretation. Endocervical cell component present.

Cytologic Diagnosis: Abnormal cells consistent with high-grade squamous intraepithelial lesion encompassing moderate to severe dysplasia, i.e., carcinoma in situ (CIN-2 to CIN-3)

Recommendations: Colposcopy and biopsy.

G.S.H., M.D.
GSH:pai
D: 7-28-95
T: 7-28-95

Discharge Summary

After a patient has reached maximum medical/surgical care in the hospital setting, discharge is the next step—either to home or an extended care institution.

The discharge summary serves a variety of needs. It is quite often used in lieu of a letter to another physician or a facility involved in the patient's medical care at a later date. Copies are usually sent to the attending physician's office for inclusion in the office records and to the referring physician who had the primary encounter with the patient for the particular illness. These summaries also may be used with the patient's authorization to substantiate disability claims.

Several forms and formats for discharge summaries may be used in various settings to meet the needs of the medical community. A sample discharge summary is shown in Figure 11.5.

Cytology Reports and Surgical Pathology Reports

Also included in patients' health records are reports for specific procedures that might be performed following an examination in the physician's office or during a hospitalization. Examples of reports that present findings from cytology or pathology procedures are shown in Figures 11.6, 11.7, and 11.8.

Radiology and Ultrasound Reports

Reports that describe findings from radiology and ultrasound procedures are shown in Figures 11.9 through 11.13.

Emergency Room Report

Another type of report that might be included in a patient's health record is shown in Figure 11.14.

Chart Notes

Brief notes describing each of the patient's problems and related progress are attached to the patient's health record. Chart notes can be made in several formats: one is the HPIP (*h*istory, *p*hysical, *i*mpression, *p*lan); another is the SOAP (see also Figure 11.2 for a more extended example); and another is the problem-oriented format. The problem-oriented format (POMR) describes the first problem the patient has with a subjective, objective, assessment, and plan of that problem. The chart notes shown in Figure 11.15 combine these three formats. Note the use of short phrases and fragmented sentences. These are widely used and accepted in chart notes, which are reports meant for the medical office records only.

Medical Correspondence

Medical office correspondence consists of letters dictated by the physician and other health care professionals. These are usually letters to physicians

Fig. 11.7   Surgical Pathology Report

Patient: F.W.
Age/Sex: 40-year-old female
Specimen Designation: Loop electrosurgical excision procedure
    (LEEP) of cervix
Date Collected: 7-13-95
Date Received: 7-14-95
Clinical Diagnosis: Low-grade squamous intraepithelial lesion (SIL)

Pathologic Diagnosis: LEEP of uterine cervix: Dysplasia, focally
    moderate (CIN-2). See comment.

Comment: Multiple sections of the cervical biopsy reveal squamous
    metaplasia and focal dysplasia. The latter is of moderate degree
    in some foci. The dysplastic changes focally extend very close
    to the internal, endocervical, surgical margin. There is no evi-
    dence of in situ or infiltrating carcinoma.

Macroscopic Description: The specimen is received in formalin and
    is designated LEEP of cervix. The clinical diagnosis is low-grade
    squamous intraepithelial lesion. The specimen consists of two
    membranous portions of tissue that have smooth, glistening,
    slightly convex epithelial surfaces. These are 1.4 x 0.65 cm and
    1.25 x 0.8 cm in greatest and least diameters. The epithelial sur-
    faces are mildly hyperemic. The first portion is cut into transverse
    sections and submitted in two cassettes as A and B, with the
    second portion sectioned transversely and submitted in two cas-
    settes as C and D.

Microscopic Diagnosis: The microscopic findings are consistent
    with the pathologic diagnosis rendered.

G.S.H., M.D.
GSH:pai
D: 7-16-95
T: 7-16-95

Fig. 11.8   Surgical Pathology Report

Patient: F.Y.
Age/Sex: 66-year-old female
Specimen Designation: Left upper lung mass.
Date Collected: 7-12-95
Date Received: 7-13-95
Clinical Diagnosis: Sarcomatous type breast cancer, no positive nodes, in
    December 1994.

Pathologic Diagnosis: Wedge resection, LUL tumor nodule: Metaplastic
    anaplastic carcinoma with sarcomatous differentiation (metaplastic car-
    cinoma). Please see comment.

Comment: Comparison of the histology of this lung lesion to the patient's
    previous metaplastic breast carcinoma (94-9230, dated 12-14-94)
    shows the cells to have essentially the same microarchitecture.

Pathology Consultation: The pathologist was called to the OR by Dr. J.K.
    for consultation on a left upper lobe tumor. The patient is a 63-year-
    old woman with a tumor nodule in the left upper lobe of the lung. She
    has a past history of anaplastic carcinoma of the breast with sarcom-
    atous differentiation in December of 1994. Dr. J.K. has performed a
    wedge biopsy of the nodule and requests pathologic evaluation. The
    specimen is received and examined by the pathologist. A representative
    portion is examined microscopically using frozen section technique,
    and a preliminary diagnosis of ''consistent with metastatic metaplastic
    carcinoma'' is rendered and reported.

Macroscopic Description: The specimen is labeled ''left upper lobe mass''
    and is received unfixed directly from the surgeon. Submitted is an
    approximate wedge-shaped portion of grey-pink pulmonary tissue con-
    taining a firm nodule. The specimen has overall dimensions of 4.8 x
    3.2 x 2.5 cm. It is covered on two sides by pleura. The pleura is grossly
    intact and without evidence of neoplasm. A line of metal staples is
    present along one edge. Sections reveal a discrete, firm, grey-white
    tumor nodule. This has overall dimensions of 2.7 x 1.9 x 1.7 cm.
    The tumor appears to ''shell out'' from the surrounding pulmonary
    parenchyma. The lesion apparently does not extend to the surgical
    margin. Section through the nodule reveals an opaque, grey-white tis-
    sue without apparent necrosis or hemorrhage. The surrounding pulmo-
    nary tissue is grossly unremarkable. A portion of the neoplasm is ob-
    tained immediately following extraction and sections are placed in

Fig. 11.8   *(continued)*

methyl-Carnoy's solution and Trump's fixative. Sections are submitted as follows: A, residual tissue from frozen section block; B and C, additional sections through tumor; and D, methyl-Carnoy's-fixed tissue from tumor.

Microscopic Diagnosis: The microscopic findings are consistent with the pathologic diagnosis.

G.S.H., M.D.
GSH:pai
D: 7-16-95
T: 7-17-95

who have referred a patient for evaluation and/or specialized treatment. Correspondence may also include letters to hospitals, insurance companies, law offices, or government offices. Letters are also written to accept a speaking engagement, plan a conference or seminar, or reply to personal letters. The extent of correspondence depends on the size and type of medical practice. Samples of some types of correspondence are shown in Figures 11.16 through 11.19.

Proofreading and Editing

Proofreading

In the medical office, the medical transcriptionist is responsible for carefully proofreading the transcribed work; this is done in stages. First, the document is checked by the spell-check device on the computer. This process will catch many typographical errors; however, words such as *two/to/too, wound/would,* and *cold/could* are examples of errors that a computer spell check would not catch. These types of contextual errors should be addressed in the second reading, while the document is on the computer screen and after the spell check has been completed. Lastly, the document should be read after being printed as a final check for accuracy. This will seem to be time-consuming at first, but with practice it can be done with accuracy and speed.

Proofreading should be done carefully and attentively. One method could be to start at the end of the document and read from back to front,

Fig. 11.9 Lumbar Spine X-ray Report

Patient: G.A.
Age/Sex: 55-year-old male
Date of X-ray: 8-16-95
X-ray No.: 556-95-LS
Referring Physician: J.K., D.O.
Indications: Low back pain

<u>Lumbar Spine Film</u>

<u>Findings:</u> Review of outside films from Exel Radiology dated 7-11-91 is accomplished. AP lateral and oblique views of the LS-spine are obtained today. There is severe degenerative disc space narrowing at the L5-S1 level with marked narrowing also seen at the L4-5 level. Subluxation of L4 anteriorly on L5 is noted and measures approximately 5 mm. Oblique views show considerable degenerative changes in the facet joints at these levels. The upper lumbar spine appears normal. No destructive lesions are seen.

<u>Impression:</u> Advanced degenerative disc disease at L4-5 and L5-S1 with pseudospondylolisthesis of L4-5.

<u>W.M., M.D.</u>
WM:ad
D: 8-16-95
T: 8-16-95

the last word to the first word. This is an excellent way to catch errors, as your eyes see each word and mark of punctuation alone, not as part of a phrase or sentence. When reading from start to finish, the brain too often "sees" what is *meant* to be there rather than what is actually there.

Editing

Editing for grammatical, punctuation, spelling, and format changes is also expected of the medical transcriptionist. However, one cardinal rule reigns: *You may never change the meaning of the person dictating.* The policies and preferences of the office as well as those of the person dictating must be clearly understood; knowing when (and when not) to edit is very important. If there is any question in your mind, always refer to the person who dictated for

Fig. 11.10   Breast Ultrasound Report

Patient: L.C.
Age/Sex: 35-year-old female
Date of X-ray: 8-21-95
X-ray No.: 484-954-BF
Referring Physician: B.M., D.O.
Indications: Breast tenderness.

Ultrasound of the Right Breast

Findings: Dynamic high resolution real-time images were carried
    out to evaluate the right breast, specifically the upper outer quad-
    rant area where the focal tenderness was noted on the prior ex-
    amination. A very small prominent duct is seen at the 7 o'clock
    2B location. No other discrete masses are seen, and there is no
    evidence for acoustic shadowing.

Impression: Negative for malignancy.

L.A., M.D.
LA:pi
D: 8-21-95
T: 8-22-95

clarification. Editing dictation is usually permitted according to the following guidelines:

1. Edit dictation that is grammatically incorrect (considered as a favor to the originator).
2. Edit dictation that is unclear, ambiguous, or could result in misreading or misunderstanding.
3. Edit dictation when there is a medical or logical inconsistency, such as different dates given for the same procedure; *left* and *right* used inconsistently; or the sex of the patient dictated inconsistently. These problems can be checked against the patient's chart or medical records for accuracy.
4. Edit dictation when slang, jargon, or inflammatory remarks are made. Consider how a lawyer, judge, juror, or insurance company employee would interpret any asides made by an exhausted, frustrated physician dictating about a noncompliant patient or an abusive/neglectful parent. If you feel you cannot fix a passage, have your supervisor or office manager listen to the dictation and offer a suggestion. As a last resort, transcribe

Fig. 11.11   Abdominal Ultrasound Report

Patient: P.M.
Age/Sex: 54-year-old male
Date of X-ray: 9-13-95
X-ray No.:   485-137-UB
Referring Physician: J.R., M.D.
Indications: Urinary bladder growth

Abdominal Ultrasound

Findings: Dynamic image was taken through the abdomen. The patient
     has had a previous cholecystectomy. The extrahepatic biliary system
     is normal. The pancreas and peripancreatic tissue planes, although diffi-
     cult to visualize, appear intact. The extrahepatic architecture is normal.
     The spleen does not appear to be enlarged. The right kidney appears
     normal in size and architecture. The left kidney shows diffuse hydrone-
     phrosis, grade 3, with poor distinction of the corticomedullary junction,
     although the exam is limited due to overlying intestinal gas and subcu-
     taneous adipose tissue. CT of the abdomen and renal regions is recom-
     mended for complete evaluation of the renal parenchymal architecture.

Impression: Grade 3 hydronephrosis, left kidney.

L.A., M.D.
LA:pi
D: 9-13-95
T: 9-13-95

---

and print it out on a separate sheet, turn it in with the report to be signed,
and query the person who dictated, "Did you intend to include this?" or
"Is this what you meant to say?"

5. Do not edit dictation if you are either unsure about the inconsistency or
   not clear about how to make a correction.
6. Do not edit if you are unsure of the meaning of the person dictating.
7. Do not edit if the changes would alter either the meaning or the style of
   the person dictating.

Problems   When problems noted in guidelines 4–7 occur, the document
should be flagged but left as dictated and referred back to the originator for
clarification. Remember that each person who dictates has a unique, individ-

Fig. 11.12   Uterine Ultrasound Report

Patient: L.D.K.
Age/Sex: 25-year-old female
Date of X-ray: 9-30-95
X-ray No.:   849-783-OB
Referring Physician: H.P., M.D.
Indications: Possible growth retardation

Obstetrics Ultrasound

Impression: The sonographic age via multiple parameters is 35 weeks.
  The most correct assessment of true gestational age is approximately
  37 weeks by previous ultrasound on the initial examination as well as
  menstrual age. The fetus is slightly small for gestational age.

Comment: A single fetus is seen in a vertex presentation. The placenta
  is posterior, showing grade 2 maturational change.
  1. The SAMP-4 is 35 weeks.
  2. The menstrual age is 37 weeks, and the age by the initial ultrasound
     examination of 9-3-91 is 37 weeks.
  3. The estimated fetal weight is 2500 grams. The fetus is slightly small
     for gestational age but well within the standard deviation from the
     mean for growth in all biometric parameters.
  4. Total intrauterine growth retardation (IUGR) score is −5 points,
     which is within normal limits.

  The graphic plots and fetal morphologic structures appear normal. There
is no evidence for oligohydramnios. Positive fetal cardiac motion is identified on real-time examination.
  For individual fetal anatomic measurements, please see the attached
computer data graphic report sheet.

R.S., M.D.
RS:bh
D: 9-30-95
T: 9-30-95

Fig. 11.13   Chest X-ray Report

Patient Name: B.R.
Age/Sex: 72-year-old female
Date of X-ray: 10-16-95
X-ray No.:   12345
Referring Physician: J.W., D.O.
Indications: Chest pain.

<u>Chest Film, PA and Lateral Views:</u>   There is increased AP diameter.
The lung fields are hyperinflated. The diaphragms are flattened.
Hyperlucencies at the left hilum consistent with vascular shadow
or calcification are noted. The cardiac silhouette is displaced
slightly to the right, obscuring the right hilum. There is a poorly
defined opacity at the right heart border, which may or may not
represent vascular shadow. Either comparison to old chest film
or obtaining further studies is indicated. The aorta is calcified and
tortuous.

<u>T.S., M.D.</u>
TS:mlg
cc: J.W., D.O.

---

ual style that should remain intact. Do not edit to reflect your own personal
writing style. You are not the author of the transcribed document, but simply
the one who transforms spoken language into written language. Many things
are acceptable in speech that are not acceptable in written language; that is
why your proofreading and editing, when appropriate, are important.

It is acceptable to leave a blank space when dictation is unclear or has
been cut off. Be sure that the person dictating realizes that a blank has been
left in the document—flag the omission or otherwise make sure it is completed before the document is signed.

The role of the medical transcriptionist is to help transform the dictation
into clear, concise, and logical documentation without reflecting the personal
style, views, or attitude of the transcriptionist. While some people who dictate
may appreciate frequent and thorough editing, others may resent such intervention. Be prepared to work with such people, and realize that they are
ultimately responsible for the content of the document, as their signatures
affirm its quality, authenticity, and accuracy. With time and understanding,
an efficient and satisfying working relationship can be attained.

Fig. 11.14   Emergency Room Report

Patient Name: H.C.
Medical Record No.:   234567
E.R. Physician: J.M.R.
Date: 7-21-95
Time of Examination: 1435 hours

<u>Chief Complaint:</u>   Motor vehicle accident.

<u>History of Present Illness:</u>   This 12-year-old male was involved in an MVA
just prior to being brought into the E.R. He was the seat-belted, shoul-
der-strapped passenger in the front seat of the car. He cannot tell me
the exact mechanism of the collision. He states there was an air bag
on his side that did not deploy. He had no head injury. He has some
mild neck pain. There is no back, arm, or leg injury. No numbness or
weakness. He has no preexisting neck problems.

<u>Physical Examination:</u>   Vital Signs: BP 118/60, pulse 72, respirations 20,
temperature 99.3 F. A well-developed male, alert and cooperative, he
is initially fully immobilized and has a normal mental status. HEENT
appear normal with scalp and face nontender. Chest, clavicles, abdomen, back, arms, and legs appear normal and are nontender. A cervical
collar is in place. Neurologic exam: His strength is 5/5 and symmetrical.
Good grip, good elbow extension/flexion, shoulder abduction, and he
has normal sensation in his fingers. Biceps brachioradialis are 1 + and
symmetric.

<u>X-ray Impression:</u>   X-rays of the cervical spine appear normal.

<u>Diagnosis:</u>   Motor vehicle accident, cervical strain.

<u>Plan:</u>   Soft collar for three days. Advil for pain. Orthopedic consultation
if pain persists past 48 hours. Return for any weakness, numbness,
lightheadedness, or other problems. Follow-up with primary care physician, Dr. J.W.

<u>V.E.E., M.D.</u>
VEE:jla
D: 7-21-95
T: 7-22-95
cc: J.W., D.O.

Fig. 11.15 Chart Notes

7-20-95—Steven—**History:** This 31-year-old male with AIDS presents for evaluation of swelling in lower anterior abdominal wall, left lower quadrant. This is the site of a previously attempted aspiration for thoracentesis while the patient was in the hospital. **Physical Exam:** Firm, tender nodular region on the left lower quadrant abdominal wall. No erythema. **Procedure:** Sterile prep and drape. Attempted aspiration after injection of local anesthesia demonstrated no frank abscess. **Plan:** Patient is currently on ´ Augmentin for a sinus infection. This was started yesterday. If this mass on the abdominal wall progresses or becomes more erythematous, I will obtain an ultrasound to evaluate for the possibility of a deep abscess, which I cannot appreciate at this time. This plan has been discussed with Dr. K.G. and Dr. A.L. SN:dd

7-20-94—Shirley—**History:** The patient is a 47-year-old female with complaints of pain and discomfort in the right leg from varicose veins. Past medical history is documented in the chart. Patient currently wears support hose but is obtaining less and less relief from the stockings. In addition, she elevates her legs frequently during the day—again without much significant relief. **Physical Exam:** Left lower extremity fairly unremarkable. Right lower extremity with large, tortuous varicosities extending over the posterior calf and posterior thigh. **Assessment:** We will evaluate for reflux to deep system. Venous Doppler studies ordered. Patient will be contacted when those results are known. SN:dd

7-20-95—David—**History:** Status post laparoscopic appendectomy for acute gangrenous appendicitis. Currently without complaints except for some mild incisional discomfort, for which he requires no pain pills. Has returned to work. Denies fevers, has a normal diet, normal bowel movements. **Physical Exam:** Incisions are healing well. Small amount of skin separation at the umbilical incision but no evidence of infection. **Assessment:** Follow-up p.r.n. SN:dd

Fig. 11.15 *(continued)*

7-20-95—Cheryl—**History:** Status post left modified radical mastectomy. Here for postop evaluation at one week. Patient has returned to normal activities and requires no further pain medication. **Physical Exam:** Resolving ecchymoses. Incision closed and intact without evidence of calor or rubor. Draining serosanguineous fluid. Drain #2 had 70 cc over 24 hours. Drain #1 had 30 cc over 24 hours. **Assessment:** Based on the patient's midcourse of chemotherapy, we will leave the suture in for about one more week. Based on drainage output, we will leave the drains in as well. Will call patient in four days to reassess drain output. SN:dd

7-20-95—Clyde—**History:** Here for reevaluation of lower extremity ulceration secondary to trauma from lack of coordination. **Physical Exam:** Posterior calf wound granulating and closing in nicely; however, now with new, deep ulcerations over lateral aspect of right foot as well as overlying ankle. Sharp debridement of these reveals that the more distal ulceration extends down to the midmetatarsal. The bone is exposed at this site. **Plan:** Due to the amount of surrounding cellulitis, we plan to admit the patient for I.V. antibiotics and further discussion of care. This has been discussed with the patient's primary care physician, Dr. P.H. SN:dd

7-20-95—Sandi—**History:** Status post right breast biopsy for intraductal papilloma. Pathology reveals same plus intraductal hyperplasia. The patient has had no postop complications. **Physical Exam:** Incision well healed without ecchymoses or erythema. Suture removed. **Assessment:** Discussed results of pathology report with patient. Hyperplasia is an indication for close follow-up, and the patient will require yearly mammograms as well as physical examination by a physician. I have encouraged Sandi to begin monthly breast self-examination. SN:dd

Accented English Be sensitive when dealing with health care professionals for whom English is not their first language. They are often well aware of their language problems, and the transcriptionist can smooth out the dictating and transcribing process. A person who dictates and speaks with an accent (even a regional U.S. accent) is often appreciative of transcriptionists' efforts. Those who are close to people from foreign countries may have developed an ear for accented English. The tone, phrasing, inflection, and sentence structure can be a challenge; however, the task of transcribing for those who dictate with a heavy accent can be learned with time, patience, understanding, and skill in editing.

Fig. 11.16   Referral Letter

27 July 1995

Reginald Garcia, M.D.
123 Red Flag Road
San Antonio, TX 78229-6016

RE: J.R.O.

Dear Reg:

This is a follow-up letter on your referred patient, J.R.O. As you will recall, she had a proctosigmoidoscopic examination on 1 May for evaluation of rectal bleeding by history. At that time, the procedure was done only up to 40 cm from the anus because the patient was very uncomfortable during the procedure.

The patient came in for repeat exam today, at which time she received 3 mg Versed I.V. prior to the procedure. After sedation with Versed, flexible proctosigmoidoscopy was done without difficulty. The scope was gradually advanced up to 60 cm from the anus. Again, as on previous endoscopy, the mucosa was normal. There was an area of narrowing of the lumen in the sigmoid and descending colon area. There were a few diverticula in the sigmoid colon. There was no gross evidence of intrinsic lesions. The small sessile polyp in the rectum seen previously was not visualized at this time. There was the presence of small hemorrhoids not described on previous endoscopy.

The patient tolerated the procedure well, and the endoscopy findings were fully explained. She was dismissed in good condition.

In view of the discrepancy between the endoscopy done in May and the one done in July as far as the small polyp in the rectum, I would like to repeat this procedure in perhaps six months—just to be sure that no such polyp exists in her rectum. It happens sometimes that what is seen one time may not be seen the next, especially if it is a small polyp.

I apologize for this discrepancy, but I hope it can be clarified the next time I am able to perform the procedure.

With warmest personal regards,

Sun F. Wu, M.D.
SFW:jn
D: 7-27-95
T: 7-30-95

Fig. 11.17   Referral Letter

19 September 1995

Clifford V. Skinner, M.D.
34124 Houston Court
San Antonio, TX 78205

RE: R.R.

Dear Dr. Skinner:

It was a pleasure to see your patient, Mr. R., for evaluation. My assessment is that he has an early inflammatory polyarthritis. As you know, his initial rheumatoid factor test by latex agglutination was negative, and his sedimentation rate was normal. He is mildly anemic. Certainly rheumatoid arthritis is the most likely diagnosis and, in fact, his prognosis if this diagnosis is confirmed is better if he is seronegative. Due to his history of peptic ulcer disease, I have asked him to begin a 2-week trial of prednisone at 7.5 mg q.a.m. I will be checking a rheumatoid factor test by nephelometry and a few other serologic and chemical evaluations. I would like to follow this patient in two weeks. If his symptoms, including morning stiffness lasting three hours, persist I may need to start a disease modifying antirheumatic drug in the very near future. I will forward copies of his lab studies to you as they become available.

Once again, thank you for referring this pleasant patient to me. If I can be of further assistance, please do not hesitate to contact me.

Sincerely,

Stanley Jenkins, M.D.
Attending Rheumatologist
SJ:ip

Fig. 11.18   Electroencephalographic Report

Patient Name: W.E.B.
Age/Sex: 16-year-old male
Patient ID No.: 95-368
Attending Physician: M.J.O'N., M.D.
Date of EEG Study: 7-20-95
Clinical Summary: History of attention-deficit hyperactivity disorder.
Current Medications: Prozac.

Stage W: The resting awake record contains a posteriorly dominant,
9 to 10 cps pattern appearing bilaterally and showing bilateral
blocking with eye opening. Lower amplitude activity mixed with
beta frequencies are present in more anterior and midhemisph-
ere derivatives. There were no diffuse focal of paroxysmal features.

Hyperventilation: Four minutes of hyperventilation, fairly well performed, produced no change in background activity.

Sleep: With drowsiness, background activity was replaced by diffuse low-amplitude 5 to 7 cps activity. With stage 1 sleep, vertex
complexes developed with normal topography. With stage 2
sleep, 15 cps spindle activity appeared in parasagittal derivatives. There were no abnormal changes in background, and no
abnormal transients appeared. Transition to arousal was normal.

Impression: Normal awake and sleep electroencephalogram.

K.J., M.D.
Consulting Neurologist
KJ:dtt
D: 7-20-95
T: 7-20-95 at 2:29 p.m.

Fig. 11.19   Laser Treatment for Emphysema

July 20, 1995

Henderson A. Thomas, M.D.
11750 S.W. 35th Court
Colby, KS 67701

RE: Claude Smythe

Dear Dr. Thomas:

Mr. Smythe was in one year after his laser treatment of emphysema. I treated him almost exclusively with a laser, but I am currently doing a lot more resection. Nonetheless, he seems to have had a significant improvement in the quality of his life. Evidently he has been well for the past year, which is a little different for him. He has required no medical care. I think the major difference with Claude is his volume reduction.

Preoperative Lung Volumes		Postoperative 3 mos.	6 mos.
TLC	138%	132%	120%
RV	347%	306%	275%
TGV	194%	174%	157%

His spirometry is about the same. I do not have his pressure volume curves at the time of this dictation; however, I will look those over and let you know. Claude is eager to get his other side done, and I have no problem with that. I told him that I would probably do a bit more resection than I did before, as this is my custom now.

Again, I was pleased to see this delightful man. I am glad he is doing so well, and I hope that doing the other side will be equally beneficial. I will keep you posted as to his progress.

Sincerely yours,

Dieter S. Besch, M.D.
Thoracic & Vascular Surgery
DSB:le
D: 7-20-95
T: 7-21-95

Frequently Confused Words

Each of the following words and phrases can be difficult or confusing for transcriptionists. Some of the words sound alike yet have different meanings, while others do not sound alike but are often used and/or spelled incorrectly. When listening to dictation, medical transcriptionists should be aware of regional pronunciations as well as foreign accents and pronunciations. Be prepared to spell, transcribe, and use the following terms correctly. (For a more general list of frequently confused words, see Appendix C.)

abduction moving or drawing away

adduction moving or drawing toward

addiction compulsive need for and use of a habit-forming substance

affect *n* a state of mind or mood, countenance

affect *vb* to influence, to produce an effect upon

effect *n* result, impression

effect *vb* to result in, bring about, to accomplish

ala nasi *n, sing* outer wall of cartilage on each side of the nose

alae nasi *n, pl* nares or openings of the nasal cavity

ante- *prefix* anterior, forward, in front of, prior to, earlier than

anti- *prefix* against, opposite

anterior in front of, forward part of, toward the head

inferior below, beneath, lower surface

interior inside, inward, inner part or cavity

approximate *see* PROXIMAL

appose to place side by side or next to; before, beside or upon

oppose to place opposite or against something, so as to provide resistance, counterbalance, or contrast

aura subjective sensation (as of voices or colored lights) experienced before an attack of some disorders (as epilepsy or migraine)

aural relating to the ear or hearing

oral relating to the mouth; spoken

auxiliary subordinate, secondary

axillary referring to the underarm area

bases plural of basis

basis the lower, basic, or fundamental part of an object; any of various anatomical parts that function as a foundation

bile fluid secreted by the liver

bowel intestine

bisect to cut in half

resect to cut out a large portion

transect to cut across

dissect to cut up, as at autopsy

caliber the internal diameter of a hollow cylinder

caliper instrument used to measure diameter or thickness (usually used in plural)

cancer malignant tumor

carcinoma malignant new growth (used as synonym for *cancer*)

CA *abbrev* carcinoma or cancer; also cardiac arrest, coronary artery, chronological age

Ca *symbol* calcium

callous *adj* hard or bony, thickened

callus *n* thickened area on skin; tissue forming around break in a bone converted into bone in healing

chord musical tones sounded together

cord slender, flexible anatomical structure (such as spinal cord)

cor the heart

cirrhosal describing a diseased liver

serosal describing a membrane covering certain cavities of the body

clavicle collarbone
pedicle stalk

coarse rough or harsh
course plan; an ordered process or succession

data *n sing or pl* factual information

defer to postpone or delay
differ to be unlike or distinct; to disagree

defuse *v* to make less harmful, potent, or tense
diffuse *adj* scattered, not concentrated

discreet showing good judgment, capable of preserving prudent silence
discrete individually distinct, not blended; (such as a discrete mass)

disease morbid process with train of symptoms
sign evidence of disease that is seen (objective)
symptom evidence of disease not seen (subjective)
syndrome a set of symptoms and signs

dissect *see* BISECT

diverticulum (*pl* **diverticula**) abnormal pouch or sac opening from a hollow organ

effect *see* AFFECT

efflux outward flow
reflux backward or return flow

elicit to draw or bring out
illicit not lawful

endogenous growing, developing, or originating from within
exogenous developing or originating from the outside, (such as exogenous obesity)

excise to cut out or off
incise to cut into

expiration process of releasing air from the lungs; synonym for death
extirpation to remove entirely (such as extirpation of varicose veins)
extubation to remove a tube from a patient

fundus bottom or base; the part of a hollow organ farthest from its opening (such as the fundus of the stomach)
fungus any one of a group of mushrooms, yeasts, or molds

glands group of cells or organ specialized to secrete or excrete materials in the body
glans conical vascular body forming the end of the penis

graft tissue for implantation
graph a written record, diagram
grasp clasp or seize

gravida a pregnant woman
multiparous having had two or more pregnancies resulting in viable offspring (para 2 or para 3, etc.)
nulligravida a woman who has never been pregnant
nulliparous never having given birth to a viable infant
(For example: gravida 5, para 3-1-1-3 refers to a woman who has been pregnant five times, resulting in three full-term deliveries, one premature birth, one abortion or miscarriage, and three living children.)

hyper- *prefix* above, beyond, or excessive
hypo- *prefix* beneath, under, or deficient

incise *see* EXCISE

illicit *see* ELICIT

inferior *see* ANTERIOR

interior *see* ANTERIOR

ileum portion of the small intestine

ileus disease (obstruction of small intestine)

ilium bone (iliac crest)

in situ in its normal place; confined to the site of origin

in toto totally

in vitro in a test tube (glass); outside the living body

in vivo in the living body

infra- *prefix* beneath, below

inter- *prefix* between or among

intra- *prefix* within, during, between layers of

incubated placed in an optimal situation for development

intubated having had a tube inserted (such as into the larynx for providing oxygen)

lienal pertaining to the spleen

renal pertaining to the kidneys

ligament a band of tissue connecting bones, supporting viscera

ligate to sew, tie, or bind with ligature

ligature a thread or wire (suture) for tying vessels

liver largest gland in the body

livid discolored as from a contusion, congestion, or cyanosis

livor discoloration of the skin on the dependent parts of a corpse

malleolus (*pl* **malleoli**) bony prominences on either side of the ankle joint

malleus (*pl* **mallei**) outermost and largest of the three bones in the ear

metacarpal relating to the hand between the wrist and the fingers

metatarsal relating to the foot between the instep and the toes

mucous pertaining to or resembling mucus

mucus viscid slippery secretion of the mucous membrane

multiparous *see* GRAVIDA

nulligravida *see* GRAVIDA

nulliparous *see* GRAVIDA

ophthalmologist a physician specializing in the care of the eyes; note the spelling, as "ophthal" is often mispronounced and misspelled

oppose *see* APPOSE

oral *see* AURAL

os (*pl* **ora**) the mouth; any opening into a hollow organ or canal such as cervical os)

os (*pl* **ossa**) bone such as *os pubis* (pubic bone) or *ossa cranii* (cranial bones)

para- *prefix* beside, beyond

peri- *prefix* around

pedicle *see* CLAVICLE

perineum genital area (between anus and scrotum or vulva)

peritoneum covering of viscera, lining of abdominopelvic wall

peroneal pertaining to the fibula, lateral side of the leg, or tissues present there

pleural referring to the pleural cavity

plural more than one

prostate male gland surrounding the urethra

prostrate overcome or lying in a horizontal position

proximal nearest, closer to any point of reference, a location

approximate bring close together (such as to approximate the edges of a wound)

pruritus an itchy skin condition

purulent containing, consisting of, or forming pus

radical going to the root or source of disease

radicle rootlike beginning of an anatomical vessel or part

renal *see* LIENAL

reflux *see* EFFLUX

resect *see* BISECT

reperitonealize to cover again with peritoneum

retroperitoneal behind the peritoneum

serosal *see* CIRRHOSAL

shoddy inferior goods; hastily or poorly done

shotty like shot or lead pellets used in shotguns; usually used in reference to lymph nodes (such as shotty nodes)

sign *see* DISEASE

sulfa sulfonamides, the sulfa drugs

sulfur nonmetallic element

symptom *see* DISEASE

syndrome *see* DISEASE

tendinitis inflammation of a tendon

tendinous resembling a tendon

tendon a band of connective tissue

tenia (*pl* **teniae**) any anatomical bandlike structure

tinea ringworm, a fungus

tinnitus abnormal noises in the ears (such as ringing, booming, or whistling)

transect *see* BISECT

ureter either of two tubes from kidney to bladder

urethra tube carrying urine out of the body

vagus the tenth cranial nerve or vagus nerve

valgus bent outward, twisted, deformed

vesical relating to the urinary bladder

vesicle small blister or sac

villous shaggy with soft hairs

villus (*pl* **villi**) small protrusion (Note: There could be a villous villus.)

Health Care Vocabulary Standards

Presently there are no standards for written prescriptions, physician's orders, consultations, standing orders, nurse's medication administration records, and other forms. Because there are many variations, medical language is not always understood and is at times misinterpreted. This can cause delays in initiating therapy, cause accidents, waste time for everyone in clarifying documents, lengthen the time it takes to train those working in the health care field, lengthen hospital stays, and waste money.

A controlled vocabulary similar to that used in the aviation industry is needed. All pilots and air traffic controllers say, *alpha, bravo,* or *charley.* They do not sometimes say *adam, beef,* or *candy!* Because precision is critical, everything possible is done to eliminate error.

Written and oral communications in the medical professions are just as critical, and establishing a controlled vocabulary is also necessary.

In the examples below are suggestions for standardizing some health care vocabulary. It is hoped that a "health care controlled vocabulary," with other suggestions from professional organizations, will evolve into an official standard.

100 mg (with space) *not* 100mg (without space)	The USP standard way of expressing a strength is to leave a space between the number and its units. Leaving this space makes it easier to read the number.
1 mg *not* 1.0 mg	This is a USP standard. When a trailing zero is used, the decimal point is sometimes not seen, thus causing a 10-fold overdose. These overdoses have caused injury and death.
0.1 mL *not* .1 mL	When the decimal point is not seen, this is read as 1 mL, causing a 10-fold overdose.
once daily (not abbreviated) *not* OD (abbreviation) *and not* QD (abbreviation)	The classic meaning for OD is right eye; thus, liquids intended to be given once daily could mistakenly be given in the right eye. When the Q is dotted too aggressively it looks like Q.I.D. and the medication is given four times daily. When a lowercase *q* is used, the tail of the *q* has come up between the *q* and the *d* to make it look like *qid*. (In the United Kingdom, Q.D. means four times daily.)
unit (not abbreviated, with a lowercase *u*) *not* U (abbreviation)	The handwritten U is mistaken for a zero when poorly written, causing a 10-fold overdose (6 U regular insulin is read as 60). The poorly written U has also been read as a *4, 6,* and *cc.* Write *unit,* leaving a space between any number and the word *unit.*
mg (lowercase *mg* with no period) *not* mg., Mg., Mg, MG, mgm, mgs	USP standard expression is mg.
mL (lowercase *m* with a capital *L,* no period) *not* mL., ml, ml., mls, mLs, cc	USP standard expression is mL.
Use generic names or trademarks *not* abbreviated drug names or combinations of drugs, such as CPZ, PBZ, NTG, MS, 5FC, MTX, 6MP, MOPP, ASA, HCTZ, etc. *and not* shortened names or chemical names	Abbreviated drug names and acronyms are not always known to the reader, at times they have more than one possible meaning, or are thought to be another drug. When the chemical name 6 mercaptopurine has been used, six doses of mercaptopurine have been mistakenly administered. The generic name, mercaptopurine, should be used. When an unofficial shortened version of the name norfloxacin, norflox, was used, Norflex was mistakenly given.

Use the metric system
not apothecary system (grains, drams, minims, ounces, etc.)

The apothecary system is so rarely used it is not usually recognized or understood. The symbol for minim (♍) can be read as mL, for example.

Use properly placed commas for numbers above 999, as in 10,000, or 5,000,000
not 5000000

Many people have difficulty in reading large numbers. The use of commas helps the reader to read these numbers correctly.

600 mg (without decimals)
not 0.6 g

USP standard; the elimination of decimals lessens the chance for error.

Do not use the term *bolus* in conjunction with the administration of potassium chloride injection. Use specific concentrations and the time in which the drug should be administered.

Some physicians erroneously indicate that potassium chloride injection should be "bolused" or be given "IV push," vaguely meaning that it should not be dripped in slowly. Many deaths have been reported when prescribers have been taken literally and the potassium chloride was given by bolus or IV push. Orders should be specific such as, "20 mEq of potassium chloride in 50 mL of 5% dextrose to run over 30 minutes."

Use *and*
not slash mark or the symbol &

A slash mark looks like 1. An order written "6 units regular insulin/20 units NPH insulin," was read as 120 units of NPH insulin. The symbol & has been read as 4.

Orally transmitted medical orders should be read back as heard for verification
not assumption that one has spoken or heard correctly

During oral communications, speakers misspeak and transcribers mishear. To minimize these errors, the transmitter must speak clearly and slowly, the transcriber must repeat what was transcribed, and the transmitter must listen attentively when this is being done. This is less likely to occur when the prescription is complete.

When prescriptions are written or orally transmitted they must be complete: specify (1) dosage form, (2) strength, (3) directions, (4) purpose or indication
not incomplete orders

Prescribers on occasion think of one drug and mistakenly order another. Nurses and pharmacists on occasion misread prescriptions because of error, poor handwriting or poor oral communications, or look-alike or sound-alike drugs.
When the prescription is complete and the purpose or indication is included, these errors are less likely to occur. Listing the purpose or indication on the prescription label will assist in increasing patient compliance.

Written communications must be legible.
not illegible handwriting

Prescribers who cannot write legibly must either print (if legible), type, use a computer, or have an employee write for them and then immediately verify and sign the document.

Prescribe specific doses
not prescribe 2 ampuls or 2 vials

There is often more than one size or concentration of drug available. Failing to be specific will lead to unintended doses being administered.

Establish a list of approved abbreviations with no abbreviation having more than one possible meaning within a context
not everyone using their own abbreviations

To understand the scope of this problem examine the contents of this book for abbreviations that have many meanings and for obscure abbreviations which would not generally be recognized. (See also list of abbreviations in Appendix C.)

Chapter 12

A Guide to Punctuation and Style

Punctuation 325
Capitals and Italics 359
Plurals and Possessives 380
Compounds 388
Abbreviations 400
Numbers 410
References 427

Punctuation

Punctuation marks are used to help clarify the structure and meaning of sentences. They separate groups of words for meaning and emphasis; they convey an idea of the variations in pitch, volume, pauses, and intonation of the spoken language; and they help avoid ambiguity. The choice of what punctuation to use, if any, will often be clear and unambiguous. In other cases, a sentence may allow for several punctuation patterns. In cases like these, varying notions of correctness have developed, and two writers might, with equal correctness, punctuate the same sentence quite differently, relying on their individual judgment and taste.

APOSTROPHE

The apostrophe is used to form most possessives and contractions as well as some plurals and inflections.

1. The apostrophe is used to indicate the possessive of nouns and indefinite pronouns. (For details, see the section beginning on page 385.)

   the girl's shoe   anyone's guess
   children's laughter   the Browns' house
   Dr. Collins's office   the AMA's convention

2. Apostrophes are sometimes used to form plurals of letters, numerals, abbreviations, symbols, and words referred to as words. (For details, see the section beginning on page 380.)

> cross your *t*'s
> three 8's   *or*   three 8s
> two L.H.D.'s   *or*   two L.H.D.s
> used &'s instead of *and*'s

3. Apostrophes mark omissions in contractions made of two or more words and in contractions of single words.

> wasn't   she'd rather not   ass'n
> they're   Jake's had it   dep't

4. The apostrophe is used to indicate that letters have been intentionally omitted from a word in order to imitate informal speech.

> "Singin' in the Rain," the popular song and movie
> "Snap 'em up" was his response.

Sometimes such words are so consistently spelled with an apostrophe that the spelling becomes an accepted variant.

> rock 'n' roll [*for* rock and roll]
> ma'am [for madam]
> sou'wester [*for* southwester]

5. Apostrophes mark the omission of digits in numerals.

> class of '98
> fashion in the '90s

If the apostrophe is used when writing the plurals of numerals, either the apostrophe that stands for the missing figures is omitted or the word is spelled out.

> 90's   *or*   nineties   *but not*   '90's

6. In informal writing, apostrophes are used to produce forms of verbs that are made of individually pronounced letters. An apostrophe or a hyphen is also sometimes used to add an *-er* ending to an abbreviation; if no confusion would result, the apostrophe is usually omitted.

> OK'd the budget   4-H'er
> X'ing out the mistakes   49er

BRACKETS

Outside of mathematics and chemistry texts, brackets are primarily used for insertions into carefully handled quoted matter. They are rarely seen in general writing but are common in historical and scholarly contexts.

1. Brackets enclose editorial comments, corrections, and clarifications inserted into quoted matter.

Surely that should have peaked [sic] the curiosity of a serious researcher.

Here they much favour the tiorba [theorbo], the arclute [archlute], and the cittarone [chitarrone], while we at home must content ourselves with the lute alone.

In Blaine's words, "All the vocal aristocracy showed up—Nat [Cole], Billy [Eckstine], Ella [Fitzgerald], Mabel Mercer—'cause nobody wanted to miss that date."

2. Brackets enclose insertions that take the place of words or phrases.

And on the next page: "Their assumption is plainly that [Durocher] would be the agent in any such negotiation."

3. Brackets enclose insertions that supply missing letters.

A postscript to a December 17 letter to Waugh notes, "If D[eutsch] won't take the manuscript, perhaps someone at Faber will."

4. Brackets enclose insertions that alter the form of a word used in an original text.

He dryly observes (p. 78) that the Gravely investors had bought stocks because "they want[ed] to see themselves getting richer."

5. Brackets are used to indicate that capitalization has been altered. This is generally optional; it is standard practice only where meticulous handling of original source material is crucial (particularly legal and scholarly contexts).

As Chief Justice Warren held for the Court, "[T]he Attorney General may bring an injunctive action . . ."
or in general contexts
"The Attorney General may bring . . . "

Brackets also enclose editorial notes when text has been italicized for emphasis.

But tucked away on page 11 we find this fascinating note: "In addition, we anticipate that *siting these new plants in marginal neighborhoods will decrease the risk of organized community opposition*" [italics added].

6. Brackets function as parentheses within parentheses, especially where two sets of parentheses could be confusing.

Posner's recent essays (including the earlier *Law and Literature* [1988]) bear this out.

7. In mathematical copy, brackets are used with parentheses to indicate units contained within larger units. They are also used with various meanings in chemical names and formulas.

$x + 5[(x + y)(2x-y)]$
$Ag[Pt(NO_2)_4]$

With Other Punctuation

8. Punctuation that marks the end of a phrase, clause, item in a series, or sentence follows any bracketed material appended to that passage.

> The report stated, "if we fail to find additional sources of supply [of oil and gas], our long-term growth will be limited."

When brackets enclose a complete sentence, closing punctuation is placed within the brackets.

> [Since this article was written, new archival evidence of document falsification has come to light.]

COLON

The colon is usually a mark of introduction, indicating that what follows it—generally a clause, a phrase, or a list—has been pointed to or described in what precedes it. (For the use of capitals following a colon, see paragraphs 7–8 on pages 360–61.)

With Phrases and Clauses

1. A colon introduces a clause or phrase that explains, illustrates, amplifies, or restates what has gone before.

> An umbrella is a foolish extravagance: if you don't leave it in the first restaurant, a gust of wind will destroy it on the way home.
> Dawn was breaking: the distant peaks were already glowing with the sun's first rays.

2. A colon introduces an appositive.

> The issue comes down to this: Will we offer a reduced curriculum, or will we simply cancel the program?
> That year Handley's old obsession was replaced with a new one: jazz.

3. A colon introduces a list or series, often following a phrase such as *the following* or *as follows.*

> She has trial experience on three judicial levels: county, state, and federal.
> Anyone planning to participate should be prepared to do the following: hike five miles with a backpack, sleep on the ground without a tent, and paddle a canoe through rough water.

It is occasionally used like a dash to introduce a summary statement following a series.

> Baseball, soccer, skiing, track: he excelled in every sport he took up.

4. Although the colon usually follows a full independent clause, it also often interrupts a sentence before the clause is complete.

> The nine proposed program topics are: offshore supply, vessel traffic, ferry services, ship repair, . . .

Information on each participant includes: name, date of birth, mailing address, . . .

For example: 58 percent of union members voted, but only 44 percent of blue-collar workers as a whole.

The association will:

Act with trust, integrity, and professionalism.

Operate in an open and effective manner.

Take the initiative in seeking diversity.

With Quotations

5. A colon usually introduces lengthy quoted material that is set off from the rest of a text by indentation but not by quotation marks.

> The *Rumpole* series has been nicely encapsulated as follows:
>
> Rumpled, disreputable, curmudgeonly barrister Horace Rumpole often wins cases despite the disdain of his more aristocratic colleagues. Fond of cheap wine ("Château Thames Embankment") and Keats's poetry, he refers to his wife as "She Who Must Be Obeyed" (an allusion to the title character of H. Rider Haggard's *She*).

6. A colon is often used before a quotation in running text, especially when (1) the quotation is lengthy, (2) the quotation is a formal statement or is being given special emphasis, or (3) a full independent clause precedes the colon.

> Said Murdoch: "The key to the success of this project is good planning. We need to know precisely what steps we will need to take, what kind of staff we will require, what the project will cost, and when we can expect completion."
>
> The inscription reads: "Here lies one whose name was writ in water."
>
> This was his verbatim response: "At this time Mr. Wilentz is still in the company's employ, and no change in his status is anticipated imminently.

Other Uses

7. A colon separates elements in bibliographic publication data and page references, in biblical citations, and in formulas used to express time and ratios. No space precedes or follows a colon between numerals.

> Stendhal, *Love* (New York: Penguin, 1975)
> *Paleobiology* 3:121
> John 4:10
> 8:30 a.m.
> a winning time of 3:43:02
> a ratio of 3:5

8. A colon separates titles and subtitles.

> *Southwest Stories: Tales from the Desert*

9. A colon follows the salutation in formal correspondence.

> Dear Judge Wright: Dear Product Manager:
> Dear Laurence: Ladies and Gentlemen:

10. A colon follows headings in memorandums, government correspondence, and general business letters.

TO:	VIA:
SUBJECT:	REFERENCE:

11. An unspaced colon separates the writer's and typist's initials in the identification lines of business letters.

>   WAL:jml

A colon also separates copy abbreviations from the initials of copy recipients. (The abbreviation *cc* stands for *carbon* or *courtesy copy; bcc* stands for *blind carbon* or *courtesy copy*.) A space follows a colon used with the fuller name of a recipient.

cc:RSP	bcc:MWK
JES	bcc: Mr. Jones

With Other Punctuation

12. A colon is placed outside quotation marks and parentheses that punctuate the larger sentence.

> The problem becomes most acute in "Black Rose and Destroying Angel": plot simply ceases to exist.
> Wilson and Hölldobler remark on the same phenomenon in *The Ants* (1990):

COMMA

The comma is the most frequently used punctuation mark in English and the one that provides the most difficulties to writers. Its most common uses are to separate items in a series and to set off or distinguish grammatical elements within sentences.

Between Main Clauses

1. A comma separates main clauses joined by a coordinating conjunction, such as *and, but, or, nor,* or *so.*

> She knew very little about the new system, and he volunteered nothing.
> The trial lasted for nine months, but the jury took only four hours to reach its verdict.
> We will not respond to any more questions on that topic this afternoon, nor will we respond to similar questions in the future.
> All the first-floor windows were barred, so he had clambered up onto the fire escape.

2. When one or both of the clauses are short or closely related in meaning, the comma is often omitted.

> They said good-bye and everyone hugged.

If commas set off another phrase that modifies the whole sentence, the comma between main clauses is often omitted.

Six thousand years ago, the top of the volcano blew off in a series of powerful eruptions and the sides collapsed into the middle.

3. Commas are sometimes used to separate short and obviously parallel main clauses that are not joined by conjunctions.

One day you're a successful corporate lawyer, the next day you're out of work.

Use of a comma to join clauses that are neither short nor obviously parallel, called *comma fault* or *comma splice*, is avoided. Clauses not joined by conjunctions are normally separated by semicolons. For details, see paragraph 1 on page 356.

4. If a sentence is composed of three or more clauses that are short and free of commas, the clauses are occasionally all separated by commas even if the last two are not joined by a conjunction. If the clauses are long or punctuated, they are separated with semicolons; the last two clauses are sometimes separated by a comma if they are joined by a conjunction. (For more details, see paragraph 5 on page 357.)

Small fish fed among the marsh weed, ducks paddled along the surface, an occasional muskrat ate greens along the bank.
The kids were tired and whiny; Napoleon, usually so calm, was edgy; Tabitha seemed to be going into heat, and even the guinea pigs were agitated.

With Compound Predicates

5. Commas are not normally used to separate the parts of a compound predicate.

The firefighter tried to enter the burning building but was turned back by the thick smoke.

However, they are often used if the predicate is long and complicated, if one part is being stressed, or if the absence of a comma could cause a momentary misreading.

The board helps to develop the financing and marketing strategies for new corporate divisions, and issues periodic reports on expenditures, revenues, and personnel appointments.
This is an unworkable plan, and has been from the start.
I try to explain to him what I want him to do, and get nowhere.

With Subordinate Clauses and Phrases

6. Adverbial clauses and phrases that begin a sentence are usually set off with commas.

Having made that decision, we turned our attention to other matters.
In order to receive a high school diploma, a student must earn 16 credits from public or private secondary schools.
In addition, staff members respond to queries, take new orders, and initiate billing.

If the sentence can be easily read without a comma, the comma may be omitted. The phrase will usually be short—four words or less—but even after a longer phrase the comma is often omitted.

> As cars age, they depreciate.   *or*   As cars age they depreciate.
> In January the firm will introduce a new line of investigative services.
> On the map the town appeared as a small dot in the midst of vast emptiness.
> If nobody comes forward by Friday I will have to take further steps.

7. Adverbial clauses and phrases that introduce a main clause other than the first main clause are usually set off with commas. If the clause or phrase follows a conjunction, one comma often precedes the conjunction and one follows the clause or phrase. Alternatively, one comma precedes the conjunction and two more enclose the clause or phrase, or a single comma precedes the conjunction. Short phrases, and phrases in short sentences, tend not to be enclosed in commas.

> They have redecorated the entire store, but[,] to the delight of their customers, it retains much of its original flavor.
> We haven't left Springfield yet, but when we get to Boston we'll call you.

8. A comma is not used after an introductory phrase if the phrase immediately precedes the main verb.

> From the next room came a loud expletive.

9. A subordinate clause or phrase that modifies a noun is not set off by commas if it is *restrictive* (or *essential*)—that is, if its removal would alter the noun's meaning.

> The man who wrote this obviously had no firsthand knowledge of the situation.
> They entered through the first door that wasn't locked.

If the meaning would not be altered by its removal, the clause or phrase is considered *nonrestrictive* (or *nonessential*) and usually is set off by commas.

> The new approach, which was based on team teaching, was well received.
> Wechsler, who has done solid reporting from other battlefronts, is simply out of his depth here.
> They tried the first door, which led nowhere.

10. Commas set off an adverbial clause or phrase that falls between the subject and the verb.

> The Clapsaddle sisters, to keep up appearances, rode to the park every Sunday in their rented carriage.

11. Commas set off modifying phrases that do not immediately precede the word or phrase they modify.

> Scarbo, intent as usual on his next meal, was snuffling around the butcher's bins.
> The negotiators, tired and discouraged, headed back to the hotel.
> We could see the importance, both long-term and short-term, of her proposal.

12. An absolute phrase (a participial phrase with its own subject that is grammatically independent of the rest of the sentence) is set off with commas.

> Our business being concluded, we adjourned for refreshments.
> We headed southward, the wind freshening behind us, to meet the rest of the fleet in the morning.
> I'm afraid of his reaction, his temper being what it is.

With Appositives

13. Commas set off a word, phrase, or clause that is in apposition to (that is, equivalent to) a preceding or following noun and that is nonrestrictive.

> It sat nursing its front paw, the injured one.
> Aleister Crowley, Britain's most infamous satanist, is the subject of a remarkable new biography.
> A cherished landmark in the city, the Hotel Sandburg has managed once again to escape the wrecking ball.
> The committee cochairs were a lawyer, John Larson, and an educator, Mary Conway.

14. Restrictive appositives are not set off by commas.

> He next had a walk-on role in the movie *The Firm.*
> Longfellow's poem *Evangeline* was a favorite of my grandmother's.
> The committee cochairs were the lawyer John Larson and the educator Mary Conway.
> Lord Castlereagh was that strange anomaly[,] a Labor-voting peer.

With Introductory and Interrupting Elements

15. Commas set off transitional words and phrases.

> Indeed, close coordination will be essential.
> Defeat may be inevitable; however, disgrace is not.
> The second report, on the other hand, shows a strong bias.

When such words and phrases fall in the middle of a clause, commas are sometimes unnecessary.

> They thus have no chips left to bargain with.
> The materials had indeed arrived.
> She would in fact see them that afternoon.

16. Commas set off parenthetical elements, such as authorial asides.

> All of us, to tell the truth, were completely amazed.
> It was, I should add, not the first time I'd seen him in this condition.

17. Commas are often used to set off words or phrases that introduce examples or explanations, such as *namely, for example,* and *that is.*

> He expects to visit three countries, namely, France, Spain, and Germany.
> I would like to develop a good, workable plan, that is, one that would outline our goals and set a timetable for accomplishing them.

Such introductory words and phrases may also often be preceded by a dash, parenthesis, or semicolon. Regardless of the punctuation that precedes the word or phrase, a comma usually follows it.

> Sports develop two valuable traits—namely, self-control and the ability to make quick decisions.
>
> In writing to the manufacturer, be as specific as possible (i.e., list the missing or defective parts, describe the malfunction, and identify the store where the unit was purchased).
>
> Most had traveled great distances to participate; for example, three had come from Australia, one from Japan, and two from China.

18. Commas set off words in direct address.

> This is our third and final notice, Mr. Sutton.
>
> The facts, my fellow Americans, are very different.

19. Commas set off mild interjections or exclamations.

> Ah, the mosaics in Ravenna are matchless.
>
> Uh-oh, His Eminence seems to be on the warpath this morning.

With Contrasting Expressions

20. A comma is sometimes used to set off contrasting expressions within a sentence.

> This project will take six months, not six weeks.

21. When two or more contrasting modifiers or prepositions, one of which is introduced by a conjunction or adverb, apply to a noun that follows immediately, the second is set off by two commas or a single comma, or not set off at all.

> A solid, if overly wordy, assessment
> *or* a solid, if overly wordy assessment
> *or* a solid if overly wordy assessment
> This street takes you away from, not toward, the capitol.
> *or* This street takes you away from, not toward the capitol.
> grounds for a civil, and maybe a criminal, case
> *or* grounds for a civil, and maybe a criminal case
> *or* grounds for a civil and maybe a criminal case

Dashes or parentheses are often used instead of commas in such sentences.

> grounds for a civil (and maybe a criminal) case

22. A comma does not usually separate elements that are contrasted through the use of a pair of correlative conjunctions such as *either . . . or, neither . . . nor,* and *not only . . . but also.*

> Neither my brother nor I noticed the error.
>
> He was given the post not only because of his diplomatic connections but also because of his great tact and charm.

When correlative conjunctions join main clauses, a comma usually separates the clauses unless they are short.

> Not only did she have to see three salesmen and a visiting reporter, but she also had to prepare for next day's meeting.
> Either you do it my way or we don't do it at all.

23. Long parallel contrasting and comparing clauses are separated by commas; short parallel phrases are not.

> The more that comes to light about him, the less savory he seems.
> The less said the better.

With Items in a Series

24. Words, phrases, and clauses joined in a series are separated by commas.

> Men, women, and children crowded aboard the train.
> Her job required her to pack quickly, to travel often, and to have no personal life.
> He responded patiently while reporters shouted questions, flashbulbs popped, and the crowd pushed closer.

When the last two items in a series are joined by a conjunction, the final comma is often omitted, especially where this would not result in ambiguity. In individual publications, the final comma is usually consistently used, consistently omitted, or used only where a given sentence would otherwise be ambiguous or hard to read. It is consistently used in most nonfiction books; elsewhere it tends to be used or generally omitted equally often.

> We are looking for a house with a big yard, a view of the harbor[,] and beach and docking privileges.

25. A comma is not generally used to separate items in a series all of which are joined with conjunctions.

> I don't understand what this policy covers or doesn't cover or only partially covers.
> They left behind the fogs and the wood storks and the lonesome soughing of the wind.

26. When the elements in a series are long or complex or consist of clauses that themselves contain commas, the elements are usually separated by semicolons, not commas. See paragraph 7 on pages 357–58.

With Coordinate Modifiers

27. A comma is generally used to separate two or more adjectives, adverbs, or phrases that modify the same word or phrase.

> She spoke in a calm, reflective manner.
> They set to their work again grimly, intently.

The comma is often omitted when the adjectives are short.

one long thin strand	skinny young waiters
a small white stone	in this harsh new light
little nervous giggles	

The comma is generally omitted where it is ambiguous whether the last modifier and the noun—or two of the modifiers—constitute a unit.

the story's stark dramatic power
a pink stucco nightclub

In some writing, especially works of fiction, commas may be omitted from most series of coordinate modifiers as a matter of style.

28. A comma is not used between two adjectives when the first modifies the combination of the second plus the noun it modifies.

the last good man	the only fresh water
a good used car	the only freshwater lake
his protruding lower lip	their black pickup truck

A comma is also not used to separate an adverb from the adjective or adverb that it modifies.

this formidably difficult task

In Quotations

29. A comma usually separates a direct quotation from a phrase identifying its source or speaker. If the quotation is a question or an exclamation and the identifying phrase follows the quotation, the comma is replaced by a question mark or an exclamation point.

She answered, "I'm afraid it's all we've got."
"The comedy is over," he muttered.
"How about another round?" Elaine piped up.
"I suspect," said Mrs. Horowitz, "we haven't seen the last of her."
"You can sink the lousy thing for all I care!" Trumbull shouted back.
"And yet . . . ," she mused.
"We can't get the door op—" Captain Hunt is heard shouting before the tape goes dead.

In some cases, a colon can replace a comma preceding a quotation; see paragraph 6 on page 329.

30. When short or fragmentary quotations are used in a sentence that is not primarily dialogue, they are usually not set off by commas.

He glad-handed his way through the small crowd with a "Looking good, Joe" or "How's the wife" for every beaming face.
Just because he said he was "about to leave this minute" doesn't mean he actually left.

Sentences that fall within sentences and do not constitute actual dialogue are not usually set off with commas. These may be mottoes or maxims, unspoken or imaginary dialogue, or sentences referred to as sentences; and they may or may not be enclosed in quotation marks. Where quotation marks are not used, a comma is often inserted to mark the beginning of the shorter sentence clearly. (For the use of quotation marks with such sentences, see paragraph 6 on page 353.)

> "The computer is down" was the response she dreaded.
> He spoke with a candor that seemed to insist, This actually happened to me and in just this way.
> The first rule is, When in doubt, spell it out.

When the shorter sentence functions as an appositive (the equivalent to an adjacent noun), it is set off with commas when nonrestrictive and not when restrictive.

> We had the association's motto, "We make waves," printed on our T-shirts.
> He was fond of the slogan "Every man a king, but no man wears a crown."

31. A comma introduces a directly stated question, regardless of whether it is enclosed in quotation marks or if its first word is capitalized. It is not used to set off indirect discourse or indirect questions introduced by a conjunction (such as *that* or *what*).

> I wondered, what is going on here?
> The question is, How do we get out of this situation?
>   *but*
> Margot replied quietly that she'd never been happier.
> I wondered what was going on here.
> The question is how do we get out of this situation.

32. The comma is usually omitted before quotations that are very short exclamations or representations of sounds.

> He jumped up suddenly and cried "I've got it!"

Replacing Omitted Words

33. A comma may indicate the omission of a word or phrase in parallel constructions where the omitted word or phrase appears earlier in the sentence. In short sentences, the comma is usually omitted.

> The larger towns were peopled primarily by shopkeepers, artisans, and traders; the small villages, by peasant farmers.
> Seven voted for the proposal, three against.
> He critiqued my presentation and I his.

34. A comma sometimes replaces the conjunction *that.*

> The smoke was so thick, they were forced to crawl.
> Chances are, there are still some tickets left.

With Addresses, Dates, and Numbers

35. Commas set off the elements of an address except for zip codes.

> Write to Bureau of the Census, Washington, DC 20233.
> In Needles, California, their luck ran out.

When a city name and state (province, country, etc.) name are used together to modify a noun that follows, the second comma may be omitted but is more often retained.

> We visited their Enid, Oklahoma plant.
> *but more commonly*
> We visited their Enid, Oklahoma, plant.

36. Commas set off the year in a full date.

> On July 26, 1992, the court issued its opinion.
> Construction for the project began on April 30, 1995.

When only the month and year are given, the first comma is usually omitted.

> In December 1903, the Wright brothers finally succeeded in keeping an airplane aloft for a few seconds.
> October 1929 brought an end to all that.

37. A comma groups numerals into units of three to separate thousands, millions, and so on.

> 2,000 case histories   a population of 3,450,000
> 15,000 units   a fee of $12,500

Certain types of numbers do not contain commas, including decimal fractions, street addresses, and page numbers. (For more on the use of the comma with numbers, see paragraphs 1–3 on pages 414–15.)

> 2.5544
> 12537 Wilshire Blvd.
> page 1415

With Names, Degrees, and Titles

38. A comma separates a surname from a following professional, academic, honorary, or religious degree or title, or an abbreviation for a branch of the armed forces.

> Amelia P. Artandi, M.D.
> Robert Hynes Menard, Ph.D., L.H.D.
> John L. Farber, Esq.
> Sister Mary Catherine, S.C.
> Admiral Herman Washington, USN

39. A comma is often used between a surname and the abbreviations *Jr.* and *Sr.*

Douglas Fairbanks, Sr. *or* Douglas Fairbanks Sr.
Dr. Martin Luther King, Jr. *or* Dr. Martin Luther King Jr.

40. A comma is often used to set off corporate identifiers such as *Incorporated, Inc., Ltd., P.C.,* and *L.P.* However, many company names omit this comma.

StarStage Productions, Incorporated
Hart International Inc.
Walsh, Brandon & Kaiser, P.C.
The sales manager from Doyle Southern, Inc., spoke at Tuesday's meeting.

Other Uses

41. A comma follows the salutation in informal correspondence and usually follows the complimentary close in both informal and formal correspondence.

Dear Rachel,
Affectionately,
Very truly yours,

42. The comma is used to avoid ambiguity when the juxtaposition of two words or expressions could cause confusion.

Under Mr. Thomas, Jefferson High School has flourished.
He scanned the landscape that opened out before him, and guided the horse gently down.

43. When normal sentence order is inverted, a comma often precedes the subject and verb. If the structure is clear without it, it is often omitted.

That we would succeed, no one doubted.
And a splendid occasion it was.

With Other Punctuation

44. Commas are used next to brackets, ellipsis points, parentheses, and quotation marks. Commas are not used next to colons, dashes, exclamation points, question marks, or semicolons. If one of the latter falls at the same point where a comma would fall, the comma is dropped. (For more on the use of commas with other punctuation, see the sections for each individual mark).

"If they find new sources [of oil and gas], their earnings will obviously rebound. . . . "
"This book takes its place among the most serious, . . . comprehensive, and enlightened treatments of its great subject."
There are only six small files (at least in this format), which take up very little disk space.
According to Hartmann, the people are "savage," their dwellings are "squalid," and the landscape is "a pestilential swamp."

DASH

The dash can function like a comma, a colon, or a parenthesis. Like commas and parentheses, dashes set off parenthetical material such as examples, supplemental facts, and explanatory or descriptive phrases. Like a colon, a dash introduces clauses that explain or expand upon something that precedes them. Though sometimes considered a less formal equivalent of the colon and parenthesis, the dash may be found in all kinds of writing, including the most formal, and the choice of which mark to use is often a matter of personal preference.

The common dash (also called the *em dash,* since it is approximately the width of a capital M in typeset material) is usually represented by two hyphens in typed and keyboarded material. (Word-processing programs make it available as a special character.)

Spacing around the dash varies. Most newspapers insert a space before and after the dash; many popular magazines do the same; but most books and journals omit spacing.

The *en dash* and the *two-* and *three-em dashes* have more limited uses, which are explained in paragraphs 13–15 on pages 342–43.

Abrupt Change or Suspension

1. The dash marks an abrupt change or break in the structure of a sentence.

> The students seemed happy enough with the new plan, but the alumni—there was the problem.

2. A dash is used to indicate interrupted speech or a speaker's confusion or hesitation.

> "The next point I'd like to bring up—" the speaker started to say.
> "Yes," he went on, "yes—that is—I guess I agree."

Parenthetical and Amplifying Elements

3. Dashes are used in place of commas or parentheses to emphasize or draw attention to parenthetical or amplifying material.

> With three expert witnesses in agreement, the defense can be expected to modify its strategy—somewhat.
> This amendment will finally prevent corporations—large and small—from buying influence through exorbitant campaign contributions.

When dashes are used to set off parenthetical elements, they often indicate that the material is more digressive than elements set off with commas but less digressive than elements set off by parentheses. For examples, see paragraph 16 on page 333 and paragraph 1 on page 347.

4. Dashes set off or introduce defining phrases and lists.

> The fund sought to acquire controlling positions—a minimum of 25% of outstanding voting securities—in other companies.
> Davis was a leading innovator in at least three styles—bebop, cool jazz, and jazz-rock fusion.

5. A dash is often used in place of a colon or semicolon to link clauses, especially when the clause that follows the dash explains, summarizes, or expands upon the preceding clause in a somewhat dramatic way.

> The results were in—it had been a triumphant success.

6. A dash or a pair of dashes often sets off illustrative or amplifying material introduced by such phrases as *for example, namely,* and *that is,* when the break in continuity is greater than that shown by a comma, or when the dash would clarify the sentence structure better than a comma. (For more details, see paragraph 17 on pages 333–34.)

> After some discussion the motion was tabled—that is, it was removed indefinitely from the board's consideration.
>
> Lawyers should generally—in pleadings, for example—attempt to be as specific as possible.

7. A dash may introduce a summary statement that follows a series of words or phrases.

> Crafts, food booths, children's activities, cider-making demonstrations—there was something for everyone.
>
> Once into bankruptcy, the company would have to pay cash for its supplies, defer maintenance, and lay off workers—moves that could threaten its future.

8. A dash often precedes the name of an author or source at the end of a quoted passage—such as an epigraph, extract, or book or film blurb—that is not part of the main text. The attribution may appear immediately after the quotation or on the next line.

> Only the sign is for sale.
> —Søren Kierkegaard
>
> "I return to her stories with more pleasure, and await them with more anticipation, than those of any of her contemporaries."—William Logan, *Chicago Tribune*

With Other Punctuation

9. If a dash appears at a point where a comma could also appear, the comma is omitted.

> Our lawyer has read the transcript—all 1,200 pages of it—and he has decided that an appeal would not be useful.
>
> If we don't succeed—and the critics say we won't—then the whole project is in jeopardy.

In a series, dashes that would force a comma to be dropped are often replaced by parentheses.

> The holiday movie crowds were being entertained by street performers: break dancers, a juggler (who doubled as a sword swallower), a steel-drummer, even a three-card-monte dealer.

10. If the second of a pair of dashes would fall where a period should also appear, the dash is omitted.

> Instead, he hired his mother—an odd choice by any standard.

Much less frequently, the second dash will be dropped in favor of a colon or semicolon.

> Valley Health announced general improvements to its practice—two to start this week: evening office hours and a voice-mail message system.
> His conduct has always been exemplary—near-perfect attendance, excellent productivity, a good attitude; nevertheless, his termination cannot be avoided.

11. When a pair of dashes sets off material ending with an exclamation point or a question mark, the mark is placed inside the dashes.

> His hobby was getting on people's nerves—especially mine!—and he was extremely good at it.
> There would be a "distinguished guest speaker"—was there ever any other kind?—and plenty of wine afterwards.

12. Dashes are used inside parentheses, and vice versa, to indicate parenthetical material within parenthetical material. The second dash is omitted if it would immediately precede the closing parenthesis; a closing parenthesis is never omitted.

> We were looking for a narrator (or narrators—sometimes a script calls for more than one) who could handle a variety of assignments.
> The wall of the Old City contains several gates—particularly Herod's Gate, the Golden Gate, and Zion Gate (or "David's Gate")—with rich histories.

En Dash and Long Dashes

13. The *en dash* generally appears only in typeset material; in typed or keyboarded material the simple hyphen is usually used instead. (Word-processing programs provide the en dash as a special character.) Newspapers similarly use the hyphen in place of the en dash. The en dash is shorter than the em dash but longer than the hyphen. It is most frequently used between numbers, dates, or other notations to signify "(up) to and including."

> pages 128–34   September 24–October 5
> 1995–97   8:30 a.m.–4:30 p.m.

The en dash replaces a hyphen in compound adjectives when at least one of the elements is a two-word compound. It replaces the word *to* between capitalized names, and is used to indicate linkages such as boundaries, treaties, and oppositions.

> post–Cold War era
> Boston–Washington train
> New Jersey–Pennsylvania border
> male–female differences   *or*   male-female differences

14. A *two-em dash* is used to indicate missing letters in a word and, less frequently, to indicate a missing word.

> The nearly illegible letter is addressed to a Mr. P—— of Baltimore.

15. A *three-em dash* indicates that a word has been left out or that an unknown word or figure is to be supplied.

> The study was carried out in ——, a fast-growing Sunbelt city.

ELLIPSIS POINTS

Ellipsis points (also known as *ellipses, points of ellipsis,* and *suspension points*) are periods, usually in groups of three, that signal an omission from quoted material or indicate a pause or trailing off of speech. A space usually precedes and follows each ellipsis point. (In newspaper style, spaces are usually omitted.)

1. Ellipsis points indicate the omission of one or more words within a quoted sentence.

> We the People of the United States . . . do ordain and establish this Constitution for the United States of America.

2. Ellipsis points are usually not used to indicate the omission of words that precede the quoted portion. However, in some formal contexts, especially when the quotation is introduced by a colon, ellipsis points are used.

> He ends with a stirring call for national resolve that "government of the people, by the people, for the people shall not perish from the earth."
>
> Its final words define the war's purpose in democratic terms: " . . . that government of the people, by the people, for the people shall not perish from the earth."

Ellipsis points following quoted material are omitted when it forms an integral part of a larger sentence.

> She maintained that it was inconsistent with "government of the people, by the people, for the people."

3. Punctuation used in the original that falls on either side of the ellipsis points is often omitted; however, it may be retained, especially if this helps clarify the sentence.

> Now we are engaged in a great civil war testing whether that nation . . . can long endure.
>
> But, in a larger sense, we can not dedicate, . . . we can not hallow this ground.
>
> We the People of the United States, in Order to . . . promote the general Welfare, and secure the Blessings of Liberty . . . , do ordain and establish this Constitution for the United States of America.

4. If an omission includes an entire sentence within a passage, the last part of a sentence within a passage, or the first part of a sentence other than the first quoted sentence, the period preceding or following the omission is retained (with no space preceding it) and is followed by three ellipsis points. When the first part of a sentence is omitted but the quoted portion acts as a sentence, the first quoted word is usually capitalized.

> We have come to dedicate a portion of that field, as a final resting place for those who here gave their lives that this nation might live. . . . But, in a larger sense, we can not dedicate—we can not consecrate—we can not hal-low—this ground.
>
> Now we are engaged in a great civil war. . . . We are met on a great battlefield of that war.
>
> The brave men, living and dead, who struggled here, have consecrated it, far above our poor power to add or detract. . . . From these honored dead we take increased devotion to that cause for which they gave the last full measure of devotion. . . .

Alternatively, the period may be dropped and all omissions may be indicated simply by three ellipsis points.

5. If the last words of a quoted sentence are omitted and the original sentence ends with punctuation other than a period, the end punctuation often follows the ellipsis points, especially if it helps clarify the quotation.

> He always ends his harangues with some variation on the question, "What could you have been thinking when you . . . ?"

6. When ellipsis points are used to indicate that a quotation has been intentionally left unfinished, the terminal period is omitted.

> The paragraph beginning "Recent developments suggest . . . " should be deleted.

7. A line of ellipsis points indicates that one or more lines have been omitted from a poem. (For more on poetry and extracts, see the section on pages 354–55.)

> When I heard the learned astronomer,
>
> . . . .
> How soon unaccountable I became tired and sick,
> Til rising and gliding out I wandered off by myself,
> In the mystical moist night-air, and from time to time,
> Looked up in perfect silence at the stars.

8. Ellipsis points are used to indicate faltering speech, especially if the faltering involves a long pause or a sentence that trails off or is intentionally left unfinished. Generally no other terminal punctuation is used.

> The speaker seemed uncertain. "Well, that's true . . . but even so . . . I think we can do better."
>
> "Despite these uncertainties, we believe we can do it, but . . . "
>
> "I mean . . . " he said, "like . . . How?"

9. Ellipsis points are sometimes used informally as a stylistic device to catch a reader's attention, often replacing a dash or colon.

> They think that nothing can go wrong . . . but it does.

10. In newspaper and magazine columns consisting of social notes, local events listings, or short items of celebrity news, ellipsis points often take the place of paragraphing to separate the items. (Ellipsis points are also often used in informal personal correspondence in place of periods or paragraphing.)

> Congratulations to Debra Morricone, our up-and-coming singing star, for her full scholarship to the Juilliard School this fall! . . . And kudos to Paul Chartier for his winning All-State trumpet performance last Friday in Baltimore! . . . Look for wit and sparkling melody when the Lions mount their annual Gilbert & Sullivan show at Syms Auditorium. This year it's . . .

EXCLAMATION POINT

The exclamation point is used to mark a forceful comment or exclamation.

1. An exclamation point can punctuate a sentence, phrase, or interjection.

> There is no alternative!
> Without a trace!
> My God! It's monstrous!

2. The exclamation point may replace the question mark when an ironic, angry, or emphatic tone is more important than the actual question.

> Aren't you finished yet!
> Do you realize what you've done!
> Why me!

Occasionally it is used *with* the question mark to indicate a very forceful question.

> How much did you say?!
> You did what!?

3. The exclamation point falls within brackets, dashes, parentheses, and quotation marks when it punctuates only the enclosed material. It is placed outside them when it punctuates the entire sentence.

> All of this proves—at long last!—that we were right from the start.
> Somehow the dog got the gate open (for the third time!) and ran into the street.
> He sprang to his feet and shouted "Point of order!"
> At this rate the national anthem will soon be replaced by "You Are My Sunshine"!

4. If an exclamation point falls where a comma could also go, the comma is dropped.

> "Absolutely not!" he snapped.
> They wouldn't dare! she told herself over and over.

If the exclamation point is part of a title, it may be followed by a comma. If the title falls at the end of a sentence, no period follows it.

Hello Dolly!, which opened in 1964, would become one of the ten longest-running shows in Broadway history.

His favorite management book is still *Up the Organization!*

HYPHEN

Hyphens have a variety of uses, the most significant of which is to join the elements of compound nouns and modifiers.

1. Hyphens are used to link elements in compound words. (For more on compound words, see the section beginning on page 388.)

   secretary-treasurer   fund-raiser
   cost-effective   spin-off

2. In some words, a hyphen separates a prefix, suffix, or medial element from the rest of the word. Consult a dictionary in doubtful cases. (For details on using a hyphen with a prefix or a suffix, see the section beginning on page 397.)

   anti-inflation
   umbrella-like
   jack-o'-lantern

3. In typed and keyboarded material, a hyphen is generally used between numbers and dates with the meaning "(up) to and including." In typeset material it is replaced by an en dash. (For details on the en dash, see paragraph 13 on page 342.)

   pages 128–34
   the years 1995–97

4. A hyphen marks an end-of-line division of a word.

   In 1975 smallpox, formerly a great scourge, was declared totally eradicated by the World Health Organization.

5. A hyphen divides letters or syllables to give the effect of stuttering, sobbing, or halting speech.

   "S-s-sammy, it's my t-toy!"

6. Hyphens indicate a word spelled out letter by letter.

   l-i-a-i-s-o-n

7. Hyphens are sometimes used to produce inflected forms of verbs made of individually pronounced letters or to add an *-er* ending to an abbreviation. However, apostrophes are more commonly used for these purposes. (For details on these uses of the apostrophe, see paragraph 6 on page 326.)

   DH-ing for the White Sox   *or*   DH'ing for the White Sox
   a dedicated UFO-er   *or*   a dedicated UFO'er

PARENTHESES

Parentheses generally enclose material that is inserted into a main statement but is not intended to be an essential part of it. For some of the cases described below, commas or dashes are frequently used instead. (For examples, see paragraph 16 on page 333 and paragraph 3 on page 340.) Parentheses are particularly used when the inserted material is only incidental. Unlike commas and dashes, an opening parenthesis is always followed by a closing one. Because parentheses are almost always used in pairs, and their shapes indicate their relative functions, they often clarify a sentence's structure better than commas or dashes.

Parenthetical Elements

1. Parentheses enclose phrases and clauses that provide examples, explanations, or supplementary facts or numerical data.

> Nominations for principal officers (president, vice president, treasurer, and secretary) were heard and approved.
>
> Four computers (all outdated models) will be replaced.
>
> First-quarter sales figures were good (up 8%), but total revenues showed a slight decline (down 1%).

2. Parentheses sometimes enclose phrases and clauses introduced by expressions such as *namely, that is, e.g.,* and *i.e.,* particularly where parentheses would clarify the sentence's structure better than commas. (For more details, see paragraph 17 on pages 333–34.)

> In writing to the manufacturer, be as specific as possible (i.e., list the defective parts, describe the malfunction, and identify the store where the unit was purchased), but also as concise.

3. Parentheses enclose definitions or translations in the main part of a sentence.

> The company announced plans to sell off its housewares (small-appliances) business.
>
> The *grand monde* (literally, "great world") of prewar Parisian society consisted largely of titled aristocracy.

4. Parentheses enclose abbreviations that follow their spelled-out forms, or spelled-out forms that follow abbreviations.

> She cited a study by the Food and Drug Administration (FDA).
>
> They attended last year's convention of the ABA (American Booksellers Association).

5. Parentheses often enclose cross-references and bibliographic references.

> Specialized services are also available (see list of stores at end of brochure).
>
> The diagram (Fig. 3) illustrates the action of the pump.
>
> Subsequent studies (Braxton 1990; Roh and Weinglass 1993) have confirmed these findings.

6. Parentheses enclose numerals that confirm a spelled-out number in a business or legal context.

> Delivery will be made in thirty (30) days.
> The fee is Four Thousand Dollars ($4,000), payable to UNCO, Inc.

7. Parentheses enclose the name of a state that is inserted into a proper name for identification.

> the Kalispell (Mont.) Regional Hospital
> the *Sacramento* (Calif.) *Bee*

8. Parentheses may be used to enclose personal asides.

> Claims were made of its proven efficacy (some of us were skeptical).
> *or*
> Claims were made of its proven efficacy. (Some of us were skeptical.)

9. Parentheses are used to enclose quotations that illustrate or support a statement made in the main text.

> After he had a few brushes with the police, his stepfather had him sent to jail as an incorrigible ("It will do him good").

Other Uses

10. Parentheses enclose unpunctuated numbers or letters indicating individual elements or items in a series within a sentence.

> Sentences can be classified as (1) simple, (2) multiple or compound, and (3) complex.

11. Parentheses indicate alternative terms.

> Please sign and return the enclosed form(s).

12. Parentheses may be used to indicate losses in accounting.

> Operating Profits
> (in millions)
> Cosmetics 26.2
> Food products 47.7
> Food services 54.3
> Transportation . . . . . . (17.7)
> Sporting goods . . . . . . (11.2)
> Total 99.3

With Other Punctuation

13. When an independent sentence is enclosed in parentheses, its first word is capitalized and a period (or other closing punctuation) is placed inside the parentheses.

> The discussion was held in the boardroom. (The results are still confidential.)

A parenthetical expression that occurs within a sentence—even if it could stand alone as a separate sentence—does not end with a period but may end with an exclamation point, a question mark, or quotation marks.

> Although several trade organizations opposed the legislation (there were at least three paid lobbyists working on Capitol Hill), the bill passed easily.
> The conference was held in Portland (Me., not Ore.).
> After waiting in line for an hour (why do we do these things?), we finally left.

A parenthetical expression within a sentence does not require capitalization unless it is a quoted sentence.

> He was totally confused ("What can we do?") and refused to see anyone.

14. If a parenthetical expression within a sentence is composed of two independent clauses, a semicolon rather than a period usually separates them. Independent sentences enclosed together in parentheses employ normal sentence capitalization and punctuation.

> We visited several showrooms, looked at the prices (it wasn't a pleasant experience; prices in this area have not gone down), and asked all the questions we could think of.
> We visited several showrooms and looked at the prices. (It wasn't a pleasant experience. Prices in this area have not gone down.)

Entire paragraphs are rarely enclosed in parentheses; instead, paragraphs of incidental material often appear as footnotes or endnotes.

15. No punctuation (other than a period after an abbreviation) is placed immediately before an opening parenthesis within a sentence; if punctuation is required, it follows the final parenthesis.

> I'll get back to you tomorrow (Friday), when I have more details.
> Tickets cost $14 in advance ($12 for seniors); the price at the door is $18.
> The relevant figures are shown below (in millions of dollars):

16. Parentheses sometimes appear within parentheses when no confusion would result; alternatively, the inner parentheses are replaced with brackets.

> Checks must be drawn in U.S. dollars. (*Please note:* We cannot accept checks drawn on Canadian banks for amounts less than four U.S. dollars ($4.00). The same regulation applies to Canadian money orders.)

17. Dashes and parentheses may be used together to set off parenthetical material. (For details, see paragraph 12 on page 342.)

> The orchestra is spirited, and the cast—an expert and enthusiastic crew of Savoyards (some of them British imports)—comes through famously.

PERIOD

Periods almost always serve to mark the end of a sentence or abbreviation.

1. A period ends a sentence or a sentence fragment that is neither a question nor an exclamation.

From the Format menu, choose Style.
Robert decided to bring champagne.
Unlikely. In fact, inconceivable.

Only one period ends a sentence.

The jellied gasoline was traced to the Trenton-based Quality Products, Inc.
Miss Toklas states categorically that "This is the best way to cook frogs' legs."

2. A period punctuates some abbreviations. No space follows an internal period within an abbreviation. (For details on punctuating abbreviations, see the section beginning on page 400.)

Assn.	Dr.	p.m.
Ph.D.	e.g.	etc.

3. Periods are used with a person's initials, each followed by a space. (Newspaper style omits the space.) If the initials replace the name, they are unspaced and may also be written without periods.

J. B. S. Haldane
L.B.J.   *or*   LBJ

4. A period follows numerals and letters when they are used without parentheses in outlines and vertical lists.

I. Objectives   Required skills are:
  A. Economy   1. Shorthand
    1. Low initial cost   2. Typing
    2. Low maintenance cost   3. Transcription
  B. Ease of operation

5. A period is placed within quotation marks, even when it did not punctuate the original quoted material. (In British practice, the period goes outside the quotation marks whenever it does not belong to the original quoted material.)

The founder was known to his employees as "the old man."
"I said I wanted to fire him," Henry went on, "but she said, 'I don't think you have the contractual privilege to do that.'"

6. When brackets or parentheses enclose an independent sentence, the period is placed inside them. When brackets or parentheses enclose a sentence that is part of a larger sentence, the period for the enclosed sentence is omitted.

Arturo finally arrived on the 23rd with the terrible news that Katrina had been detained by the police. [This later proved to be false; see letter 255.]
I took a good look at her (she was standing quite close to me).

QUESTION MARK

The question mark always indicates a question or doubt.

1. A question mark ends a direct question.

What went wrong?
"When do they arrive?" she asked.

A question mark follows a period only when the period punctuates an abbreviation. No period follows a question mark.

> Is he even an M.D.?
> "Will you arrive by 10 p.m.?"
> A local professor would be giving a paper with the title "Economic Stagnation or Equilibrium?"

2. Polite requests that are worded as questions usually take periods, because they are not really questions. Conversely, a sentence that is intended as a question but whose word order is that of a statement is punctuated with a question mark.

> Could you please send the necessary forms.
> They flew in yesterday?

3. The question mark ends a question that forms part of a sentence. An indirect question is not followed by a question mark.

> What was her motive? you may be asking.
> I naturally wondered, Will it really work?
> I naturally wondered whether it would really work.
> He asked when the report was due.

4. The question mark punctuates each element of a series of questions that share a single beginning and are neither numbered nor lettered. When the series is numbered or lettered, only one question mark is generally used.

> Can you give us a reasonable forecast? Back up your predictions? Compare them with last year's earnings?
> Can you (1) give us a reasonable forecast, (2) back up your predictions, and (3) compare them with last year's earnings?

5. The question mark indicates uncertainty about a fact or the accuracy of a transcription.

> Homer, Greek epic poet (9th–8th? cent. B.C.)
> He would have it that Farjeon[?] is the onlie man for us.

6. The question mark is placed inside brackets, dashes, parentheses, or quotation marks when it punctuates only the material enclosed by them and not the sentence as a whole. It is placed outside them when it punctuates the entire sentence.

> I took a vacation in 1992 (was it really that long ago?), but I haven't had time for one since.
> What did Andrew mean when he called the project "a fiasco from the start"?
> Williams then asks, "Do you realize the extent of the problem [the housing shortage]?"

QUOTATION MARKS

The following paragraphs describe the use of quotation marks to enclose quoted matter in regular text, and for other, less frequent uses. For the use of quotation marks to enclose titles, see paragraph 70 on pages 375–76.

Basic Uses

1. Quotation marks enclose direct quotations but not indirect quotations or paraphrases.

> Dr. Mee added, "We'd be grateful for anything you could do."
> "We just got the lab results," he crowed, "and the blood types match!"
> "I'm leaving," she whispered. "This meeting could go on forever."
> "Mom, we *tried* that already!" they whined in unison.
> "Ssshh!" she hissed.
> She said she was leaving.
> Algren once said something like, Don't ever play poker with anyone named Doc, and never eat at a diner called Mom's.

2. Quotation marks enclose fragments of quoted matter.

> The agreement makes it clear that he "will be paid only upon receipt of an acceptable manuscript."
> As late as 1754, documents refer to him as "yeoman" and "husbandman."

3. Quotation marks enclose words or phrases borrowed from others, and words of obvious informality introduced into formal writing. Words introduced as specialized terminology are sometimes enclosed in quotation marks but more often italicized.

> Be sure to send a copy of your résumé—or as some folks would say, your "biodata summary."
> They were afraid the patient had "stroked out"—had had a cerebrovascular accident.
> referred to as "closed" or "privately held" corporations
> *but more frequently*
> referred to as *closed* or *privately held* corporations
> New Hampshire's only "green" B&B

4. Quotation marks are sometimes used to enclose words referred to as words. Italics are also frequently used for this purpose.

> changed every "he" to "she"
> *or*
> changed every *he* to *she*

5. Quotation marks may enclose representations of sounds, though these are also frequently italicized.

> If it sounds like "quank, quank" [*or* like *quank, quank*], it may be the green treefrog.

6. Quotation marks often enclose short sentences that fall within longer sentences, especially when the shorter sentence is meant to suggest spoken dialogue. Mottoes and maxims, unspoken or imaginary dialogue, and sentences referred to as sentences may all be treated in this way.

> On the gate was the inscription "Arbeit macht frei" [or *Arbeit macht frei*]—"Work will make you free."
> The fact was, the poor kid didn't know "C'mere" from "Sic 'em."
> In effect, the voters were saying "You blew it, and you don't get another chance."
> Their reaction could only be described as "Kill the messenger."
> She never got used to their "That's the way it goes" attitude.
> *or*
> She never got used to their that's-the-way-it-goes attitude.

Quotation marks are often omitted in sentences of this kind when the structure is clear without them. (For the use of commas in such sentences, see paragraphs 29–30 on pages 336–37.)

> The first rule is, When in doubt, spell it out.

7. Direct questions are enclosed in quotation marks when they represent quoted dialogue, but usually not otherwise.

> She asked, "What went wrong?"
> The question is, What went wrong?
> We couldn't help wondering, Where's the plan?
> *or*
> We couldn't help wondering, "Where's the plan?"

8. Quotation marks enclose translations of foreign or borrowed terms.

> This is followed by the Dies Irae ("Day of Wrath"), a climactic movement in many settings of the Requiem.
> The term comes from the Latin *sesquipedalis,* meaning "a foot and a half long."

They also frequently enclose definitions.

> *Concupiscent* simply means "lustful."
> *or*
> *Concupiscent* simply means lustful.

9. Quotation marks sometimes enclose letters referred to as letters.

> The letter "m" is wider than the letter "i."
> Put an "x" in the right spot

However, such letters are more frequently italicized (or underlined), or left undifferentiated from the surrounding text where no confusion would result.

> How many *e*'s are in her name?
> a V-shaped blade
> He was happy to get a B in the course.

With Longer Quotations

10. Quotation marks are not used with longer passages of prose or poetry that are indented as separate paragraphs, called *extracts* or *block quotations.* Quoted text is usually set as an extract when it is longer than a sentence or runs to at least four lines, but individual requirements of consistency, clarity, or emphasis may alter these limits. Extracts are set off from the normal text by (1) indenting the passage on the left, and often on the right as well, and (2) usually setting it in smaller type. Extracts are usually preceded by a sentence ending with a colon, and they usually begin with a capitalized first word. The first line of an extract has no added indention; however, if the extract consists of more than one paragraph, the subsequent paragraphs are indented. (For the use of ellipsis points to show omissions within extracts, see the section beginning on page 343.)

> The chapter begins with a general description of memos:
>
> > The interoffice memorandum or memo is a means of informal communication within a firm or organization. It replaces the salutation, complimentary close, and written signature of the letter with identifying headings.

If the extract continues the flow of an incomplete sentence, no punctuation is required and the extract begins with a lowercase letter.

> They describe the memo as
>
> > a means of informal communication within a firm or organization. It replaces the salutation, complimentary close, and written signature of the letter with identifying headings.

If the sentence preceding the extract does not refer directly to it, the sentence usually ends with a period, though a colon is also common.

> As of the end of April she believed that the product stood a good chance of success.
>
> > Unit sales are strong, revenues are better than forecast, shipments are being made on schedule, and inventory levels are stable.

11. When an extract itself includes quoted material, double quotation marks enclose the material.

> The authors recommend the following procedure:
>
> > The presiding officer will call for the appropriate report from an officer, board member, standing committee, or special committee by saying, "Will the chairperson of the Ways and Means Committee please present the committee's report?'

12. When poetry is set as an extract, the lines are divided exactly as in the original. A spaced slash separates lines of run-in poetry.

> The experience reminded them of Pope's observation:
>
> > A little learning is a dang'rous thing;
> > Drink deep, or taste not the Pierian spring:
> > There shallow draughts intoxicate the brain,
> > And drinking largely sobers us again.

When Gerard Manley Hopkins wrote that "Nothing is so beautiful as spring— / When weeds, in wheels, shoot long and lovely and lush," he probably had my yard in mind.

13. Quotation marks are not used with epigraphs. However, they are generally used with advertising blurbs.

The whole of science is nothing more than a refinement of everyday thinking.
—Albert Einstein
"A brutal irony, a slam-bang humor and a style of writing as balefully direct as a death sentence."—*Time*

With Other Punctuation

14. When a period or comma follows text enclosed in quotation marks, it is placed within the quotation marks, even if the original language quoted was not followed by a period or comma.

He smiled and said, "I'm happy for you."
But perhaps Pound's most perfect poem was "The Return."
The cameras were described as "waterproof," but "moisture-resistant" would have been a better description.

In British usage, the period or comma goes outside the quoted matter whenever the original text did not include the punctuation.

15. When a colon or semicolon follows text enclosed in quotation marks, the colon or semicolon is placed outside the quotation marks.

But they all chimed in on "O Sole Mio": raw adolescents, stately matrons, decrepit old pensioners, their voices soaring in passion together.
She spoke of her "little cottage in the country"; she might better have called it a mansion.

16. The dash, question mark, and exclamation point are placed inside quotation marks when they punctuate the quoted matter only, but outside the quotation marks when they punctuate the whole sentence.

"I can't see how—" he started to say.
He thought he knew where he was going—he remembered her saying, "Take two lefts, then stay to the right"—but the streets didn't look familiar.
He asked, "When did they leave?"
What is the meaning of "the open door"?
She collapsed in her seat with a stunned "Good God!"
Save us from his "mercy"!

Single Quotation Marks

17. Single quotation marks replace double quotation marks when the quoted material occurs within quoted material.

The witness said, "I distinctly heard him say, 'Don't be late,' and then I heard the door close."

> "We'd like to close tonight with that great Harold Arlen wee-hours standard, 'One for My Baby.'"
>
> This analysis is indebted to Del Banco's "Elizabeth Bishop's 'Insomnia': An Inverted View."

When both single and double quotation marks occur at the end of a sentence, the period falls within both sets of marks.

> The witness said, "I distinctly heard him say, 'Don't be late.'"

British usage often reverses American usage, enclosing quoted material in single quotation marks, and enclosing quotations within quotations in double quotation marks. In British usage, commas and periods following quoted material go inside only those quotation marks that enclose material that originally included the period or comma.

18. A quotation within a quotation within a quotation is usually enclosed in double quotation marks. (Such constructions are usually avoided by rewriting.)

> As the *Post* reported it, "Van Houten's voice can be clearly heard saying, 'She said "You wouldn't dare" and I said "I just did."'"
>
> *or*
>
> The *Post* reported that Van Houten's voice was clearly heard saying, "She said 'You wouldn't dare' and I said 'I just did.'"

SEMICOLON

The semicolon may be used much like the comma, period, or colon, depending on the context. Like a comma, it may separate elements in a series. Like a period or colon, it frequently marks the end of a complete clause, and like a colon it signals that the remainder of the sentence is closely related to the first part. However, in each case the semicolon is normally used in a distinctive way. It serves as a higher-level comma; it connects clauses, as a period does not; and it does not imply any following exemplification, amplification, or description, as a colon generally does.

Between Clauses

1. A semicolon separates related independent clauses joined without a coordinating conjunction.

> Cream the shortening and sugar; add the eggs and beat well.
>
> The river rose and overflowed its banks; roads became flooded and impassable; freshly plowed fields disappeared from sight.

2. A semicolon often replaces a comma between two clauses joined by a coordinating conjunction if the sentence might otherwise be confusing—for example, because of particularly long clauses or the presence of other commas.

> In a society that seeks to promote social goals, government will play a powerful role; and taxation, once simply a means of raising money, becomes, in addition, a way of furthering those goals.

3. A semicolon joins two clauses when the second includes a conjunctive adverb such as *accordingly, however, indeed,* or *thus,* or a phrase that acts like a conjunctive adverb such as *in that case, as a result,* or *on the other hand.*

> Most people are covered by insurance of some kind; indeed, many don't even see their medical bills.
>
> It won't be easy to sort out the facts; a decision must be made, however.
>
> The case could take years to work its way through the courts; as a result, many plaintiffs will accept settlements.

When *so* and *yet* are treated as conjunctive adverbs, they are often preceded by a semicolon and followed by a comma. When treated as coordinating conjunctions, as they usually are, they are generally only preceded by a comma.

> The new recruits were bright, diligent, and even enthusiastic; yet[,] the same problems persisted.
>
> His grades improved sharply, yet the high honor roll still eluded him.

4. A semicolon may join two statements when the second clause is elliptical, omitting essential words that are supplied by the first. In short sentences, a comma often replaces the semicolon.

> The conference sessions, designed to allow for full discussions, were much too long; the breaks between them, much too short.
>
> The aged Scotch was haunting, the Asiago piquant.

5. When a series of clauses are separated by semicolons and a coordinating conjunction precedes the final clause, the final semicolon is sometimes replaced with a comma.

> The bars had all closed hours ago; a couple of coffee shops were open but deserted[; *or* ,] and only a few lighted upper-story windows gave evidence of other victims of insomnia.

6. A semicolon is often used before introductory expressions such as *for example, that is,* and *namely,* in place of a colon, comma, dash, or parenthesis. (For more details, see paragraph 17 on pages 333–34.)

> On one point only did everyone agree; namely, too much money had been spent already.
>
> We were fairly successful on that project; that is, we made our deadlines and met our budget.

In a Series

7. A semicolon is used in place of a comma to separate phrases or items in a series when the phrases or items themselves contain commas. A comma may replace the semicolon before a conjunction that precedes the last item in a series.

> The assets in question include $22 million in land, buildings, and equipment; $34 million in cash, investments, and accounts receivable; and $8 million in inventory.

> The votes against were: Precinct 1, 418; Precinct 2, 332; Precinct 3, 256.
>
> The debate about the nature of syntactic variation continues to this day (Labov 1991; Dines 1991, 1993; Romaine 1995).
>
> The Pissarro exhibition will travel to Washington, D.C.; Manchester, N.H.; Portland, Ore., and Oakland, Calif.

When the items in a series are long or are sentences themselves, they are usually separated by semicolons even if they lack internal commas.

> Among the committee's recommendations were the following: more hospital beds in urban areas where there are waiting lines for elective surgery; smaller staff size in half-empty rural hospitals; and review procedures for all major purchases.

With Other Punctuation

8. A semicolon that punctuates the larger sentence is placed outside quotation marks and parentheses.

> I heard the senator on yesterday's "All Things Considered"; his views on Medicare are encouraging.
>
> She found him urbane and entertaining (if somewhat overbearing); he found her charmingly ingenuous.

SLASH

The slash (also known as the *virgule, diagonal, solidus, oblique,* and *slant*) is most commonly used in place of a short word or a hyphen or en dash, or to separate numbers or text elements. There is generally no space on either side of the slash.

1. A slash represents the words *per* or *to* when used between units of measure or the terms of a ratio.

> 40,000 tons/year
> 29 mi/gal
> price/earnings ratio   *or*   price–earnings ratio
> cost/benefit analysis   *or*   cost–benefit analysis
> a 50/50 split   *or*   a 50–50 split
> 20/20 vision

2. A slash separates alternatives, usually representing the words *or* or *and/or.*

> alumni/ae
> his/her
> the *affect/effect* problem   *or*   the *affect-effect* problem

3. A slash replaces the word *and* in some compound terms.

> air/sea cruise   *or*   air-sea cruise
> the May/June issue   *or*   the May-June issue

1996/97   *or*   1996–97
travel/study trip   *or*   travel-study trip

4. A slash is sometimes used to replace certain prepositions such as *at, versus,* and *for.*

U.C./Berkeley   *or*   U.C.–Berkeley
parent/child issues   *or*   parent–child issues
Vice President/Editorial   *or*   Vice President, Editorial

5. A slash punctuates a few abbreviations.

w/o [*for* without]
c/o [*for* care of]
I/O [*for* input/output]
d/b/a [*for* doing business as]
w/w [*for* wall-to-wall]
o/a [*for* on or about]

6. The slash separates the elements in a numerical date, and numerators and denominators in fractions.

11/29/95
2 3/16 inches wide   *or*   2 $\frac{3}{16}$ inches wide
a 7/8-mile course   *or*   a $\frac{7}{8}$-mile course

7. The slash separates lines of poetry that are run in with the text around them. A space is usually inserted before and after the slash.

Alexander Pope once observed: "'Tis with our judgments as our watches, none / Go just alike, yet each believes his own."

Capitals and Italics

Words and phrases are capitalized or italicized (underlining takes the place of italics in typed or handwritten text) to indicate that they have a special significance in particular contexts. (Quotation marks sometimes perform the same functions; see paragraphs 69–71 on pages 375–76 and the section on quotation marks beginning on page 352.)

BEGINNINGS

1. The first word of a sentence or sentence fragment is capitalized.

They make a desert and call it peace.
So many men, so many opinions.
O times! O customs!

2. The first word of a sentence contained within parentheses is capitalized. However, a parentheticalal sentence occurring inside another sentence is not capitalized unless it is a complete quoted sentence.

> No one answered the telephone. (They were probably on vacation.)
> The road remains almost impassable (the locals don't seem to care), and the journey is only for the intrepid.
> After waiting in line for an hour (what else could we do?), we finally left.
> In the primary election Evans placed third ("My campaign started late").

3. The first word of a direct quotation is capitalized. However, if the quotation is interrupted in mid- sentence, the second part does not begin with a capital.

> The department manager explained, "We have no budget for new computers."
> "We have no budget for new computers," explained the department manager, "but we may next year."

4. When a quotation, whether a sentence fragment or a complete sentence, is syntactically dependent on the sentence in which it occurs, the quotation does not begin with a capital.

> The brochure promised a tour of "the most exotic ancient sites."
> His first response was that "there is absolutely no truth to the reports."

5. The first word of a sentence within a sentence that is not a direct quotation is usually capitalized. Examples include mottoes and rules, unspoken or imaginary dialogue, sentences referred to as sentences, and direct questions. (For the use of commas and quotation marks with such sentences, see paragraphs 30–31 on pages 336–37 and paragraphs 6–7 on page 353.)

> You know the saying "Fools rush in where angels fear to tread."
> The first rule is, When in doubt, spell it out.
> One ballot proposition sought to enforce the sentencing rule of "Three strikes and you're out."
> My question is, When can we go?

6. The first word of a line of poetry is traditionally capitalized. However, in the poetry of this century line beginnings are often lowercased. The poem's original capitalization is always reproduced.

> Death is the mother of beauty, mystical,
> Within whose burning bosom we devise
> Our earthly mothers waiting, sleeplessly.
>
> > —Wallace Stevens

> > If tributes cannot
> be implicit,
> give me diatribes and the fragrance of iodine,
> the cork oak acorn grown in Spain . . .
>
> > —Marianne Moore

7. The first word following a colon is lowercased when it begins a list and usually lowercased when it begins a complete sentence. However, when

the sentence introduced is lengthy and distinctly separate from the preceding clause, it is often capitalized.

> In the early morning they broadcast an urgent call for three necessities: bandages, antibiotics, and blood.
> The advantage of this system is clear: it's inexpensive.
> The situation is critical: This company cannot hope to recoup the fourth-quarter losses that were sustained in five operating divisions.

8. If a colon introduces a series of sentences, the first word of each sentence is capitalized.

> Consider the steps we have taken: A subcommittee has been formed to evaluate past performance. New sources of revenue are being explored. Several candidates have been interviewed for the new post of executive director.

9. The first words of items that form complete sentences in run-in lists are usually capitalized, as are the first words of items in vertical lists. However, numbered phrases within a sentence are lowercased. For details, see the section beginning on page 421.

10. The first word in an outline heading is capitalized.

> I. Editorial tasks
> II. Production responsibilities
>   A. Cost estimates
>   B. Bids

11. In minutes and legislation, the introductory words *Whereas* and *Resolved* are capitalized (and *Resolved* is also italicized). The word immediately following is also capitalized.

> Whereas, Substantial benefits . . .
> *Resolved,* That . . .

12. The first word and certain other words of the salutation of a letter and the first word of a complimentary close are capitalized.

> Dear Sir or Madam: Sincerely yours,
> Ladies and Gentlemen: Very truly yours,
> To whom it may concern:

13. The first word and each subsequent major word following a SUBJECT or TO heading in a memorandum are capitalized.

> SUBJECT: Pension Plans
> TO: All Department Heads and Editors

PROPER NOUNS AND ADJECTIVES

The following paragraphs describe the ways in which a broad range of proper nouns and adjectives are styled. Capitals are always employed, sometimes in conjunction with italics or quotation marks.

Abbreviations

1. Abbreviated forms of proper nouns and adjectives are capitalized, just as the spelled-out forms would be. (For details on capitalizing abbreviations, see the section beginning on page 402.)

> Jan. [*for* January]
> NATO [*for* North Atlantic Treaty Organization]

Abstractions and Personifications

2. Abstract concepts and qualities are sometimes capitalized when the concept or quality is being personified. If the term is simply used in conjunction with other words that allude to human characteristics or qualities, it is not capitalized.

> as Autumn paints each leaf in fiery colors
> the statue of Justice with her scales
> hoping that fate would lend a hand

Academic Degrees

3. The names of academic degrees are capitalized when they follow a person's name. The names of specific degrees used without a person's name are usually lowercased. More general names for degrees are lowercased.

> Lawton I. Byrne, Doctor of Laws
> earned his associate in science degree   *or*   earned his Associate in Science degree
> completed course work for his doctorate
> working for a master's degree

Abbreviations for academic degrees are always capitalized. (For details, see paragraphs 11–12 on page 406.)

> Susan L. Wycliff, M.S.W.
> received her Ph.D. in clinical psychology

Animals and Plants

4. The common names of animals and plants are not capitalized unless they contain a proper noun, in which case the proper noun is usually capitalized and any name element preceding (but not following) it is often capitalized. When in doubt, consult a dictionary. (For scientific names, see the section on pages 373–74.)

> the springer spaniel   Queen Anne's lace
> Holstein cows   black-eyed Susan
> California condor   mayflower
> a Great Dane   jack-in-the-pulpit

Awards and Prizes

5. Names of awards and prizes are capitalized. Words and phrases that are not actually part of the award's name are lowercased.

Academy Award	Nobel Prize winner
Emmy	Nobel Prize in medicine
Rhodes Scholarship	*but*
Rhodes scholar	Nobel Peace Prize
Pulitzer Prize–winning novelist	

Derivatives of Proper Names

6. Derivatives of proper names are capitalized when used in their primary sense. If the derived term has taken on a specialized meaning, it is often lowercased. Consult a dictionary when in doubt.

Roman sculpture	pasteurized milk
Viennese culture	french fries
Victorian prudery	*but*
a Britishism	American cheese
Hodgkins disease	Dutch door
chinaware	

Geographical and Topographical References

7. Terms that identify divisions of the earth's surface and distinct areas, regions, places, or districts are capitalized, as are derivative nouns and adjectives.

the Pacific Rim	Burgundy
the Great Lakes	Burgundians
Arnhem Land	the Highlands
the Golan Heights	Highland attitudes

8. Popular names of localities are capitalized.

| Little Italy | the Sunbelt |
| the Left Bank | the Big Easy |

9. Compass points are capitalized when they refer to a geographical region or form part of a street name. They are lowercased when they refer to a simple direction.

the Southwest	North Pole
West Coast	north of the Rio Grande
North Atlantic	born in the East
East Pleasant Street	driving east on I-90

10. Nouns and adjectives that are derived from compass points and that designate or refer to a specific geographical region are usually capitalized.

| Southern hospitality | Southwestern recipes |
| Easterners | Northern Europeans |

11. Words designating global, national, regional, and local political divisions are capitalized when they are essential elements of specific names. They are usually lowercased when they precede a proper name or are not part of a specific name.

the Roman Empire	the state of New York
British Commonwealth nations	the Third Precinct
New York State	voters in three precincts

In legal documents, such words are often capitalized regardless of position.

the State of New York

12. Common geographical terms (such as *lake, mountain, river,* or *valley*) are capitalized if they are part of a proper name.

Lake Tanganyika	Cape of Good Hope
Great Salt Lake	Massachusetts Bay
Atlas Mountains	Cayman Islands
Mount Everest	Yosemite Valley

13. Common geographical terms preceding names are usually capitalized.

Lakes Huron and Erie
Mounts McKinley and Whitney

When *the* precedes the common term, the term is lowercased.

the river Nile

14. Common geographical terms that are not used as part of a single proper name are not capitalized. These include plural terms that follow two or more proper names, and terms that are used descriptively or alone.

the Indian and South Pacific oceans
the Mississippi and Missouri rivers
the Pacific coast of Mexico
Caribbean islands
the river delta

15. The names of streets, monuments, parks, landmarks, well-known buildings, and other public places are capitalized. However, common terms that are part of these names (such as *street, park,* or *bridge*) are lowercased when they occur after multiple names or are used alone.

State Street	Golden Gate Bridge
the Lincoln Memorial	Empire State Building
Statue of Liberty	Beverly Hills Hotel
the Pyramids	back to the hotel
Grant Park	Main and Oak streets

Well-known shortened forms of place-names are capitalized.

the Hill [*for* Capitol Hill]
the Channel [*for* English Channel]
the Street [*for* Wall Street]

Governmental, Judicial, and Political Bodies

16. Full names of legislative, deliberative, executive, and administrative bodies are capitalized, as are easily recognizable short forms of these names. However, nonspecific noun and adjective references to them are usually lowercased.

United States Congress	the Fed
Congress	congressional hearings
the House	a federal agency

    When words such as *department, committee,* or *agency* are used in place of a full name, they are most often capitalized when the department or agency is referring to itself, but otherwise usually lowercased.

    This Department welcomes constructive criticism . . .
    The department claimed to welcome such criticism . . .

    When such a word is used in the plural to describe more than one specific body, it is usually capitalized when it precedes the names and lowercased when it follows them.

    involving the Departments of State and Justice
    a briefing from the State and Justice department

17. Full names of high courts are capitalized. Short forms of such names are often capitalized in legal documents but lowercased otherwise.

    . . . in the U.S. Court of Appeals for the Ninth Circuit
    International Court of Justice
    The court of appeals [*or* Court of Appeals] held . . .
    the Virginia Supreme Court
    a federal district court
    the state supreme court

    However, both the full and short names of the U.S. Supreme Court are capitalized.

    the Supreme Court of the United States
    the Supreme Court
    the Court

18. Names of city and county courts are usually lowercased.

the Springfield municipal court	the county court
small-claims court	juvenile court

19. The noun *court,* when it applies to a specific judge or presiding officer, is capitalized in legal documents.

    It is the opinion of this Court that . . .
    The Court found that . . .

20. The terms *federal* and *national* are capitalized only when they are essential elements of a name or title. (*Federal* is also capitalized when it refers to

a historical architectural style, to members of the original Federalist party, or to adherents of the Union in the Civil War.)

Federal Election Commission   National Security Council
a federal commission   national security
Federalist principles

21. The word *administration* is sometimes capitalized when it refers to the administration of a specific U.S. president, but is more commonly lowercased. Otherwise, it is lowercased except when it is a part of the official name of a government agency.

the Reagan administration   *or*   the Reagan Administration
the administration   *or*   the Administration
from one administration to the next
the Social Security Administration

22. Names of political organizations and their adherents are capitalized, but the word *party* is often lowercased.

the Democratic National Committee
the Republican platform
the Christian Coalition
most Republicans
the Democratic party   *or*   the Democratic Party
party politics

Names of less-distinct political groupings are usually lowercased, as are their derivative forms.

the right wing
the liberals
the conservative agenda
  but often
the Left
the Right

23. Terms describing political and economic philosophies are usually lowercased; if derived from proper names, they are usually capitalized. Consult a dictionary for doubtful cases.

authoritarianism   nationalism
democracy   social Darwinist
fascism *or* Fascism   Marxist

Historical Periods and Events

24. The names of some historical and cultural periods and movements are capitalized. When in doubt, consult a dictionary or encyclopedia.

Bronze Age   Third Reich
Middle Ages   the atomic age
Prohibition   Victorian era

the Renaissance   age of Pericles
New Deal   the baby boom
Fifth Republic

25. Century and decade designations are normally lowercased.

the nineteenth century
the twenties
the turn of the century
a 12th-century manuscript
   but
Gay Nineties
Roaring Twenties

26. The names of conferences, councils, expositions, and specific sporting, cultural, and historical events are capitalized.

Fourth World Conference on   Cannes Film Festival
  Women   Miss America Contest
Council of Trent   San Francisco Earthquake
New York World's Fair   Johnstown Flood
Super Bowl

27. Full names of specific treaties, laws, and acts are capitalized.

Treaty of Versailles
the Nineteenth Amendment
the Bill of Rights
Clean Air Act of 1990
   but
gun-control laws
an equal-rights amendment

28. The words *war, revolution,* and *battle* are capitalized when they are part of a full name. Official names of actions are capitalized. Descriptive terms such as *assault* and *siege* are usually lowercased even when used in conjunction with a place-name.

War of the Roses
World War II
the French Revolution
Battle of Gettysburg
Operation Desert Storm
between the two world wars
the American and French revolutions
the siege of Leningrad
Washington's winter campaign

Hyphenated Compounds

29. The second (third, etc.) element of a hyphenated compound is generally capitalized only if it is itself a proper noun or adjective. (For hyphenated titles, see paragraph 65 below.)

Arab-Israeli negotiations
East-West trade agreements
French-speaking peoples

Forty-second street
twentieth-century architecture

30. When joined to a proper noun or adjective, common prefixes (such as *pre-* or *anti-*) are usually lowercased, but geographical and ethnic combining forms (such as *Anglo-* or *Sino-*) are capitalized. (For details, see paragraphs 45 and 52 on pages 397 and 398–99.)

anti-Soviet forces
Sino-Japanese relations

Legal Material

31. The names of the plaintiff and defendant in legal case titles are italicized. The *v.* (for *versus*) may be roman or italic. Cases that do not involve two opposing parties are also italicized. When the party involved rather than the case itself is being discussed, the reference is not italicized. In running text, a case name involving two opposing parties may be shortened.

Jones v. *Massachusetts*
Smith et al. v. Jones
In re Jones
She covered the Jones trial for the newspaper.
The judge based his ruling on a precedent set in the *Jones* decision.

Medical Terms

32. Proper names that are elements in terms designating diseases, symptoms, syndromes, and tests are capitalized. Common nouns are lowercased; however, abbreviations of such nouns are all-capitalized.

Alzheimer's disease
Tourette's syndrome
Schick test

black lung disease
mumps
AIDS

33. Scientific names of disease-causing organisms follow the rules discussed in paragraph 58 on page 373. The names of diseases or conditions derived from scientific names of organisms are lowercased and not italicized.

a neurotoxin produced by *Clostridium botulinum*
nearly died of botulism

34. Generic names of drugs are lowercased; trade names should be capitalized.

retinoic acid
Retin-A

Military Terms

35. The full titles of branches of the U.S. armed forces are capitalized, as are standard short forms.

| U.S. Marine Corps | the Marines |
| the Marine Corps | the Corps |

Those of other countries are capitalized when the precise title is used; otherwise they are usually lowercased. The plurals of *army, navy, air force,* and *coast guard* are lowercased.

Royal Air Force
the Guatemalan army
the tiny armies of both countries

The modifiers *army, navy, marine coast, guard,* and *air force* are usually lowercased; *naval* is lowercased unless it is part of an official name. The noun *marine* is usually lowercased.

an army helicopter	the first naval engagement
a career navy man	the Naval Reserves
the marine barracks	a former marine

Full or shortened names of specific units of a branch are usually capitalized.

U.S. Army Corps of Engineers
the Third Army
the Eighty-second [*or* 82nd] Airborne
the U.S. Special Forces, or Green Berets
. . . of the First Battalion. The battalion commander . . .

36. Military ranks are capitalized when they precede the names of their holders, or replace the name in direct address. Otherwise they are lowercased.

Major General Smedley Butler
Please be seated, Admiral.
The major arrived precisely on time.

37. The names of decorations, citations, and medals are capitalized.

Medal of Honor
Purple Heart

Numerical Designations

38. A noun introducing a reference number is usually capitalized. The abbreviation *No.* is usually omitted.

| Order 704 | Form 2E |
| Flight 409 | Policy 118–4-Y |

39. Nouns used with numbers or letters to refer to major reference entities or actual captions in books or periodicals are usually capitalized. Nouns that designate minor reference entities and do not appear in captions are lowercased.

| Book II | Figure D.4 |
| Volume 5 | page 101 |

Chapter 2   line 8
Table 3   paragraph 6.1
Example 16.2   question 21

Organizations

40. Names of organizations, corporations, and institutions, and terms derived from those names to designate their members, are capitalized.

> the League of Women Voters
> General Motors Corporation
> the Smithsonian Institution
> the University of the South
> the Rotary Club
> all Rotarians

Common nouns used descriptively or occurring after the names of two or more organizations are lowercased.

> enrolled at the university
> Yale and Harvard universities
>   *but*
> the Universities of Utah and Nevada

41. Words such as *agency, department, division, group,* or *office* that designate corporate and organizational units are capitalized only when used as part of a specific proper name. (For governmental units, see paragraph 16 on page 365.)

> head of the Sales Division of K2 Outfitters
> a memo to the sales divisions of both companies

42. Nicknames for organizations are capitalized.

> the Big Six accounting firms
> referred to IBM as Big Blue
> trading on the Big Board

People

43. The names and initials of persons are capitalized. If a name is hyphenated, both elements are capitalized. Particles forming the initial elements of surnames (such as *de, della, der, du, l', la, le, ten, ter, van,* and *von*) may or may not be capitalized, depending on the practice of the family or individual. However, the particle is always capitalized at the beginning of a sentence. The prefixes *Mac, Mc,* and *O'* are always capitalized.

> Cecil Day-Lewis
> Agnes de Mille
> Cecil B. DeMille
> Walter de la Mare

Mark deW. Howe
Martin Van Buren
. . . of van Gogh's life. Van Gogh's technique is . .

44. A nickname or epithet that either is added to or replaces the name of a person or thing is capitalized.

Babe Ruth   the Sun King
Stonewall Jackson   Deep Throat
Billy the Kid   Big Mama Thornton

A nickname or epithet placed between a person's first and last name is enclosed in quotation marks or parentheses or both. If it precedes the first name, it is sometimes enclosed in quotation marks but more often not.

Charlie "Bird" [*or* ("Bird") *or* (Bird)] Parker
Mother Maybelle Carter

45. Words of family relationship preceding or used in place of a person's name are capitalized; otherwise, they are lowercased.

Uncle Fred   her uncle's book
Mother's birthday   my mother's legacy

46. Words designating languages, nationalities, peoples, races, religious groups, and tribes are capitalized. Designations based on color are usually lowercased.

Spanish   Muslims
Spaniards   Assiniboin
Chinese   both blacks and whites
Asians   white, black, and Hispanic jurors

47. Corporate, professional, and governmental titles are capitalized when they immediately precede a person's name, unless the name is being used as an appositive.

President John Tyler
Professor Wendy Doniger of the University of Chicago
Senator William Fulbright of Arkansas
Arkansas's late former senator, William Fulbright

48. When corporate or governmental titles are used as part of a descriptive phrase to identify a person rather than as part of the name itself, the title is lowercased.

Marcia Ramirez, president of Logex Corp.
the president of Logex Corp., Marcia Ramirez
    but
Logex Corp.'s prospects for the coming year were outlined by President Marcia Ramirez.

49. High governmental titles may be capitalized when used in place of individuals' names. In minutes and official records of proceedings, corporate or organizational titles are capitalized when used in place of individuals' names.

> The Secretary of State objected.
> The Judge will respond to questions in her chambers.
> The Treasurer then stated his misgivings about the project.
> > *but*
> The report reached the senator's desk yesterday.
> The judge's rulings were widely criticized.
> The co-op's treasurer, it turned out, had twice been convicted of embezzlement.

50. The word *president* may be capitalized whenever it refers to the U.S. presidency, but more commonly is capitalized only when it refers to a specific U.S. president.

> It is the duty of the president [*or* President] to submit a budget to Congress.
> The President's budget, due out on Wednesday, is being eagerly awaited.

51. Titles are capitalized when they are used in direct address.

> Is it very contagious, Doctor?
> You may call your next witness, Counselor.

Religious Terms

52. Words designating the supreme being are capitalized. Plural forms such as *gods, goddesses,* and *deities* are not.

> Allah   the Almighty
> Brahma   the Trinity
> Jehovah   in the eyes of God
> Yahweh   the angry gods

53. Personal pronouns referring to the supreme being are often capitalized, especially in religious writing. Relative pronouns (such as *who, whom,* and *whose*) usually are not.

> God gave His [*or* his] Son
> Allah, whose Prophet, Muhammad . . .

54. Traditional designations of apostles, prophets, and saints are capitalized.

> the Madonna   the Twelve
> the Prophet   St. John of the Cross
> Moses the Lawgiver   John the Baptist

55. Names of religions, denominations, creeds and confessions, and religious orders are capitalized, as are adjectives and nouns derived from these names.

Judaism	Eastern Orthodox
Church of England	Islamic
Apostles' Creed	Jesuit teachers
Society of Jesus	a Buddhist

Full names of specific places of worship are capitalized, but terms such as *church, synagogue,* and *mosque* are lowercased when used alone. The word *church* is sometimes capitalized when it refers to the worldwide Catholic Church.

Hunt Memorial Church	Beth Israel Synagogue
the local Baptist church	services at the synagogue

56. Names of the Bible and other sacred works, their books and parts, and versions or editions of them are capitalized but not italicized. Adjectives derived from the names of sacred books are capitalized, except for the words *biblical* and *scriptural.*

Bible	biblical
the Scriptures	Talmud
Revised Standard Version	Talmudic
Old Testament	Koran *or* Qur'an
Book of Revelation	Koranic *or* Qur'anic

57. The names of prayers and well-known passages of the Bible are capitalized.

the Ave Maria	Ten Commandments
Lord's Prayer	Sermon on the Mount
the Our Father	the Beatitudes

Scientific Terms

58. Genus names in biological binomial nomenclature are capitalized; species names are lowercased, even when derived from a proper name. Both names are italicized.

Both the wolf and the domestic dog are included in the genus *Canis.*
The California condor (*Gymnogyps californianus*) is facing extinction.

The names of races, varieties, or subspecies are lowercased and italicized.

Hyla versicolor chrysoscelis
Otis asio naevius

59. The New Latin names of classes, families, and all groups above the genus level in zoology and botany are capitalized but not italicized. Their derivative nouns and adjectives are lowercased.

Gastropoda	gastropod
Thallophyta	thallophytic

60. The names, both scientific and informal, of planets and their satellites, stars, constellations, and other specific celestial objects are capitalized.

However, except in technical writing, the words *sun, earth,* and *moon* are usually lowercased unless they occur with other astronomical names. A generic term that follows the name of a celestial object is usually lowercased.

Jupiter   Mars, Venus, and Earth
the North Star   life on earth
Andromeda   a voyage to the moon
Ursa Major   Halley's comet
the Little Dipper

Names of meterorological phenomena are lowercased.

aurora australis
northern lights
parhelic circle

61. Terms that identify geological eons, eras, periods, systems, epochs, and strata are capitalized. The generic terms that follow them are lowercased.

Mesozoic era   in the Middle Ordovician
Upper Cretaceous epoch   the Age of Reptiles
Quaternary period

62. Proper names that are elements of the names of scientific laws, theorems, and principles are capitalized, but the common nouns *law, theorem, theory,* and the like are lowercased. In the names of popular or fanciful theories or observations, such words are usually capitalized as well.

Mendel's law   Einstein's theory of relativity
the Pythagorean theorem   Murphy's Law
Occam's razor   the Peter Principle

63. The names of computer services and databases are capitalized. Some names of computer languages are written with an initial capital letter, some with all letters capitalized, and some commonly both ways. When in doubt, consult a dictionary.

America Online   BASIC
World Wide Web   Pascal   *or*   PASCAL
CompuServe   Internet   *or*   internet
Microsoft Word

Time Periods and Dates

64. The names of the days of the week, months of the year, and holidays and holy days are capitalized. Names of the seasons are lowercased.

Tuesday   Ramadan
June   Holy Week
Yom Kippur   last winter's storm
Veterans Day

Titles of Works

65. Words in titles of books, magazines, newspapers, plays, movies, long poems, and works of art such as paintings and sculpture are capitalized except for internal articles, coordinating conjunctions, prepositions, and the *to* of infinitives. Prepositions of four or more letters are often capitalized. The entire title is italicized. For sacred works, see paragraph 56 on page 373.

> *Far from* [or *From*] *the Madding Crowd*
> Wolfe's *Of Time and the River*
> *Publishers Weekly*
> *USA Today*
> the original play *A Streetcar Named Desire*
> *All about* [or *About*] *Eve*, with Bette Davis
> Monet's *Water-Lily Pool*, in the Louvre
> Rodin's *Thinker*

The elements of hyphenated compounds in titles are usually capitalized, but articles, coordinating conjunctions, and prepositions are lowercased.

> *The Post-Physician Era: Medicine in the Twenty-First Century*
> *Politics in Early Seventeenth-Century England*

66. The first word following a colon in a title is capitalized.

> *Jane Austen: A Literary Life*

67. An initial article that is part of a title is capitalized and italicized. It is often omitted if it would be awkward in context.

> *The Oxford English Dictionary*
> the 20-volume *Oxford English Dictionary*

68. In the titles of newspapers, the city or local name is usually italicized, but the preceding *the* is usually not italicized or capitalized.

> reported in the *New York Times*
> last Thursday's *Atlanta Constitution*

69. Many periodicals, especially newspapers, do not use italics for titles, but instead either simply capitalize the important words of the title or, more commonly, capitalize the words and enclose the title in quotation marks.

> the NB. column in the Times Literary Supplement
> The Nobel committee singled out Walcott's book-length epic "Omeros."

70. The titles of articles in periodicals, short poems, short stories, essays, lectures, dissertations, chapters of books, radio and television programs, and novellas published in a collection are capitalized and enclosed in quotation marks. The capitalization of articles, conjunctions, and prepositions follows the rules explained in paragraph 65 above.

an article on Rwanda, "After the Genocide," in the *New Yorker*
Robert Frost's "The Death of the Hired Man"
O'Connor's story "Good Country People"
"The Literature of Exhaustion," John Barth's seminal essay
last Friday's lecture, "Labor's Task: A View for the Nineties"
The Jungle Book's ninth chapter is the well-known "Rikki-tikki-tavi."
listening to "All Things Considered"
watched "Good Morning America"

71. The titles of long musical compositions are generally capitalized and italicized; the titles of songs and other short compositions are capitalized and enclosed in quotation marks, as are the popular names of longer works. The titles of compositions identified primarily by their musical forms (such as *quartet, sonata,* or *mass*) are capitalized only, as are movements identified by their tempo markings.

Mozart's *The Magic Flute*
Frank Loesser's *Guys and Dolls*
"The Lady Is a Tramp"
Beethoven's "Für Elise"
the Piano Sonata in C-sharp minor, Op. 27, No. 2, or "Moonlight" Sonata
Symphony No. 104 in D major
Brahms's Violin Concerto in D
the Adagietto movement from Mahler's Fifth Symphony

72. Common titles of book sections (such as *preface, introduction,* or *index*) are usually capitalized when they refer to a section of the same book in which the reference is made. Otherwise, they are usually lowercased. (For numbered sections of books, see paragraph 39 on pages 369–70).

See the Appendix for further information.
In the introduction to her book, the author explains her goals.

Trademarks

73. Registered trademarks, service marks, collective marks, and brand names are capitalized. They do not normally require any further acknowledgment of their special status.

Frisbee	Jacuzzi	Levi's
Coke	Kleenex	Vaseline
College Board	Velcro	Dumpster
Realtor	Xerox	Scotch tape
Walkman	Band-Aid	Teflon

Transportation

74. The names of individual ships, submarines, airplanes, satellites, and space vehicles are capitalized and italicized. The designations *U.S.S., S.S., M.V.,* and *H.M.S.* are not italicized.

Challenger
Enola Gay
H.M.S. *Bounty*

OTHER STYLING CONVENTIONS

1. Foreign words and phrases that have not been fully adopted into English are italicized. In general, any word that appears in the main section of *Merriam-Webster's Collegiate Dictionary* does not need to be italicized.

> These accomplishments will serve as a monument, *aere perennius,* to the group's skill and dedication.
> "The cooking here is *wunderbar!*"
> The prix fixe lunch was $20.
> The committee meets on an ad hoc basis.

A complete foreign-language sentence (such as a motto) can also be italicized. However, long sentences are usually treated as quotations; that is, they are set in roman type and enclosed in quotation marks. (For details, see paragraph 6 on page 353.)

> The inscription *Honi soit qui mal y pense* encircles the seal.

2. In nonfiction writing, unfamiliar words or words that have a specialized meaning are set in italics on their first appearance, especially when accompanied by a short definition. Once these words have been introduced and defined, they are not italicized in subsequent references.

> *Vitiligo* is a condition in which skin pigment cells stop making pigment. Vitiligo usually affects . . .
> Another method is the *direct-to-consumer* transaction, in which the publisher markets directly to the individual by mail or door-to-door.

3. Italics are often used to indicate words referred to as words. However, if the word was actually spoken, it is usually enclosed in quotation marks instead.

> Purists still insist that *data* is a plural noun.
> *Only* can also be an adverb, as in "I *only* tried to help."
> We heard his warning, but we weren't sure what "repercussions" meant in that context.

4. Italics are often used for letters referred to as letters, particularly when they are shown in lowercase.

> You should dot your *i*'s and cross your *t*'s.

If the letter is being used to refer to its sound and not its printed form, slashes or brackets are used instead of italics in technical contexts.

> The pure /p/ sound is rarely heard in the mountain dialect.

A letter used to indicate a shape is capitalized but not italicized. Such letters are often set in sans-serif type.

an A-frame house   Churchill's famous V sign
the I beam   forming a giant X

5. Italics are often used to show numerals referred to as numerals. However, if there is no chance of confusion, they are usually not italicized.

The first *2* and the last *1* are barely legible.
Anyone whose ticket number ends in 4 or 6 will win a door prize.

6. Italics are used to emphasize or draw attention to words in a sentence.

Students must notify the dean's office *in writing* of any added or dropped courses.
It was not *the* model for the project, but merely *a* model.

7. Italics are used to indicate a word created to suggest a sound.

Its call is a harsh, drawn-out *kreee-awww.*

8. Individual letters are sometimes italicized when used for lists within sentences or for identifying elements in an illustration.

providing information about *(a)* typing, *(b)* transcribing, *(c)* formatting, and *(d)* graphics
located at point A on the diagram

9. Commas, colons, and semicolons that follow italicized words are usually italicized.

the Rabbit tetralogy (*Rabbit Run, Rabbit Redux, Rabbit Is Rich,* and *Rabbit at Rest); Bech: A Book; S;* and others

However, question marks, exclamation points, quotation marks, and apostrophes are not italicized unless they are part of an italicized title.

Did you see the latest issue of *Newsweek?*
Despite the greater success of *Oklahoma!* and *South Pacific,* Rodgers was fondest of *Carousel.*
"Over Christmas vacation he finished *War and Peace.*"
Students always mistake the old script *s*'s for *f*'s.

Parentheses and brackets may be italicized if most of the words they enclose are also italicized, or if both the first and last words are italicized.

(see also Limited Partnership)
[German, *wunderbar*]
(and is replaced throughout by *&)*

10. Full capitalization is occasionally used for emphasis or to indicate that a speaker is talking very loudly. It is avoided in formal writing, where italics are far more often used for emphasis.

Term papers received after Friday, May 18, WILL BE RETURNED UNREAD.
Scalpers mingled in the noisy crowd yelling "SIXTY DOLLARS!"

11. The text of signs, labels, and inscriptions may be reproduced in various ways.

> a poster reading SPECIAL THRILLS COMING SOON
> a gate bearing the infamous motto "Arbeit macht frei"
> a Do Not Disturb sign
> a barn with an old CHEW MAIL POUCH ad on the side
> the stop sign

12. *Small capitals,* identical to large capitals but usually about the height of a lowercase *x,* are commonly used for era designations and computer commands. They may also be used for cross-references, for headings in constitutions and bylaws, and for speakers in a dramatic dialogue.

> The dwellings date from A.D. 200 or earlier.
> Press ALT + CTRL + PLUS + SIGN on the numeric keyboard.
> (See LETTERS AS LETTERS, page 162.)
> SECTION IV. The authority for parliamentary procedure in meetings of the Board . . .
> LADY WISHFORT. O dear, has my Nephew made his Addresses to Millamant? I order'd him.
> FOIBLE. Sir Wilfull is set in to drinking, Madam, in the Parlour.

13. *Underlining* indicates italics in typed material. It is almost never seen in typeset text.

14. *Boldface* type has traditionally been used primarily for headings and captions. It is sometimes also used in place of italics for terminology introduced in the text, especially for terms that are accompanied by definitions; for cross-references; for headwords in listings such as glossaries, gazetteers, and bibliographies; and for page references in indexes that locate a specific kind of material, such as illustrations, tables, or the main discussions of a given topic. (In mathematical texts, arrays, tensors, vectors, and matrix notation are standardly set bold as well.)

> **Application Forms and Tests** Many offices require applicants to fill out an employment form. Bring a copy . . .
> **Figure 4.2: The Electromagnetic Spectrum**
> The two axes intersect at a point called the **origin**.
> See **Medical Records**, page 123.
> **antecedent:** the noun to which a pronoun refers
> **appositive:** a word, phrase, or clause that is equivalent to a preceding noun
> Records, medical, **123–37**, 178, 243
> Referrals, **38–40**, 139

Punctuation that follows boldface type is set bold when it is part of a heading or heading-like text; otherwise it is generally set roman.

> **Table 9:** Metric Conversion
> **Warning:** This and similar medications . . .

Excellent fourth-quarter earnings were reported by the pharmaceutical giants **Abbott Laboratories**, **Burroughs Wellcome**, and **Merck**.

Plurals and Possessives

The next sections describe the ways in which plurals, possessives, and compounds are most commonly formed.

In regard to plurals and compounds, consulting a dictionary will solve many of the problems discussed in this chapter. A good college dictionary, such as *Merriam-Webster's Collegiate Dictionary*, will provide plural forms for any common word, as well as a large number of permanent compounds. Any dictionary much smaller than the *Collegiate* will often be more frustrating in what it fails to show than helpful in what it shows.

PLURALS

The basic rules for writing plurals of English words, stated in paragraph 1, apply in the vast majority of cases. The succeeding paragraphs treat the categories of words whose plurals are most apt to raise questions.

Most good dictionaries give thorough coverage to irregular and variant plurals, and many of the rules provided here are reflected in the dictionary entries.

The symbol → is used here to link the singular and plural forms.

1. The plurals of most English words are formed by adding *-s* to the singular. If the noun ends in *-s*, *-x*, *-z*, *-ch*, or *-sh*, so that an extra syllable must be added in order to pronounce the plural, *-es* is added. If the noun ends in a *-y* preceded by a consonant, the *-y* is changed to *-i* and *-es* is added.

voter → voters	blowtorch → blowtorches
anticlimax → anticlimaxes	calabash → calabashes
blitz → blitzes	allegory → allegories

Abbreviations

2. The plurals of abbreviations are commonly formed by adding *-s* or *-'s;* however, there are some significant exceptions. (For details, see paragraphs 1–5 on pages 402–3.)

yr. → yrs.	M.B.A. → M.B.A.'s
TV → TVs	p. → pp.

Animals

3. The names of many fishes, birds, and mammals have both a plural formed with a suffix and one that is identical with the singular. Some have only one or the other.

bass → bass *or* basses   lion → lions
partridge → partridge *or* partridges   sheep → sheep
sable → sables *or* sable

Many of the animals that have both plural forms are ones that are hunted, fished, or trapped; those who hunt, fish for, and trap them are most likely to use the unchanged form. The *-s* form is often used to emphasize diversity of kinds.

caught three bass
but
basses of the Atlantic Ocean
a place where antelope feed
but
antelopes of Africa and southwest Asia

Compounds and Phrases

4. Most compounds made up of two nouns—whether they appear as one word, two words, or a hyphenated word—form their plurals by pluralizing the final element only.

courthouse → courthouses
judge advocate → judge advocates
player-manager → player-managers

5. The plural form of a compound consisting of an *-er* noun and an adverb is made by pluralizing the noun element only.

runner-up → runners-up   diner-out → diners-out
onlooker → onlookers   passerby → passersby

6. Nouns made up of words that are not nouns form their plurals on the last element.

show-off → show-offs
pushover → pushovers
tie-in → tie-ins
lineup → lineups

7. Plurals of compounds that consist of two nouns separated by a preposition are normally formed by pluralizing the first noun.

sister-in-law → sisters-in-law   chief of staff → chiefs of staff
attorney-at-law → attorneys-at-law   grant-in-aid → grants-in-aid
power of attorney → powers of
  attorney

8. Compounds that consist of two nouns separated by a preposition and a modifier form their plurals in various ways.

snake in the grass → snakes in the grass
justice of the peace → justices of the peace

jack-in-the-box → jack-in-the-boxes   *or*   jacks-in-the-box
will-o'-the wisp → will-o'-the-wisps

9. Compounds consisting of a noun followed by an adjective are usually pluralized by adding *-s* to the noun. If the adjective tends to be understood as a noun, the compound may have more than one plural form.

attorney general → attorneys general   *or*   attorney generals
sergeant major → sergeants major   *or*   sergeant majors
poet laureate → poets laureate   *or*   poet laureates
heir apparent → heirs apparent
knight-errant → knights-errant

Foreign Words and Phrases

10. Many nouns of foreign origin retain the foreign plural. However, most also have a regular English plural.

alumnus → alumni
genus → genera
crisis → crises
criterion → criteria
appendix → appendixes   *or*   appendices
concerto → concerti   *or*   concertos
symposium → symposia   *or*   symposiums

11. Phrases of foreign origin may have a foreign plural, an English plural, or both.

pièce de résistance → pièces de résistance
hors d'oeuvre → hors d'oeuvres
beau monde → beau mondes   *or*   beaux mondes

Irregular Plurals

12. A few English nouns form their plurals by changing one or more of their vowels, or by adding *-en* or *-ren.*

foot → feet	woman → women
goose → geese	tooth → teeth
louse → lice	ox → oxen
man → men	child → children
mouse → mice	

13. Some nouns do not change form in the plural. (See also paragraph 3 above.)

series → series	corps → corps
politics → politics	species → species

14. Some nouns ending in *-f, -fe,* and *-ff* have plurals that end in *-ves.* Some of these also have regularly formed plurals.

elf → elves
loaf → loaves
scarf → scarves   *or*   scarfs

wife → wives
staff → staffs   *or*   staves

Italic Elements

15. Italicized words, phrases, abbreviations, and letters are usually pluralized by adding -*s* or -*'s* in roman type. (See also paragraphs 16, 21, and 26 below.)

three *Fortunes* missing from the stack
a couple of *Gravity's Rainbows* in stock
used too many *etc.*'s in the report
a row of *x*'s

Letters

16. The plurals of letters are usually formed by adding -*'s*, although capital letters are often pluralized by adding -*s* alone.

p's and q's
V's of migrating geese   *or*   Vs of migrating geese
dot your *i*'s
straight As   *or*   straight A's

Numbers

17. Numerals are pluralized by adding -*s* or, less commonly, -*'s*.

two par 5s   *or*   two par 5's
1990s   *or*   1990's
in the 80s   *or*   in the 80's   *or*   in the '80s
the mid-$20,000s   *or*   the mid-$20,000's

18. Written-out numbers are pluralized by adding -*s*.

all the fours and eights
scored three tens

Proper Nouns

19. The plurals of proper nouns are usually formed with -*s* or -*es*.

Clarence → Clarences
Jones → Joneses
Fernandez → Fernandezes

20. Plurals of proper nouns ending in -*y* usually retain the -*y* and add -*s*.

Sunday → Sundays
Timothy → Timothys
Camry → Camrys

Words ending in -*y* that were originally proper nouns are usually pluralized by changing -*y* to -*i* and adding -*es*, but a few retain the -*y*.

bobby → bobbies   Tommy → Tommies
johnny → johnnies   Bloody Mary → Bloody Marys

Quoted Elements

21. The plural of words in quotation marks are formed by adding *-s* or *-'s* within the quotation marks, or *-s* outside the quotation marks. (See also paragraph 26 below.)

> too many "probably's" [*or* "probablys"] in the statement
> one "you" among millions of "you"s
> a record number of "I can't recall"s

Symbols

22. When symbols are referred to as physical characters, the plural is formed by adding either *-s* or *-'s.*

> printed three *s
> used &'s instead of *and*'s
> his π's are hard to read

Words Ending in *-ay, -ey,* and *-oy*

23. Words that end in *-ay, -ey,* or *-oy,* unlike other words ending in *-y,* are pluralized by simply adding *-s.*

> castaways
> donkeys
> envoys

Words Ending in *-ful*

24. Any noun ending in *-ful* can be pluralized by adding *-s,* but most also have an alternative plural with *-s-* preceding the suffix.

> handful → handfuls
> teaspoonful → teaspoonfuls
> armful → armfuls *or* armsful
> bucketful → bucketfuls *or* bucketsful

Words Ending in *-o*

25. Most words ending in *-o* are normally pluralized by adding *-s.* However, some words ending in *-o* preceded by a consonant take *-es* plurals.

> solo → solos   cargo → cargoes *or* cargos
> photo → photos   proviso → provisos *or* provisoes
> tomato → tomatoes   halo → haloes *or* halos
> potato → potatoes   echo → echoes
> hobo → hoboes   motto → mottoes
> hero → heroes

Words Used as Words

26. Words referred to as words and italicized usually form their plurals by adding *-'s* in roman type. (See also paragraph 21 above.)

five *and*'s in one sentence
all those *wherefore*'s and *howsoever*'s

When a word referred to as a word has become part of a fixed phrase, the plural is usually formed by adding -*s* without the apostrophe.

oohs and aahs
dos and don'ts   *or*   do's and don'ts

POSSESSIVES
Common Nouns
1. The possessive of singular and plural common nouns that do not end in an *s* or *z* sound is formed by adding -'*s* to the end of the word.

the child's skates	this patois's range
women's voices	people's opinions
the cat's dish	the criteria's common theme

2. The possessive of singular nouns ending in an *s* or *z* sound is usually formed by adding -'*s*. A less common alternative is to add -'*s* only when it is easily pronounced; if it would create a word that is difficult to pronounce, only an apostrophe is added.

the witness's testimony
the disease's course
the race's sponsors
the prize's recipient
rickets's symptoms   *or*   rickets' symptoms

A multisyllabic singular noun that ends in an *s* or *z* sound drops the -*s* if it is followed by a word beginning with an *s* or *z* sound.

for appearance' sake
for goodness' sake

3. The possessive of plural nouns ending in an *s* or *z* sound is formed by adding only an apostrophe. However, the possessive of one-syllable irregular plurals is usually formed by adding -'*s*.

dogs' leashes	buyers' guarantees
birds' migrations	lice's lifespans

Proper Names
4. The possessives of proper names are generally formed in the same way as those of common nouns. The possessive of singular proper names is formed by adding -'*s*.

Jane's rules of behavior	Tom White's presentation
three books of Carla's	Paris's cafes

The possessive of plural proper names, and of some singular proper names ending in an *s* or *z* sound, is made by adding just an apostrophe.

the Stevenses' reception	New Orleans' annual festival
the Browns' driveway	the United States' trade deficit
Massachusetts' capital	Protosystems' president

5. The possessive of singular proper names ending in an *s* or *z* sound may be formed by adding either -'*s* or just an apostrophe. Adding -'*s* to all such names, without regard for the pronunciation of the resulting word, is more common than adding just the apostrophe. (For exceptions see paragraph 6 below).

Jones's car   *or*   Jones' car
Bliss's statue   *or*   Bliss' statue
Dickens's novels   *or*   Dickens' novels

6. The possessive form of classical and biblical names of two or more syllables ending in -*s* or -*es* is usually made by adding just an apostrophe. If the name has only one syllable, the possessive form is made by adding -'*s.*

Socrates' students	Elias' prophecy
Claudius' reign	Zeus's warnings
Ramses' kingdom	Cis's sons

The possessives of the names *Jesus* and *Moses* are always formed with just an apostrophe.

Jesus' disciples
Moses' law

7. The possessive of names ending in a silent -*s*, -*z*, or -*x* are usually formed with -'*s.*

Des Moines's recreation department
Josquin des Prez's music
Delacroix's painting

8. When the possessive ending is added to an italicized name, it is not italicized.

East of Eden's main characters
the *Spirit of St. Louis*'s historic flight
Brief Encounter's memorable ending

Pronouns

9. The possessive of indefinite pronouns is formed by adding -'*s.*

anyone's rights	somebody's wedding
everybody's money	one's own
someone's coat	either's preference

Some indefinite pronouns usually require an *of* phrase to indicate possession.

the rights of each
the inclination of many
the satisfaction of all

10. Possessive pronouns do not include apostrophes.

mine	hers
ours	his
yours	theirs
its	

Miscellaneous Styling Conventions

11. No apostrophe is generally used today with plural nouns that are more descriptive than possessive.

weapons systems	steelworkers union
managers meeting	awards banquet
singles bar	

12. The possessive form of a phrase is made by adding an apostrophe or -'s to the last word in the phrase.

his father-in-law's assistance
board of directors' meeting
from the student of politics' point of view
after a moment or so's though

Constructions such as these are often rephrased.

from the point of view of the student of politics
after thinking for a moment or so

13. The possessive form of words in quotation marks can be formed in two ways, with -'s placed either inside the quotation marks or outside them.

the "Marseillaise"'s [*or* "Marseillaise's"] stirring melody

Since both arrangements look awkward, this construction is usually avoided.

the stirring melody of the "Marseillaise"

14. Possessives of abbreviations are formed like those of nouns that are spelled out. The singular possessive is formed by adding -'s; the plural possessive, by adding an apostrophe only.

the IRS's ruling
AT&T's long-distance service
IBM Corp.'s annual report
Eli Lilly & Co.'s chairman
the HMOs' lobbyists

15. The possessive of nouns composed of numerals is formed in the same way as for other nouns. The possessive of singular nouns is formed by adding -'s; the possessive of plural nouns is formed by adding an apostrophe only.

>1996's commencement speaker
>the 1920s' greatest jazz musicians

16. Individual possession is indicated by adding -'s to each noun in a sequence. Joint possession may be indicated in the same way, but is most commonly indicated by adding an apostrophe or -'s to the last noun in the sequence.

>Joan's and Emily's friends
>Jim's, Ed's, and Susan's reports
>her mother and father's anniversary
>Peter and Jan's trip   *or*   Peter's and Jan's trip

Compounds

A compound is a word or word group that consists of two or more parts that work together as a unit to express a specific concept. Compounds can be formed by combining two or more words (as in *double-check, cost-effective, farmhouse, graphic equalizer, park bench, around-the-clock,* or *son of a gun*), by combining prefixes or suffixes with words (as in *ex-president, shoeless, presorted,* or *uninterruptedly*), or by combining two or more word elements (as in *macrophage* or *photochromism*). Compounds are written in one of three ways: solid (as in *cottonmouth*), hyphenated (*screenwriter-director*), or open (*health care*). Because of the variety of standard practice, the choice among these styles for a given compound represents one of the most common and vexing of all style issues that writers encounter.

A good dictionary will list many *permanent compounds,* compounds so commonly used that they have become permanent parts of the language. It will not list *temporary compounds,* those created to meet a writer's need at a particular moment. Most compounds whose meanings are self-evident from the meanings of their component words will not be listed, even if they are permanent and quite widely used. Writers thus cannot rely wholly on dictionaries to guide them in writing compounds.

One approach is to hyphenate all compounds not in the dictionary, since hyphenation immediately identifies them as compounds. But hyphenating all such compounds runs counter to some well-established American practice and can therefore call too much attention to the compound and momentarily distract the reader. Another approach (which applies only to compounds whose elements are complete words) is to leave open any compound not in the dictionary. Though this is widely done, it can result in the reader's failing to recognize a compound for what it is. A third approach is to pattern the compound after other similar ones. Though this approach is likely to be more complicated, it can make the compound look more familiar and thus less distracting or confusing. The paragraphs that follow are intended to help you use this approach.

As a general rule, writing meant for readers in specialized fields usually does not hyphenate compounds, especially technical terminology.

Compound Nouns

Compound nouns are combinations of words that function in a sentence as nouns. They may consist of two or more nouns, a noun and a modifier, or two or more elements that are not nouns.

Short compounds consisting of two nouns often begin as open compounds but tend to close up as they become familiar.

1. **noun + noun** Compounds composed of two nouns that are short and commonly used, of which the first is accented, are usually written solid.

farmhouse	lifeboat	football
hairbrush	paycheck	workplace

2. When a noun + noun compound is short and common but pronounced with nearly equal stress on both nouns, it is more likely to be open.

fuel oil	health care
park bench	desk lamp

3. Noun + noun compounds that consist of longer nouns and are self-evident or temporary are usually written open.

   costume designer
   computer terminal
   billiard table

4. When a noun + noun compound describes a double title or double function, the compound is hyphenated.

   hunter-gatherer
   secretary-treasurer
   bar-restaurant

   Sometimes a slash is used in place of the hyphen.

   bar/restaurant

5. Compounds formed from a noun or adjective followed by *man, woman, person,* or *people* and denoting an occupation are normally solid.

anchorman	spokesperson
congresswoman	salespeople

6. Compounds that are units of measurement are hyphenated.

foot-pound	column-inch
kilowatt-hour	light-year

7. adjective + noun   Most adjective + noun compounds are written open.

municipal court	minor league
genetic code	nuclear medicine
hazardous waste	basic training

8. Adjective + noun compounds consisting of two short words are often written solid when the first word is accented. However, some are usually written open, and a few are hyphenated.

notebook	shortcut	steel mill
bluebird	dry cleaner	two-step

9. participle + noun   Most participle + noun compounds are written open.

landing craft	sounding board	preferred stock
frying pan	barbed wire	informal consent

10. noun's + noun   Compounds consisting of a possessive noun followed by another noun are usually written open; a few are hyphenated. Compounds of this type that have become solid have lost the apostrophe.

fool's gold	Queen Anne's lace	foolscap
hornet's nest	cat's-paw	menswear
seller's market	bull's-eye	

11. noun + verb + -er or -ing   Compounds in which the first noun is the object of the verb or gerund to which the suffix has been added are most often written open but sometimes hyphenated. Permanent compounds like these are sometimes written solid.

problem solver	street-sweeping	air conditioner
deal making	fund-raiser	lifesaving
ticket-taker	gene-splicing	

12. object + verb   Noun compounds consisting of a verb preceded by a noun that is its object are written in various ways.

fish fry	bodyguard
eye-opener	roadblock

13. verb + object   A few, mostly older compounds are formed from a verb followed by a noun that is its object; they are written solid.

cutthroat	carryall
breakwater	pickpocket

14. noun + adjective   Compounds composed of a noun followed by an adjective are written open or hyphenated.

sum total	president-elect
consul general	secretary-general

15. particle + noun   Compounds consisting of a particle (usually a preposition or adverb) and a noun are usually written solid, especially when they are short and the first syllable is accented.

downturn	outpatient	afterthought
outfield	undertone	onrush
input	upswing	

A few particle + noun compounds, especially when composed of longer elements or having equal stress on both elements, are hyphenated or open.

on-ramp	off year
cross-reference	cross fire

16. verb + particle; verb + adverb   These compounds may be hyphenated or solid. Compounds with particles such as *to, in,* and *on* are often hyphenated. Compounds with particles such as *up, off,* and *out* are hyphenated or solid with about equal frequency. Those with longer particles or adverbs are usually solid.

lean-to	backup	time-out
trade-in	spin-off	turnout
add-on	payoff	hideaway
start-up		

17. verb + -er + particle; verb + -ing + particle   Except for *passerby,* these compounds are hyphenated.

runner-up	listener-in	talking-to
diners-out	carrying-on	falling-out

18. letter + noun   Compounds formed from a single letter (or sometimes a combination of them) followed by a noun are either open or hyphenated.

T square	T-shirt
B vitamin	*f*-stop
V neck	H-bomb
Rh factor	A-frame
D major	E-mail *or* e-mail

19. Compounds of three or four elements   Compounds of three or four words may be either hyphenated or open. Those incorporating prepositional phrases are more often open; others are usually hyphenated.

editor in chief	right-of-way
power of attorney	jack-of-all-trades
flash in the pan	give-and-take
base on balls	rough-and-tumble

20. Reduplication compounds   Compounds that are formed by reduplication and so consist of two similar-sounding elements are hyphenated if each element has more than one syllable. If each element has only one syllable, the compound is often written solid. Very short words and newly coined words are more often hyphenated.

namby-pamby	crisscross	sci-fi
razzle-dazzle	singsong	hip-hop

Compound Adjectives

Compound adjectives are combinations of words that work together to modify a noun—that is, they work as *unit modifiers*. As unit modifiers they can be distinguished from other strings of adjectives that may also precede a noun.

For instance, in "a low, level tract of land" the two adjectives each modify the noun separately; the tract is both low and level. These are *coordinate* (i.e., equal) *modifiers*. In "a low monthly fee" the first adjective modifies the noun plus the second adjective; the phrase denotes a monthly fee that is low. It could not be revised to "a monthly and low fee" without altering or confusing its meaning. Thus, these are *noncoordinate modifiers*. However, "low-level radiation" does not mean radiation that is low and level or level radiation that is low, but rather radiation that is at a low level. Both words work as a unit to modify the noun.

Unit modifiers are usually hyphenated, in order to help readers grasp the relationship of the words and to avoid confusion. The hyphen in "a call for more-specialized controls" removes any ambiguity as to which word *more* modifies. By contrast, the lack of a hyphen in a phrase like "graphic arts exhibition" may give it an undesirable ambiguity.

21. Before the noun (attributive position)   Most two-word compound adjectives are hyphenated when placed before the noun.

> the fresh-cut grass
> its longer-lasting effects
> her lace-trimmed dress
> a made-up excuse
> his best-selling novel
> projected health-care costs

22. Compounds whose first word is an adverb ending in *-ly* are usually left open.

> a privately chartered boat
> politically correct opinions
> its weirdly skewed perspective
> a tumultuously cascading torrent

23. Compounds formed of an adverb not ending in *-ly* followed by a participle (or sometimes an adjective) are usually hyphenated when placed before a noun.

> the well-worded statement
> more-stringent measures

his less-exciting prospects
their still-awaited assignments
her once-famous uncle

24. The combination of *very* + adjective is not a unit modifier. (See also paragraph 33 below.)

a very happy baby

25. When a compound adjective is formed by using a compound noun to modify another noun, it is usually hyphenated.

a hazardous-waste site
the basic-training period
a minor-league pitcher
a roll-call vote
their problem-solving abilities

Some familiar open compound nouns are frequently left open when used as adjectives.

a high school diploma   *or*   a high-school diploma
a real estate license   *or*   a real-estate license
an income tax refund   *or*   an income-tax refund

26. A proper name used as a modifier is not hyphenated. A word that modifies the proper name is attached by a hyphen (or an en dash in typeset material).

the Civil War era
a New England tradition
a *New York Times* article
the Supreme Court decision
the splendid *Gone with the Wind* premiere
a Los Angeles-based company
a Pulitzer Prize–winning author
pre–Bull Run skirmishes

27. Compound adjectives composed of foreign words are not hyphenated when placed before a noun unless they are hyphenated in the foreign language itself.

per diem expenses
an ad hoc committee
her *faux-naïf* style
a comme il faut arrangement
the a cappella chorus
a ci-devant professor

28. Compounds that are quoted, capitalized, or italicized are not hyphenated.

> a "Springtime in Paris" theme
> the book's "I'm OK, you're OK" tone
> his AMERICA FIRST sign
> the *No Smoking* notice

29. Chemical names and most medical names used as modifiers are not hyphenated.

> a sodium hypochlorite bleach
> the amino acid sequence
> a new Parkinson's disease medication

30. Compound adjectives of three or more words are hyphenated when they precede the noun.

> step-by-step instructions
> state-of-the-art equipment
> a wait-and-see attitude
> a longer-than-expected list
> turn-of-the-century medicine

31. Following the noun When a compound adjective follows the noun it modifies, it usually ceases to be a unit modifier and is therefore no longer hyphenated.

> instructions that guide you step by step
> a list that was longer than expected

However, a compound that follows the noun it modifies often keeps its hyphen if it continues to function as a unit modifier, especially if its first element is a noun.

> hikers who were ill-advised to cross the glacier
> an actor too high-strung to relax
> industries that could be called low-tech
> metals that are corrosion-resistant
> tends to be accident-prone

32. Permanent compound adjectives are usually written as they appear in the dictionary even when they follow the noun they modify.

> for reasons that are well-known
> a plan we regarded as half-baked
> The problems are mind-boggling.

However, compound adjectives of three or more words are normally not hyphenated when they follow the noun they modify, since they usually cease to function as adjectives.

> These remarks are off the record.
> medical practice of the turn of the century

When compounds of three or more words appear as hyphenated adjectives in dictionaries, the hyphens are retained as long as the phrase is being used as a unit modifier.

> The candidate's position was middle-of-the-road

33. When an adverb modifies another adverb that is the first element of a compound modifier, the compound may lose its hyphen. If the first adverb modifies the whole compound, however, the hyphen is retained.

> a very well developed idea
> *but*
> a delightfully well-written book
> a most ill-timed event

34. Adjective compounds that are color names in which each element can function as a noun are almost always hyphenated.

> red-orange fabric
> The fabric was red-orange.

Color names in which the first element can only be an adjective are often unhyphenated before a noun and usually unhyphenated after.

> a bright red tie
> the pale yellow-green chair
> reddish orange fabric *or* reddish-orange fabric
> The fabric was reddish orange.

35. Compound modifiers that include a number followed by a noun (except for the noun *percent*) are hyphenated when they precede the noun they modify, but usually not when they follow it. (For details on measurement, see paragraph 42 on page 426.)

> the four-color press
> a 12-foot-high fence
> a fence 12 feet high
> a 300-square-mile area
> an area of 300 square miles
> *but*
> a 10 percent raise

If a currency symbol precedes the number, the hyphen is omitted.

> an $8.5 million deficit

36. An adjective composed of a number followed by a noun in the possessive is not hyphenated.

> a nine days' wonder
> a two weeks' wait
> *but*
> a two-week wait

Compound Adverbs

37. Adverb compounds consisting of preposition + noun are almost always written solid. However, there are a few important exceptions.

> downstairs
> uphill
> offshore
> overnight
> > *but*
> in-house
> off-key
> on-line

38. Compound adverbs of more than two words are usually written open, and they usually follow the words they modify.

> here and there
> more or less
> head and shoulders
> hand in hand
> every which way
> once and for all
> > *but*
> a more-or-less certain result

A few three-word adverbs are usually hyphenated, but many are written open even if the corresponding adjective is hyphenated.

> placed back-to-back
> met face-to-face
> > *but*
> a word-for-word quotation
> quoted word for word
> software bought off the shelf

Compound Verbs

39. Two-word verbs consisting of a verb followed by an adverb or a preposition are written open.

follow up	strike out	run across
roll back	take on	set back

40. A compound composed of a particle followed by a verb is written solid.

overlook	undercut
outfit	download

41. A verb derived from an open or hyphenated compound noun is hyphenated.

double-space	water-ski
rubber-stamp	field-test

42. A verb derived from a solid noun is written solid.

mastermind	brainstorm
highlight	sideline

Compounds Formed with Word Elements

Many new and temporary compounds are formed by adding word elements to existing words or by combining word elements. There are three basic kinds of word elements: prefixes (such as *anti-, non-, pre-, post-, re-, super-*), suffixes (such as *-er, -fold, -ism, -ist, -less, -ness*), and combining forms (such as *mini-, macro-, pseudo-, -graphy, -logy*). Prefixes and suffixes are usually attached to existing words; combining forms are usually combined to form new words.

43. prefix + word   Except as specified in the paragraphs below, compounds formed from a prefix and a word are usually written solid.

anticrime	subzero
nonaligned	superheroine
premedical	transnational
reorchestration	postdoctoral

44. If the prefix ends with a vowel and the word it is attached to begins with the same vowel, the compound is usually hyphenated.

anti-incumbent	semi-independent
de-escalate	intra-arterial
co-organizer	pre-engineered

However, there are many exceptions.

reelect
preestablished
cooperate

45. If the base word or compound to which a prefix is added is capitalized, the resulting compound is almost always hyphenated.

pre-Victorian
anti-Western
post-Darwinian
non-English-speaking
   but
transatlantic
transalpine

If the prefix and the base word together form a new proper name, the compound may be solid with the prefix capitalized.

Postimpressionists
Precambrian
   but
Pre-Raphaelite

46. Compounds made with *ex-*, in its "former" sense, and *self-* are hyphenated.

ex-mayor self-control
ex-husband self-sustaining

Compounds formed from *vice-* are usually hyphenated. Some permanent compounds are open.

vice-chair vice president
vice-consul vice admiral

A temporary compound with *quasi(-)* or *pseudo(-)* may be written open (if *quasi* or *pseudo* is being treated as a modifier) or hyphenated (if it is being treated as a combining form).

quasi intellectual *or* quasi-intellectual
pseudo liberal *or* pseudo-liberal

47. If a prefix is added to a hyphenated compound, it may be either followed by a hyphen or closed up solid to the next element. Permanent compounds of this kind should be checked in a dictionary.

unair-conditioned non-self-governing
ultra-up-to-date unself-confident

48. If a prefix is added to an open compound, the hyphen is often replaced by an en dash in typeset material.

ex–campaign treasurer
post–World War I era

49. A compound that would be identical with another word if written solid is usually hyphenated to prevent misreading.

a re-creation of the setting
shopped at the co-op
multi-ply fabric

50. Compounds that might otherwise be solid are often hyphenated in order to clarify their formation, meaning, or pronunciation.

tri-city re-oil anti-fur
de-iced non-news pro-choice

51. When prefixes are attached to numerals, the compounds are hyphenated.

pre-1995 models
post–1945 economy
non-19th-century architecture

52. Compounds created from proper ethnic or national combining forms are hyphenated when the second element is an independent word, but solid when it is a combining form.

Anglo-Saxon	Anglophile
Judeo-Christian	Francophone
Sino-Japanese	Sinophobe

53. Prefixes that are repeated in the same compound are separated by a hyphen.

re-refried
post-postmodern

54. Compounds consisting of different prefixes or adjectives with the same base word which are joined by *and* or *or* are shortened by pruning the first compound back to a hyphenated prefix.

pre- and postoperative care
anti- or pro-Revolutionary sympathies
over- and underachievers
early- and mid-20th-century painters
4-, 6-, and 8-foot lengths

55. word + suffix Except as noted in the paragraphs below, compounds formed by adding a suffix to a word are written solid.

Fourierism	characterless
benightedness	custodianship
yellowish	easternmost

56. Compounds made with a suffix or a terminal combining form are often hyphenated if the base word is more than two syllables long, if it ends with the same letter the suffix begins with, or if it is a proper name.

industry-wide	jewel-like
recession-proof	Hollywood-ish
American-ness	Europe-wide

57. Compounds made from a number + *-odd* are hyphenated. A number + *-fold* is written solid if the number is spelled out but hyphenated if it is in numerals.

fifty-odd	tenfold
50-odd	10-fold

58. Most compounds formed from an open or hyphenated compound + a suffix do not separate the suffix with a hyphen. But combining forms that also exist as independent words, such as *-like, -wide, -worthy,* and *-proof,* are attached by a hyphen.

self-righteousness
middle-of-the-roadism
bobby-soxer
a Red Cross-like approach
a New York-wide policy

Open compounds often become hyphenated when a suffix is added unless they are proper nouns.

> flat-taxer
> Ivy Leaguer
> World Federalist

59. combining form + combining form   New terms in technical fields created with one or more combining forms are normally written solid.

> cyberworld
> macrographic

Abbreviations

Abbreviations may be used to save space and time, to avoid repetition of long words and phrases, or simply to conform to conventional usage.

The contemporary styling of abbreviations is inconsistent and arbitrary, and no set of rules can hope to cover all the possible variations, exceptions, and peculiarities encountered in print. The form abbreviations take—capitalized vs. lowercased, punctuated vs. unpunctuated—often depends on a writer's preference or a publisher's or organization's policy. However, the following paragraphs provide a number of useful guidelines to contemporary practice. In doubtful cases, a good general dictionary or a dictionary of abbreviations will usually show standard forms for common abbreviations.

The present discussion deals largely with general, nontechnical writing. In scientific writing, abbreviations are almost never punctuated.

An abbreviation is not divided at the end of a line.

Abbreviations are almost never italicized. An abbreviation consisting of single initial letters, whether punctuated or not, never standardly has spacing between the letters. (Initials of personal names, however, normally are separated by spaces.)

The first reference to any frequently abbreviated term or name that could be confusing or unfamiliar is commonly spelled out, often followed immediately by its abbreviation in parentheses. Later references employ the abbreviation alone.

PUNCTUATION

1. A period follows most abbreviations that are formed by omitting all but the first few letters of a word.

> cont. [*for* continued]   Oct. [*for* October]
> enc. [*for* enclosure]   univ. [*for* university]

Former abbreviations that are now considered words do not need a period.

lab   photo
gym   ad

2. A period follows most abbreviations that are formed by omitting letters from the middle of a word.

govt. [*for* government]   bros. [*for* brothers]
atty. [*for* attorney]   .   Dr. [*for* Doctor]

Some abbreviations, usually called *contractions,* replace the omitted letters with an apostrophe. Such contractions do not end with a period. (In American usage, very few contractions other than two-word contractions involving verbs are in standard use.)

ass'n   *or*   assn. [*for* association]
dep't   *or*   dept. [*for* department]
nat'l   *or*   natl. [*for* national]
can't [*for* cannot]

3. Periods are usually omitted from abbreviations made up of single initial letters. However, for some of these abbreviations, especially uncapitalized ones, the periods are usually retained. No space follows an internal period.

GOP [*for* Grand Old Party]
PR [*for* public relations]
CEO   *or*   C.E.O. [*for* chief executive officer]
a.m. [*for* ante meridiem]

4. A few abbreviations are punctuated with one or more slashes in place of periods. (For details on the slash, see the section beginning on page 358.)

c/o [*for* care of]
d/b/a   *or*   d.b.a. [*for* doing business as]
w/o [*for* without]
w/w [*for* wall-to-wall]

5. Terms in which a suffix is added to a numeral are not genuine abbreviations and do not require a period. (For details on ordinal numbers, see the section on page 413.)

1st   3d
2nd   8vo

6. Isolated letters of the alphabet used to designate a shape or position in a sequence are not abbreviations and are not punctuated.

T square
A1
F minor

7. When a punctuated abbreviation ends a sentence, its period becomes the terminal period.

For years she claimed she was "the oldest living fossil at Briggs & Co."

CAPITALIZATION

1. Abbreviations are capitalized if the words they represent are proper nouns or adjectives.

F [*for* Fahrenheit]
IMF [*for* International Monetary Fund]
Jan. [*for* January]
Amer. [*for* American]
LWV [*for* League of Women Voters]

2. Abbreviations are usually all-capitalized when they represent initial letters of lowercased words. However, some common abbreviations formed in this way are often lowercased.

IQ [*for* intelligence quotient]
U.S. [*for* United States]
COLA [*for* cost-of-living allowance]
FYI [*for* for your information]
f.o.b.   *or*   FOB [*for* free on board]
c/o [*for* care of]

3. Most abbreviations formed from single initial letters that are pronounced as words, rather than as a series of letters, are capitalized. Those that are not proper nouns and have been assimilated into the language as words in their own right are most often lowercased.

OSHA	snafu
NATO	laser
CARE	sonar
NAFTA	scuba

4. Abbreviations that are ordinarily capitalized are commonly used to begin sentences, but abbreviations that are ordinarily uncapitalized are not.

Dr. Smith strongly disagrees.
OSHA regulations require these new measures.
Page 22 [*not* P. 22] was missing.

PLURALS, POSSESSIVES, AND COMPOUNDS

1. Punctuated abbreviations of single words are pluralized by adding *-s* before the period.

yrs. [*for* years]
hwys. [*for* highways]
figs. [*for* figures]

2. Punctuated abbreviations that stand for phrases or compounds are usually pluralized by adding *-'s* after the last period.

M.D.'s   *or*   M.D.s
Ph.D.'s   *or*   Ph.D.s

LL.B.'s   *or*   LL.B.s
v.p.'s

3. All-capitalized, unpunctuated abbreviations are usually pluralized by adding a lowercase -*s*.

IRAs	CPAs
PCs	SATs

4. The plural form of a few lowercase one-letter abbreviations is made by repeating the letter.

ll. [*for* lines]
pp. [*for* pages]
nn. [*for* notes]
vv. [*for* verses]
ff.   *or*   ff [*for* and the following ones *or* folios]

5. The plural form of abbreviations of units of measurement (including one-letter abbreviations) is the same as the singular form. (For more on units of measurement, see the section beginning on page 426.)

10 cc   *or*   cc. [*for* cubic centimeters]
30 m   *or*   m. [*for* meters]
15 mm   *or*   mm. [*for* millimeters]
24 h. [*for* hours]
10 min. [*for* minutes]
45 mi. [*for* miles]

However, in informal nontechnical text several such abbreviations are pluralized like other single-word abbreviations.

lbs.	qts.
gals.	hrs.

6. Possessives of abbreviations are formed like those of spelled-out nouns: the singular possessive is formed by adding -'*s*, the plural possessive simply by adding an apostrophe.

the CEO's speech	the PACs' influence
Apex Co.'s profits	Brown Bros.' ads

7. Compounds that consist of an abbreviation added to another word are formed in the same way as compounds that consist of spelled-out nouns.

an FDA-approved drug
an R&D-driven company
the Eau Claire, Wisc.–based publisher

Compounds formed by adding a prefix or suffix to an abbreviation are usually hyphenated.

pre-CD recordings	a CIA-like operation
non-IRA deductions	a PCB-free product

SPECIFIC STYLING CONVENTIONS

A and *An*

1. The choice of the article *a* or *an* before abbreviations depends on the sound, rather than the actual letter, with which the abbreviation begins. If it begins with a consonant sound, *a* is normally used; if with a vowel sound, *an* is used.

a CD-ROM version	an FDA-approved drug
a YAF member	an M.D. degree
a U.S. Senator	an ABA convention

A.D. and B.C.

2. The abbreviations A.D. and B.C. and other abbreviated era designations usually appear in books and journals as small capitals; in newspapers and in typed or keyboarded material, they usually appear as full capitals. The abbreviation B.C. follows the date; A.D. usually precedes the date, though in many publications A.D. follows the date as well. In references to whole centuries, A.D. follows the century. (For more on era designations, see paragraph 12 on page 419.)

    A.D. 185   *but also*   185 A.D.
    41 B.C.
    the fourth century A.D.

Agencies, Associations, Organizations, and Companies

3. The names of agencies, associations, and organizations are usually abbreviated after being spelled out on their first occurrence in a text. If a company is easily recognizable from its initials, the abbreviation is likewise usually employed after the first mention. The abbreviations are usually all-capitalized and unpunctuated. (In contexts where the abbreviation will be recognized, it often replaces the full name throughout.)

    Next, the president of the Pioneer Valley Transit Authority presented the annual PVTA award.
    . . . at the American Bar Association (ABA) meeting in June. The ABA's new officers . . .
    International Business Machines released its first-quarter earnings figures today. An IBM spokesperson . . .

4. The words *Company, Corporation, Incorporated,* and *Limited* in company names are commonly abbreviated even at their first appearance, except in quite formal writing.

    Procter & Gamble Company   *or*   Procter & Gamble Co.
    Brandywine Corporation   *or*   Brandywine Corp.

Ampersand

5. The ampersand (&), representing the word *and,* is often used in the names of companies.

H&R Block
Standard & Poor's
Ogilvy & Mather

It is not used in the names of federal agencies.

U.S. Fish and Wildlife Service
Office of Management and Budget

Even when a spelled-out *and* appears in a company's official name, it is often replaced by an ampersand in writing referring to the company, whether for the sake of consistency or because of the writer's inability to verify the official styling.

6. When an ampersand is used in an abbreviation, there is usually no space on either side of the ampersand.

The Barkers welcome all guests to their B&B at 54 West Street.
The S&P 500 showed gains in technology stocks.
The Texas A&M Aggies prevailed again on Sunday.

7. When an ampersand is used between the last two elements in a series, the comma is omitted.

Jones, Kuhn & Malloy, Attorneys at Law

Books of the Bible

8. Books of the Bible are spelled out in running text but generally abbreviated in references to chapter and verse.

The minister based his first Advent sermon on Matthew.
Ye cannot serve God and mammon.—Matt. 6:24

Compass Points

9. Compass points are normally abbreviated when they follow street names; these abbreviations may be punctuated and are usually preceded by a comma.

1600 Pennsylvania Avenue[,] NW [N.W.]

When a compass point precedes the word *Street, Avenue,* etc., or when it follows the word but forms an integral part of the street name, it is usually spelled out.

230 West 43rd Street
50 Park Avenue South

Dates

10. The names of days and months are spelled out in running text.

at the Monday editorial meeting
the December issue of *Scientific American*
a meeting held on August 1, 1995

The names of months usually are not abbreviated in datelines of business letters, but they are often abbreviated in government and military correspondence.

> *business dateline:* November 1, 1995
> *military dateline:* 1 Nov 95

Degrees and Professional Ratings

11. Abbreviations of academic degrees are usually punctuated; abbreviations of professional ratings are slightly more commonly unpunctuated.

> Ph.D.
> B.Sc.
> M.B.A.
> PLS *or* P.L.S. [*for* Professional Legal Secretary]
> CMA *or* C.M.A. [*for* Certified Medical Assistant]
> FACP *or* F.A.C.P. [*for* Fellow of the American College of Physicians]

12. Only the first letter of each element in abbreviations of degrees and professional ratings is generally capitalized.

> D.Ch.E. [*for* Doctor of Chemical Engineering]
> Litt.D. [*for* Doctor of Letters]
> D.Th. [*for* Doctor of Theology]
> *but*
> LL.B. [*for* Bachelor of Laws]
> LL.M. [*for* Master of Laws]
> LL.D. [*for* Doctor of Laws]

Geographical Names

13. When abbreviations of state names are used in running text immediately following the name of a city or county, the traditional state abbreviations are often used.

> Ellen White of 49 Lyman St., Saginaw, Mich., has been chosen . . .
> the Dade County, Fla., public schools
> *but*
> Grand Rapids, in western Michigan, . . .

Official postal service abbreviations for states are used in mailing addresses.

> 6 Bay Rd.
> Gibson Island, MD 21056

14. Terms such as *Street, Road,* and *Boulevard* are often written as punctuated abbreviations in running text when they form part of a proper name.

> an accident on Windward Road [*or* Rd.]
> our office at 1234 Cross Blvd. [*or* Boulevard]

15. Names of countries are usually spelled in full in running text.

> South Africa's president urged the United States to impose meaningful sanctions.

Abbreviations for country names (in tables, for example), are usually punctuated. When formed from the single initial letters of two or more individual words, they are sometimes unpunctuated.

Mex.	Ger.	U.K. *or* UK
Can.	Scot.	U.S. *or* US

16. *United States* is normally abbreviated when used as an adjective or attributive. When used as a noun, it is generally spelled out.

> the U.S. Department of Justice
> U.S. foreign policy
> The United States has declined to participate.

17. *Saint* is usually abbreviated when it is part of a geographical or topographical name. *Mount, Point,* and *Fort* may be either spelled out or abbreviated. (For the abbreviation of *Saint* with personal names, see paragraph 25 below.)

> St. Paul, Minnesota   *or*   Saint Paul, Minnesota
> St. Thomas, U.S.V.I.   *or*   Saint Thomas
> Mount Vernon   *or*   Mt. Vernon
> Point Reyes   *or*   Pt. Reyes
> Fort Worth   *or*   Ft. Worth
> Mt. Kilimanjaro   *or*   Mount Kilimanjaro

Latin Words and Phrases

18. Several Latin words and phrases are almost always abbreviated. They are punctuated, lowercased, and usually not italicized.

etc.	viz.	q.v.
i.e.	et al.	c. *or* ca.
e.g.	ibid.	fl.
cf.	op. cit.	et seq.

Versus is usually abbreviated *v.* in legal writing, *vs.* otherwise.

> *Da Costa* v. *United States*
> good vs. evil   *or*   good versus evil

Latitude and *Longitude*

19. The words *latitude* and *longitude* are abbreviated in tables and in technical contexts but often written out in running text.

> *in a table:*   lat. 10°20′N *or* lat. 10–20N
> *in text:*   from 10°20′ north latitude to 10°30′ south latitude
> *or*   from lat. 10°20′N to lat. 10°30′S

Military Ranks and Units

20. Official abbreviations for military ranks follow specific unpunctuated styles for each branch of the armed forces. Nonmilitary writing usually employs a punctuated and less concise style.

in the military:	BG Carter R. Stokes, USA
	LCDR Dawn Wills-Craig, USN
	Col S. J. Smith, USMC
	LTJG Carlos Ramos, USCG
	Sgt Bernard P. Brodkey, USAF
outside the military:	Brig. Gen. Carter R. Stokes
	Lt. Comdr. Dawn Wills-Craig
	Col. S. J. Smith
	Lt. (j.g.) Carlos Ramos
	Sgt. Bernard P. Brodkey

21. Outside the military, military ranks are usually given in full when used with a surname only but abbreviated when used with a full name.

Major Mosby
Maj. John S. Mosby

Number

22. The word *number,* when followed by a numeral, is usually abbreviated to *No.* or *no.*

The No. 1 priority is to promote profitability.
We recommend no. 6 thread.
Policy No. 123–5-X
Publ. Nos. 12 and 1

Personal Names

23. When initials are used with a surname, they are spaced and punctuated. Unspaced initials of a few famous persons, which may or may not be punctuated, are sometimes used in place of their full names.

E. M. Forster
C. P. E. Bach
JFK   *or*   J.F.K.

24. The abbreviations *Jr.* and *Sr.* may or may not be preceded by a comma.

Martin Luther King Jr.   *or*   Martin Luther King, Jr.

Saint

25. The word *Saint* is often abbreviated when used before the name of a saint. When it forms part of a surname or an institution's name, it follows the style used by the person or institution. (For the styling of *Saint* in geographical names, see paragraph 17 above.)

St. [*or* Saint] Teresa of Avila   St. Martin's Press

Augustus Saint-Gaudens   St. John's College
Ruth St. Denis

Scientific Terms

26. In binomial nomenclature, a genus name may be abbreviated to its initial letter after the first reference. The abbreviation is always capitalized, punctuated, and italicized.

> . . . its better-known relative *Atropa belladonna* (deadly nightshade).
> Only *A. belladonna* is commonly found in . . .

27. Abbreviations for the names of chemical compounds and the symbols for chemical elements and formulas are unpunctuated.

MSG	Pb	NaCl
PCB	O	FeS

28. Abbreviations in computer terms are usually unpunctuated.

PC	I/O	Ctrl
RAM	DOS	ASCII
MB	Esc	EBCDIC
CD-ROM	Alt	

Time

29. When time is expressed in figures, the abbreviations *a.m. (ante meridiem)* and *p.m. (post meridiem)* are most often written as punctuated lowercase letters, sometimes as punctuated small capital letters. In newspapers, they usually appear in full-size capitals. (For more on *a.m.* and *p.m.*, see paragraph 39 on page 425.)

> 8:30 a.m.   *or*   8:30 A.M.   *or*   8:30 A.M.
> 10:00 p.m.   *or*   10:00 P.M.   *or*   10:00 P.M.

Time-zone designations are usually capitalized and unpunctuated.

> 9:22 a.m. EST [*for* eastern standard time]
> 4:45 p.m. CDT [*for* central daylight time]

Titles and Degrees

30. The courtesy titles *Mr., Ms., Mrs.,* and *Messrs.* occur only as abbreviations today. The professional titles *Doctor, Professor, Representative,* and *Senator* are often abbreviated.

> Ms. Lee A. Downs
> Messrs. Lake, Mason, and Nambeth
> Doctor Howe   *or*   Dr. Howe

31. Despite some traditional objections, the honorific titles *Honorable* and *Reverend* are often abbreviated, with and without *the* preceding the titles.

> the Honorable Samuel I. O'Leary   *or*   [the] Hon. Samuel I. O'Leary
> the Reverend Samuel I. O'Leary   *or*   [the] Rev. Samuel I. O'Leary

32. When an abbreviation for an academic degree, professional certification, or association membership follows a name, no courtesy or professional title precedes it.

> Dr. Jesse Smith   *or*   Jesse Smith, M.D.   *but not*   Dr. Jesse Smith, M.D.
> Katherine Fox Derwinski, CLU
> Carol W. Manning, M.D., FACPS
> Michael B. Jones II, J.D.
> Peter D. Cohn, Jr., CPA

33. The abbreviation *Esq.* (for *Esquire*) often follows attorneys' names in correspondence and in formal listings, and less often follows the names of certain other professionals, including architects, consuls, clerks of court, and justices of the peace. It is not used if a degree or professional rating follows the name, or if a courtesy title or honorific (*Mr., Ms., Hon., Dr.,* etc.) precedes the name.

> Carolyn B. West, Esq.   *not*   Ms. Carolyn B. West, Esq.   *and not*   Carolyn
>   B. West, J.D., Esq.

Units of Measurement

34. A unit of measurement that follows a figure is often abbreviated, especially in technical writing. The figure and abbreviation are separated by a space. If the numeral is written out, the unit should also be written out.

> 15 cu. ft.   *but*   fifteen cubic feet
> What is its capacity in cubic feet?

35. Abbreviations for metric units are usually unpunctuated; those for traditional units are usually punctuated in nonscientific writing. (For more on units of measurement, see the section on page 426.)

14 ml	50 m	4 sec.
12 km	8 ft.	20 min.

Numbers

The treatment of numbers presents special difficulties because there are so many conventions to follow, some of which may conflict in a particular passage. The major issue is whether to spell out numbers or to express them in figures, and usage varies considerably on this point.

NUMBERS AS WORDS OR FIGURES

At one style extreme—usually limited to proclamations, legal documents, and some other types of very formal writing—all numbers (sometimes even including dates) are written out. At the other extreme, some types of technical writing may contain no written-out numbers. Figures are generally easier to read than spelled-out numbers; however, the spelled-out forms are helpful in certain circumstances, and are often felt to be less jarring than figures in nontechnical writing.

Basic Conventions

1. Two alternative basic conventions are in common use. The first and more widely used system requires that numbers up through nine be spelled out, and that figures be used for exact numbers greater than nine. (In a variation of this system, the number ten is spelled out.) Round numbers that consist of a whole number between one and nine followed by *hundred, thousand, million,* etc., may either be spelled out or expressed in figures.

> The museum includes four rooms of early American tools and implements, 345 pieces in all.
> He spoke for almost three hours, inspiring his audience of 19,000 devoted followers.
> They sold more than 700 [*or* seven hundred] TVs during the 10-day sale.
> She'd told him so a thousand times.

2. The second system requires that numbers from one through ninety-nine be spelled out, and that figures be used for all exact numbers above ninety-nine. (In a variation of this system, the number one hundred is spelled out.) Numbers that consist of a whole number between one and ninety-nine followed by *hundred, thousand, million,* etc., are also spelled out.

> Audubon's engraver spent nearly twelve years completing these four volumes, which comprise 435 hand-colored plates.
> In the course of four hours, she signed twenty-five hundred copies of her book.

3. Written-out numbers only use hyphens following words ending in *-ty.* The word *and* before such words is usually omitted.

> twenty-two
> five-hundred ninety-seven
> two thousand one hundred forty-nine

Sentence Beginnings

4. Numbers that begin a sentence are written out. An exception is occasionally made for dates. Spelled-out numbers that are lengthy and awkward are usually avoided by restructuring the sentence.

> Sixty-two new bills will be brought before the committee.
>   *or* There will be 62 new bills brought before the committee.
> Nineteen ninety-five was our best earnings year so far.
>   *or occasionally* 1995 was our best earnings year so far.
> One hundred fifty-seven illustrations, including 86 color plates, are contained in the book.
>   *or* The book contains 157 illustrations, including 86 color plates.

Adjacent Numbers and Numbers in Series

5. Two separate figures are generally not written adjacent to one another in running text unless they form a series. Instead, either the sentence is rephrased or one of the figures is spelled out—usually the figure with the shorter written form.

> sixteen ½-inch dowels
> worked five 9-hour days in a row
> won twenty 100-point games
> lost 15 fifty-point matches
> By 1997, thirty schools . . .

6. Numbers paired at the beginning of a sentence are usually written alike. If the first word of the sentence is a spelled-out number, the second number is also spelled out. However, each number may instead be styled independently, even if that results in an inconsistent pairing.

> Sixty to seventy-five copies will be required.
> *or*   Sixty to 75 copies will be required.

7. Numbers that form a pair or a series within a sentence or a paragraph are often treated identically even when they would otherwise be styled differently. The style of the largest number usually determines that of the others. If one number is a mixed or simple fraction, figures are used for all the numbers in the series.

> She wrote one proposal and thirteen [*or* 13] memos that week.
> His total record sales came to a meager 8 [*or* eight] million; Bing Crosby's, he mused, may have surpassed 250 million.
> The three jobs took 5, 12, and 4½ hours, respectively.

Round Numbers

8. Approximate or round numbers, particularly those that can be expressed in one or two words, are often spelled out in general writing. In technical and scientific writing, they are expressed as numerals.

> seven hundred people   *or*   700 people
> five thousand years   *or*   5,000 years
> four hundred thousand volumes   *or*   400,000 volumes
> *but not*   400 thousand volumes
>   *but in technical writing*
> 200 species of fish
> 50,000 people per year
> 300,000 years

9. Round (and round-appearing) numbers of one million and above are often expressed as figures followed by the word *million, billion,* and so forth. The figure may include a one- or two-digit decimal fraction; more exact numbers are written entirely in figures.

the last 600 million years
about 4.6 billion years old
1.2 million metric tons of grain
$7.25 million
$3,456,000,000

Ordinal Numbers

10. Ordinal numbers generally follow the styling rules for cardinal numbers. In technical writing, ordinal numbers are usually written as figure-plus-suffix combinations. Certain ordinal numbers—for example, those for percentiles and latitudes—are usually set as figures even in nontechnical contexts.

entered the seventh grade
wrote the 9th [*or* ninth] and 12th [*or* twelfth] chapters
in the 21st [*or* twenty-first] century
the 7th percentile
the 38th parallel

11. In figure-plus-suffix combinations where the figure ends in 2 or 3, either a one- or a two-letter suffix may be used. A period does not follow the suffix.

2d   *or*   2nd
33d   *or*   33rd
102d   *or*   102nd

Roman Numerals

12. Roman numerals are traditionally used to differentiate rulers and popes with identical names.

King George III
Henri IV
Innocent X

13. When Roman numerals are used to differentiate related males with the same name, they are used only with the full name. Ordinals are sometimes used instead of Roman numerals. The possessive is formed in the usual way. (For the use of *Jr.* and *Sr.,* see paragraph 24 on page 408.)

James R. Watson II
James R. Watson 2nd *or* 2d
James R. Watson II's [*or* 2nd's *or* 2d's] alumni gift

14. Lowercase Roman numerals are generally used to number book pages that precede the regular Arabic sequence (often including a table of contents, acknowledgments, foreword, or other material).

on page iv of the preface
See Introduction, pp. ix–xiii.

15. Roman numerals are used in outlines; see paragraph 23 on page 422.

16. Roman numerals are found as part of a few established scientific and technical terms. Chords in the study of music harmony are designated by capital and lowercase Roman numerals (often followed by small Arabic numbers). Most technical terms that include numbers, however, express them in Arabic form.

> blood-clotting factor VII
> quadrant III
> the cranial nerves II and IX
> HIV-III virus
> Population II stars
> type I error
> vii$_6$ chord
> > *but*
> adenosine 3′,5′-monophosphate
> cesium 137
> PL/1 programming language

17. Miscellaneous uses of Roman numerals include the Articles, and often the Amendments, of the Constitution. Roman numerals are still sometimes used for references to the acts and scenes of plays and occasionally for volume numbers in bibliographic references.

> Article IX
> Act III, Scene ii   *or*   Act 3, Scene 2
> (III, ii)   *or*   (3, 2)
> Vol. XXIII, No. 4   *but usually*   Vol. 23, No. 4

PUNCTUATION

These paragraphs provide general rules for the use of commas, hyphens, and en dashes with compound and large numbers. For specific categories of numbers, such as dates, money, and decimal fractions, see Specific Styling Conventions, beginning on page 417.

Commas in Large Numbers

1. In general writing, figures of four digits may be written with or without a comma; including the comma is more common. If the numerals form part of a tabulation, commas are necessary so that four-digit numerals can align with numerals of five or more digits.

> 2,000 cases   *or less commonly*   2000 cases

2. Whole numbers of five digits or more (but not decimal fractions) use a comma to separate three-digit groups, counting from the right.

> a fee of $12,500
> 15,000 units
> a population of 1,500,000

3. Certain types of numbers of four digits or more do not contain commas. These include decimal fractions and the numbers of policies and contracts, checks, street addresses, rooms and suites, telephones, pages, military hours, and years.

2.5544	Room 1206
Policy 33442	page 145
check 34567	1650 hours
12537 Wilshire Blvd.	in 1929

4. In technical writing, the comma is frequently replaced by a thin space in numerals of five or more digits. Digits to the right of the decimal point are also separated in this way, counting from the decimal point.

28 666 203
209.775 42

Hyphens

5. Hyphens are used with written-out numbers between 21 and 99.

forty-one years old
his forty-first birthday
Four hundred twenty-two visitors were counted.

6. A hyphen is used in a written-out fraction employed as a modifier. A nonmodifying fraction consisting of two words only is usually left open, although it may also be hyphenated. (For details on fractions, see the section beginning on page 420.)

a one-half share
three fifths of her paycheck   *or*   three-fifths of her paycheck
   but
four five-hundredths

7. Numbers that form the first part of a modifier expressing measurement are followed by a hyphen. (For units of measurement, see the section on page 426.)

a 5-foot board
a 28-mile trip
an eight-pound baby
   but
a $6 million profit

8. Serial numbers, Social Security numbers, telephone numbers, and extended zip codes often contain hyphens that make lengthy numerals more readable or separate coded information.

020–42–1691
413–734–3134   *or*   (413) 734–3134
01102–2812

9. Numbers are almost never divided at the end of a line. If division is unavoidable, the break occurs only after a comma.

Inclusive Numbers

10. Inclusive numbers—those that express a range—are usually separated either by the word *to* or by a hyphen or en dash, meaning "(up) to and including."

> spanning the years 1915 to 1941
> the fiscal year 1994–95
> the decade 1920–1929
> pages 40 to 98
> pp. 40–98

Inclusive numbers separated by a hyphen or en dash are not used after the words *from* or *between*.

> from page 385 to page 419   *not*   from page 385–419
> from 9:30 to 5:30   *not*   from 9:30–5:30
> between 1997 and 2000   *not*   between 1997–2000
> between 80 and 90 percent   *not*   between 80–90 percent

11. Inclusive page numbers and dates may be either written in full or elided (i.e., shortened) to save space or for ease of reading.

> pages 523–526   *or*   pages 523–26
> 1955–1969   *or*   1955–69

However, inclusive dates that appear in titles and other headings are almost never elided. Dates that appear with era designations are also not elided.

> *England and the French Revolution 1789–1797*
> 1900–1901   *not*   1900–01   *and not*   1900–1
> 872–863 B.C.   *not*   872–63 B.C.

12. The most common style for the elision of inclusive numbers is based on the following rules: Never elide inclusive numbers that have only two digits.

> 24–28   *not*   24–8
> 86–87   *not*   86–7

Never elide inclusive numbers when the first number ends in 00.

> 100–103   *not*   100–03   *and not*   100–3
> 300–329   *not*   300–29

In other numbers, do not omit the tens digit from the higher number. *Exception:* Where the tens digit of both numbers is zero, write only one digit for the higher number.

> 234–37   *not*   234–7
> 3,824–29   *not*   3,824–9
> 605–7   *not*   605–07

13. Units of measurement expressed in words or abbreviations are usually used only after the second element of an inclusive number. Symbols, however, are repeated.

> ten to fifteen dollars
> 30 to 35 degrees Celsius
> an increase in dosage from 200 to 500 mg
>> *but*
> 45° to 48° F
> $50–$60 million   *or* $50 million to $60 million

14. Numbers that are part of an inclusive set or range are usually styled alike: figures with figures, spelled-out words with other spelled-out words.

> from 8 to 108 absences
> five to twenty guests
> 300,000,000 to 305,000,000   *not*   300 million to 305,000,00

SPECIFIC STYLING CONVENTIONS

The following paragraphs, arranged alphabetically, describe styling practices commonly followed for specific situations involving numbers.

Addresses

1. Numerals are used for all building, house, apartment, room, and suite numbers except for *one,* which is usually written out.

> 6 Lincoln Road   Apartment 609   Suite 2000
> 1436 Fremont Street   Room 982   One Bayside Drive

When the address of a building is used as its name, the number in the address is often written out.

> the sophisticated elegance of Ten Park Avenue

2. Numbered streets have their numbers written as ordinals. Street names from First through Tenth are usually written out, and numerals are used for all higher-numbered streets. Less commonly, all numbered street names up to and including One Hundredth are spelled out.

> 167 Second Avenue
> 19 South 22nd Street   *or less commonly*   19 South Twenty-second Street
> 145 East 145th Street
> in the 60s   *or*   in the Sixties [streets from 60th to 69th]
> in the 120s [streets from 120th to 129th]

When a house or building number immediately precedes the number of a street, a spaced hyphen may be inserted between the two numbers, or the street number may be written out, for the sake of clarity.

> 2018 - 14th Street
> 2018 Fourteenth Street

3. Arabic numerals are used to designate highways and, in some states, county roads.

Interstate 90 *or* I-90	Texas 23
U.S. Route 1 *or* U.S. 1	County 213

Dates

4. Year numbers are written as figures. If a year number begins a sentence, it may be left as a figure but more often is spelled out; the sentence may also be rewritten to avoid beginning it with a figure.

the 1997 edition
Nineteen thirty-seven marked the opening of the Golden Gate Bridge.
  or   The year 1937 marked the opening of the Golden Gate Bridge.
  or   The Golden Gate Bridge opened in 1937.

5. A year number may be abbreviated to its last two digits when an event is so well known that it needs no century designation. In these cases an apostrophe precedes the numerals.

the blizzard of '88
class of '91   *or*   class of 1991
the Spirit of '76

6. Full dates are traditionally written in the sequence month-day-year, with the year set off by commas that precede and follow it. An alternative style, used in the military and in U.S. government publications, is the inverted sequence day-month-year, which does not require commas.

traditional:	July 8, 1976, was a warm, sunny day in Philadelphia.
	the explosion on July 16, 1945, at Alamogordo
military:	the explosion on 16 July 1945 at Alamogordo
	the amendment ratified on 18 August 1920

7. Ordinal numbers are not used in full dates. Ordinals are sometimes used, however, for a date without an accompanying year, and they are always used when preceded in a date by the word *the.*

December 4, 1829
on December 4th   *or*   on December 4
on the 4th of December

8. All-figure dating, such as 6–8-95 or 6/8/95, is usually avoided except in informal writing. For some readers, such dates are ambiguous; the examples above generally mean June 8, 1995, in the United States, but in almost all other countries mean August 6, 1995.

9. Commas are usually omitted from dates that include the month and year but not the day. The word *of* is sometimes inserted between the month and year.

in October 1997
back in January of 1981

10. References to specific centuries may be either written out or expressed in figures.

in the nineteenth century   *or*   in the 19th century
a sixteenth-century painting   *or*   a 16th-century painting

11. The name of a specific decade often takes a short form, usually with no apostrophe and uncapitalized. When the short form is part of a set phrase, it is capitalized.

a song from the sixties
   occasionally   a song from the 'sixties   *or*   a song from the Sixties
tunes of the Gay Nineties

The name of a decade is often expressed in numerals, in plural form. The figure may be shortened, with an apostrophe to indicate the missing numerals; however, apostrophes enclosing the figure are generally avoided. Any sequence of such numbers is generally styled consistently.

the 1950s and 1960s   *or*   the '50s and '60s
   but not
the '50's and '60's
the 1950s and '60s
the 1950s and sixties

12. Era designations precede or follow words that specify centuries or numerals that specify years. Era designations are unspaced abbreviations, punctuated with periods. They are usually typed or keyboarded as regular capitals, and typeset in books as small capitals and in newspapers as full-size capitals. The abbreviation B.C. (before Christ) is placed after the date, while A.D. (*anno Domini,* "in the year of our Lord") is usually placed before the date but after a century designation. Any date given without an era designation or context is understood to mean A.D.

1792–1750 B.C.
between 600 and 400 B.C.
from the fifth or fourth millennium to c. 250 B.C.
between 7 B.C. and A.D. 22
c. A.D. 100 to 300
the second century A.D.
the 17th century

13. Less common era designations include A.H. (*anno Hegirae,* "in the year of [Muhammad's] Hegira," or *anno Hebraico,* "in the Hebrew year"); B.C.E. (before the common era; a synonym for B.C.); C.E. (of the common era; a synonym for A.D.); and B.P. (before the present; often used by geologists and archeologists, with or without the word *year*). The abbrevia-

tion A.H. is usually placed before a specific date but after a century designation, while B.C.E., C.E., and B.P.,. are placed after both a date and a
century.

> the tenth of Muharram, A.H. 61 (October 10, A.D. 680)
> the first century A.H.
> from the 1st century B.C.E. to the 4th century C.E.
> 63 B.C.E.
> the year 200 C.E.
> 5,000 years B.P.
> two million years B.P.

Degrees of Temperature and Arc

14. In technical writing, a quantity expressed in degrees is generally written
as a numeral followed by the degree symbol ($°$). In the Kelvin scale,
neither the word *degree* nor the symbol is used with the figure.

> a 45° angle
> 6°40′10″N
> 32° F
> 0° C
> Absolute zero is zero kelvins or 0 K.

15. In general writing, the quantity expressed in degrees may or may not be
written out. A figure may be followed by either the degree symbol or the
word *degree;* a spelled-out number is always followed by the word *degree.*

> latitude 43°19″N
> latitude 43 degrees N
> a difference of 43 degrees latitude
> The temperature has risen about thirty degrees.

Fractions and Decimal Fractions

16. In nontechnical prose, fractions standing alone are usually written out.
Common fractions used as nouns are usually unhyphenated, although
the hyphenated form is also common. When fractions are used as modifiers, they are hyphenated.

> lost three quarters of its value   *or*   lost three-quarters of its value
> had a two-thirds chance of winning

Multiword numerators and denominators are usually hyphenated, or written as figures.

> one one-hundredth of an inch   *or*   1/100 of an inch

17. Mixed fractions (fractions with a whole number, such as 3½) and fractions that form part of a modifier are usually expressed in figures in
running text.

waiting 2½ hours
a 7/8-mile course
2½-pound weights

Fractions that are not on the keyboard or available as special characters on a computer may be typed in full-sized digits; in mixed fractions, a space is left between the whole number and the fraction.

a 7/8-mile course
waiting 2 3/4 hours

18. Fractions used with units of measurement are usually expressed in figures, but common short words are often written out.

¹⁄₁₀ km	half a mile
⅓ oz.	a half-mile walk
⅞ inch	a sixteenth-inch gap

19. Decimal fractions are always set as figures. In technical writing, a zero is placed to the left of the decimal point when the fraction is less than a whole number; in general writing, the zero is usually omitted. Commas are not used in numbers following a decimal point.

An example of a pure decimal fraction is 0.375, while 1.402 is classified as a mixed decimal fraction.
a .22-caliber rifle
0.142857

20. Fractions and decimal fractions are usually not mixed in a text.

weights of 5½ lbs., 3¼ lbs., and ½ oz.
or weights of 5.5 lbs., 3.25 lbs., and .5 oz.
not weights of 5.5 lbs., 3¼ lbs., and ½ oz.

Lists and Outlines

21. Both run-in and vertical lists are often numbered. In run-in numbered lists—that is, numbered lists that form part of a normal-looking sentence—each item is preceded by a number (or, less often, an italicized letter) enclosed in parentheses. The items are separated by commas if they are brief and unpunctuated; if they are complex or punctuated, they are separated by semicolons. The entire list is introduced by a colon if it is preceded by a full clause, and often when it is not.

I will try to establish (1) the immediate historical background, (2) the chronological sequence of events in the critical two days, and (3) the likely cause-and-effect relations of the key decisions and actions.

The new medical dictionary has several special features: *(a)* common variant spellings; *(b)* examples of words used in context; *(c)* abbreviations, combining forms, prefixes, and suffixes; and *(d)* brand names for drugs and their generic equivalents.

22. In vertical lists, each number is followed by a period; the periods align vertically. Run-over lines usually align under the item's first word. Each item may be capitalized, especially if the items are syntactically independent of the words that introduce them.

> The English peerage consists of five ranks, listed here in descending order:
> 1. Duke (duchess)
> 2. Marquess (marchioness)
> 3. Earl (countess)
> 4. Viscount (viscountess)
> 5. Baron (baroness)

The listed items end with periods (or question marks) when they are complete sentences, and also often when they are not.

> We require answers to the following questions:
> 1. Does the club intend to engage heavy-metal bands to perform in the future?
> 2. Will any such bands be permitted to play past midnight on weekends?
> 3. Are there plans to install proper acoustic insulation?

Items that are syntactically dependent on the words that introduce them often begin with a lowercase letter and end with a comma or semicolon just as in a run-in series in an ordinary sentence.

> The signed consent may be given by
> 1. the patient,
> 2. a legally qualified representative (such as a parent or guardian) of the patient,
> 3. an executor or administrator of an estate, or
> 4. an agency designated by the court as a guardian.

A vertical list may also be unnumbered, or may use bullets (•) in place of numerals, especially where the order of the items is not important.

> Chief among the important advances in communication were these 19th-century inventions:
>   Morse's telegraph
>   Daguerre's camera
>   Bell's telephone
>   Edison's phonograph

> This book covers in detail:
> • Punctuation
> • Capitalization and italicization
> • Numbers
> • Abbreviations
> • Grammar and composition

23. Outlines standardly use Roman numerals, capitalized letters, Arabic numerals, and lowercase letters, in that order. Each numeral or letter is followed by a period, and each item is capitalized.

> I. Using health information
>   A. Confidentiality
>   B. Insurance billing
>   1. Requirements for health information

    2. Diagnosis coding
    3. Procedure coding

 II. Managing health information
   A. Storage and retrieval
     1. Filing systems
       a. Numerical
       b. Color-coded
     2. Retrieval systems
   B. Record disposal

Money

24. A sum of money that can be expressed in one or two words is usually written out in running text, as is the unit of currency. But if several sums are mentioned in the sentence or paragraph, all are usually expressed as figures and are used with the unspaced currency symbol.

> The scalpers were asking eighty dollars.
> Grandfather remembered the days of the five-cent cigar.
> The shoes on sale are priced at $69 and $89.
> Jill wanted to sell the lemonade for 25¢, 35¢, and 45¢.

25. Monetary units of mixed dollars-and-cents amounts are expressed in figures.

> $16.75
> $307.02

26. Even-dollar amounts are often expressed in figures without a decimal point and zeros. But when even-dollar amounts appear near amounts that include cents, the decimal point and zeros are usually added for consistency. The dollar sign is repeated before each amount in a series or inclusive range.

> They paid $500 for the watercolor.
> The price had risen from $8.00 to $9.95.
> bids of $80, $90, and $100
> in the $80–$100 range

27. Sums of money in the millions or above rounded to no more than one decimal place are usually expressed in a combination of figures and words.

> a $10-million building program
> $4.5 billion

28. In legal documents a sum of money is usually written out fully, often capitalized, with the corresponding figures in parentheses immediately following.

> Twenty-five Thousand Dollars ($25,000)

Organizations and Governmental Entities

29. Ordinal numbers in the names of religious organizations and churches are usually written out.

> Seventh-Day Adventists
> Third Congregational Church

30. Local branches of labor unions and fraternal organizations are generally identified by a numeral, usually placed after the name.

> Motion Picture Studio Mechanics Local 476
> Loyal Order of Moose No. 220
> Local 4277 Communications Workers of America

31. In names of governmental bodies and electoral, judicial, and military units, ordinal numbers of one hundred or below are usually written out but often not.

> Second Continental Congress
> Fifth Republic
> First Congressional District
> Court of Appeals for the Third Circuit
> U.S. Eighth Army
> Twelfth Precinct   *or*   12th Precinct
> Ninety-eighth Congress   *or*   98th Congress

Percentages

32. In technical writing, and often in business and financial writing, percentages are written as a figure followed by an unspaced % symbol. In general writing, the word *percent* normally replaces the symbol, and the number may either be written out (if it does not include a decimal) or expressed as a figure.

> *technical:*   15%
>   13.5%
> *general:*   15 percent
>   87.2 percent
>   Fifteen percent of the applicants were accepted.
>   a four percent increase   *or*   a 4% increase

33. In a series or range, the percent sign is usually included with all numbers, even if one of the numbers is zero.

> rates of 8.3%, 8.8%, and 9.1%
> a variation of 0% to 10% *or* a 0%–10% variation

Plurals

34. The plurals of written-out numbers, including fractions, are formed by adding -*s* or -*es*.

> at sixes and sevens   ever since the thirties
> divided into eighths   still in her thirties

35. The plurals of figures are formed by adding -*s* or less commonly -'*s*, especially where the apostrophe can prevent a confusing typographic appearance.

> in the '80s
> since the 1980s [*or less commonly* 1980's]
> temperatures in the 80s and 90s [*or* 80's and 90's]
> the *I*'s looked like *l*'s

Ratios

36. Ratios are generally expressed in figures, usually with the word *to*; in technical writing the figures may be joined by a colon or a slash instead. Ratios expressed in words use a hyphen (or en dash) or the word *to*.

> odds of 10 to 1   29 mi/gal
> a proportion of 1 to 4   a fifty-fifty chance
> a 3:1 ratio   a ratio of ten to four

Time of Day

37. In running text, the time of day is usually spelled out when expressed in even, half, or quarter hours or when it is followed by *o'clock*.

> around four-thirty
> arriving by ten
> planned to leave at half past five
> now almost a quarter to two
> arrived at nine o'clock

38. Figures are generally used when specifying a precise time.

> an appointment at 9:30 tomorrow morning
> buses at 8:42, 9:12, and 10:03 a.m.

39. Figures are also used when the time of day is followed by *a.m.* and *p.m.* These are usually written as punctuated lowercase letters, sometimes as small capital letters. They are not used with *o'clock* or with other words that specify the time of day.

> 8:30 a.m.   *or*   8:30 A.M.
> 10:30 p.m.   *or*   10:30 P.M.
> 8 a.m.   *or*   8 A.M.
> home by nine o'clock
> 9:15 in the morning
> eleven in the evening

With *twelve o'clock* or *12:00*, it is helpful to specify *midnight* or *noon* rather than the ambiguous *a.m.* or *p.m.*

> The third shift begins at 12:00 (midnight).

40. Even-hour times are generally written with a colon and two zeros when used in a series or pairing with any times not ending in two zeros.

> started at 9:15 a.m. and finished at 2:00 p.m.
> worked from 8:30 to 5:00

41. The 24-hour clock system—also called *military time*—uses no punctuation and omits *o'clock, a.m., p.m.* or any other additional indication of the time of day. The word *hours* sometimes replaces them.

> from 0930 to 1100
> at 1600 hours

Units of Measurement

42. In technical writing, all numbers used with units of measurement are written as numerals. In nontechnical writing, such numbers often simply follow the basic conventions explained on page 411; alternatively, even in nontechnical contexts all such numbers often appear as numerals.

> In the control group, only 8 of the 90 plants were affected.
> picked nine quarts of berries
> chugging along at 9 [*or* nine] miles an hour
> a pumpkin 5 [*or* five] feet in diameter
> weighing 7 pounds 9 ounces
> a journey of 3 hours and 45 minutes

The singular form of units of measurement is used in a modifier before a noun, the plural form in a modifier that follows a noun.

> a 2- by 9-inch board   *or*   a two-inch by nine-inch board   *or*   a two- by nine-inch board
> measured 2 inches by 9 inches   *or*   measured two inches by nine inches
> a 6-foot 2-inch man
> is 6 feet 2 inches tall   *or*   is six feet two inches tall
> is six feet two   *or*   is 6 feet 2

43. When units of measurement are written as abbreviations or symbols, the adjacent numbers are always figures. (For abbreviations with numerals, see the section on page 410.)

6 cm	$4.25	4′
1 mm	67.6 fl. oz.	98.6°

44. When two or more quantities are expressed, as in ranges or dimensions or series, an accompanying symbol is usually repeated with each figure.

> 4″ × 6″ cards
> temperatures of 30°, 55°, 43°, and 58°
> $450–$500 suits

Other Uses

45. Figures are generally used for precise ages in newspapers and magazines, and often in books as well.

Taking the helm is Colin Corman, 51, a risk-taking high roller.

At 9 [*or* nine] she mastered the Mendelssohn Violin Concerto.

the champion 3[*or* three]-year-old filly

for anyone aged 62 and over

46. Figures are used to refer to parts of a book, such as volume, chapter, illustration, and table numbers.

vol. 5, p. 202

Chapter 8   *or*   Chapter Eight

Fig. 4

47. Serial, policy, and contract numbers use figures. (For punctuation of these numbers, see paragraph 3 on page 415.)

Serial No. 5274

Permit No. 63709

48. Figures are used to express stock-market quotations, mathematical calculations, scores, and tabulations.

Industrials were up 4.23.

$3 \times 15 = 45$

a score of 8 to 2   *or*   a score of 8–2

the tally: 322 ayes, 80 nays

References

Writers give credit to other authors' published work in several ways. One is by the use of reference numbers within the text that are keyed to numbered references listed at the end of the article, as shown below.

Numbered reference: As some researchers noted, "New morphological, biochemical, and karyological studies suggest that *P. boylii* actually comprises several distinct species,"[12] and . . .

Alternatively, parenthetical references within the text are used; these are placed immediately after the quotation or piece of information whose source it refers to. Such references direct the reader to a list of references at the end of the article, chapter, or book, alphabetically arranged by author. The facts included in a parenthetical reference are the author's last name and date of publication; a volume and/or page number is also sometimes included, as shown below.

Parenthetical reference: As some researchers noted, "New morphological, biochemical, and karyological studies suggest that *P. boylii* actually comprises several distinct species" (Nowak 1991, 2:661) and . . .

In a carefully documented work, an alphabetically ordered bibliography or list of references normally follows the entire text (including any endnotes). Different publishers and journals have adopted varying styles, and their specific styles should be followed when submitting a manuscript for publication. However, the following examples illustrate a fairly standard format for a list of references. For more extensive treatment than can be provided here, consult *Merriam-Webster's Standard American Style Manual, The Chicago Manual of Style,* or the *American Medical Association Manual of Style.*

The principal features of a reference entry are these: (1) the author or list of authors is placed first; (2) the names of more than three authors are indicated by *et al.* after the first author's name; (3) initials are used for the author's first and middle names, and these are often closed up without any punctuation; (4) the date is usually placed directly after the author's name; (5) words in titles are lowercased except for the first word, the first word of any subtitle, and proper nouns and adjectives; (6) article titles are not enclosed in quotation marks; (7) book and journal titles may or may not be italicized; and (8) in journals, volume and page numbers are separated by a colon. The following examples include both books and periodical articles. They would be arranged in alphabetical order by author in an unannotated list.

Books

One author:	Creighton, T.E. 1983. *Proteins: Structures and molecular properties.* New York: W.H. Freeman.
Two or three authors:	Clayton, D., and M. Hills. 1993. *Statistical models in epidemiology.* Oxford, England: Oxford University Press.
Four or more authors:	Alberts, B., et al. 1989. *Molecular biology of the cell.* 2d ed. New York: Garland.
Corporate author:	American Psychiatric Association. 1987. *Diagnostic and statistical manual of mental disorders.* 3d ed. Washington, D.C.: American Psychiatric Association.
No author:	*Effects of managed care: An update.* 1994. Washington, D.C.: Congressional Budget Office.
Editor:	Clemente, C.E., ed. 1984. *Gray's anatomy of the human body.* 30th ed. Baltimore: Williams & Wilkins
Part of a book:	Mayr, E. 1982. Processes of speciation in animals. *Mechanisms of speciation.* Ed. C. Barigozzi. New York: Alan R. Liss.
Second or later edition:	Stryer, L. *Biochemistry.* 1988. 3d ed. New York: W.H. Freeman.
Two or more volumes:	Jubb, K.V., et al. 1992. *Pathology of domestic animals.* 4th ed. 2 vols. San Diego, Calif.: Academic Press.

Articles

Weekly magazine:	Preston, R. 1992. A reporter at large: Crisis in the hot zone. *New Yorker,* 26 Oct.:58-81.

Monthly magazine:	Weindruch, R. 1996. Caloric restriction and aging. *Scientific American* 274 (Jan.): 46–52.
Journal paginated by issue:	McPherson, D.D. 1996. Three-dimensional arterial imaging. *Science & Medicine* 3, no.2:22–31.
Journal paginated by volume:	Gould, S. J., and N. Eldredge. 1977. Punctuated equilibria: The tempo and mode of evolution reconsidered. *Paleobiology* 3:115–51.
Newspaper:	Broad, W.J. 1992. Big science squeezes small-scale researchers. *New York Times,* 29 Dec.:C1.

Appendix A

Career Development

You as the Job Applicant   431
Sources for Jobs   436
Interviewing   440
On the Job   444

The preceding chapters document procedures and information that you need for the daily activities in a medical office. This appendix presents information about developing your career.

You as the Job Applicant

Whether you are a novice or experienced medical office worker, there will be times during your career when you will be changing jobs or places of employment. The need to seek employment can be looked upon as an opportunity to assess current skills and personal characteristics. Employers want to hire individuals who have many of the characteristics listed below. Ideal candidates for a medical office staff should be:

- Dependable
- Punctual
- Friendly
- Cooperative
- Well-groomed
- Responsible
- Enthusiastic
- Self-controlled
- Honest
- Flexible
- Sensitive to handling confidential information

The various ways in which you can obtain a medical office position will differ according to (1) your educational background and the professional contacts you have made during your studies or past employment, (2) your past or current on-the-job experience, and (3) the nature of your geographical area. If you live in a city or large suburb, you will undoubtedly rely more often on medical and general employment agencies and on newspaper ads as you search for the right position. If you live in a small town where most of the residents know each other, you will probably depend on personal contacts with the local physicians and their staff.

Starting Your Search for a Job

Explore and evaluate every possible opportunity. Do not settle for the first offer that comes along unless you are absolutely certain that it is right for you. Visit places where you would like to work. For example, look at the roster of physicians on the board in the lobby of a medical building to see if you should investigate openings in some of these offices.

Consider nontraditional employment opportunities for medical office workers. Besides the ambulatory care setting, your skills could be useful in emergency care centers, hospitals, medical schools, foundations, nursing homes, pharmaceutical and chemical companies, medical-claims departments of insurance companies, and medical publishers.

Résumés

A current, up-to-date résumé is an essential tool to use in your job search. The résumé is the complete statement of your professional advancement and accomplishments to date. As such, it is a key factor in achieving your employment objectives.

Essential information Although many books have been written on this subject, there are several elements essential to all well-written résumés. These include the following:

1. Personal identification—your full name, address, and telephone number (home and/or office) placed at the top of the résumé
2. Employment experience—each job that you have held, listed chronologically from present to past, including the name and address of each doctor, practice, or organization (such as a clinic, hospital, or HMO); applicable employment dates; your job title and a brief job description or concise summary of your special accomplishments in each position
3. Educational background—a list of the institutions you have attended or from which you have graduated, starting with the highest level and concluding with high school
4. Special skills—a list of special skills (such as medical transcription or phlebotomy) that might prove a valuable asset to a prospective employer
5. References—summarized by the phrase "References provided on request" at the end of your résumé

Additional information If you have no previous employment experience, you can supplement your education category with a list of business and secretarial courses you have successfully completed; your transcription rates; and any academic or professional honors. If you have completed any special projects (such as typing a manuscript or participating in a research project), you can mention them under the heading "Special Projects" after the educational section.

While employers are prohibited by federal law from asking certain questions, you as a candidate can present in a résumé any information that you feel will put you in a positive light. For example, while an employer cannot ask you about church activities, you may wish to explain how you successfully lead a youth group in your church, thus demonstrating an experience in both leadership and organizational skills.

The résumé will not only give you an opportunity to demonstrate some of your best work, it will help you to complete the application form at the interview. By having your polished résumé on hand, you will have anticipated most of the application's questions and be able to simply and neatly copy this information onto the application form.

Excluded information   The following information should *not* be given on the résumé itself:

- Names and addresses of references—List on a separate sheet and provide them at the interview or in an interview follow-up letter.
- Salary—Discuss salary requirements and ranges during the interview itself, since you do not want to undersell yourself ahead of time or price yourself out of a job market with which you may be unfamiliar.
- Your reasons, if any, for changing jobs—Since wording can often be misunderstood without personal clarification, it is best to discuss this matter with the interviewer, and only if you are asked, rather than committing yourself on paper.
- Your reasons for present unemployment, if applicable—This topic is also best dealt with in person or in a telephone conversation.
- Photograph—This can work for or against you, depending on the subjectivity of the person evaluating your application. (It is illegal for an employer to request a photograph.)

Format   Your résumé normally should not exceed one or two pages. For maximum brevity as well as comprehensiveness, plan the material and then compose a draft before keyboarding or typing the final version. All facts should be double-checked. Use plain, straightforward English, devoid of technical jargon and superlatives. Check and recheck your résumé for any misspelling. An error on a résumé is a sign of a careless employee.

The résumé should be typed or printed out on plain standard bond paper. Margins should be balanced. Although there are many acceptable résumé formats, the simplest is to block all material flush left without indention. Entries should be single-spaced, with double- or triple-spacing between entries, depending on the available space on the page. Underline or capitalize main and secondary headings. Copies must be clean and legible; for this purpose, offset copies or photocopies are suggested. (See Figure A.1 for a sample résumé.)

Fig. A.1   Résumé

Joan Bramwell Connor
1216 Philadelphia St., S.E.
Grand Rapids, MI 49506
(616) 555-1212 (home)
(616) 555-1000 (office)

EMPLOYMENT EXPERIENCE

1993 to present	Towers Internal Medicine Associates, P.C. 21 Michigan St., N.E. Grand Rapids, MI 49503 Medical Assistant
1989 to 1993	Grand Valley Medical Group 350 Clement St. S.E. Fort Haven, MI 49375 Medical Assistant
1985 to 1989	Dickinson Hospital Records Department Grand Rapids, MI 49503 Records Clerk

EDUCATION

1981-1982	University of Michigan Ann Arbor, MI
1982-1984	Springfield College Grand Rapids, MI A.S. in Medical Assisting
1988 to present	150 Continuing Education Units

NATIONAL CERTIFICATION

1987	CMA credential
1988	CMA-Administrative specialist

SKILLS	Windows 95 Lotus 1-2-3 Proficient in Spanish

References provided on request

References

When you include a list of references, follow the general format and style that you have used for your résumé. Do not change paper size or color and do not use a different type style. Again, white bond paper is appropriate. Head the list "References." Single-space each entry and double- or triple-space between entries.

List the full name, address, and telephone number of each person who has agreed to recommend you. Include at least one supervisor and/or doctor from each former place of employment. Include one former instructor, if applicable. Personal character references can be listed at the bottom of the sheet, if necessary. Give the physician or interviewer the reference list when it is asked for but do not attach this list to your résumé. (See Figure A.2 for a sample list of references.)

Fig. A.2 References

Joan Bramwell Connor

REFERENCES

Helen P. Thornton, M.D.
Towers Internal Medicine Associates
21 Michigan St., N.E.
Grand Rapids, MI 49503
(616) 555-1000

John L. Stimson, M.D.
Dickinson Hospital
129 Main St.
Grand Rapids, MI 49503
(616) 555-2121

Mary Jones Applegate, R.N.
Grand Valley Medical Group
350 Clement St. S.E.
Fort Haven, MI 49375
(616) 555-3434

Personal Reference
The Reverend Donald O'Leary
The Rectory
Grace Episcopal Church
6 Northwood St.
Spring Green, MI 48765
(616) 555-6767

Contacting references   Contact the people you are listing to make sure they agree to your using them as a reference, so they can be prepared for a phone call. Even friends who think highly of you may stumble if they receive a reference check that they are not expecting. Alerting the people you list as references will enable them to mentally prepare their responses if they are contacted. Many employers do not contact personal references any more, but most should contact business references.

If you are entering the job market from school, references from teachers and your grade point average will be the most important items the employer will use to evaluate your technical skills.

Cover Letter

You may be asked to submit a cover letter along with your résumé. This letter will greatly assist in preselling you to a prospective employer if it is properly formatted and well-written. This type of letter is a concrete indication of your verbal and technical skills and your general personality and intelligence.

Unless a handwritten letter is requested, you should type or print out the letter on plain bond paper. Do not use social stationery or personalized letterhead. Exotic typefaces should be avoided. The block or the semiblock format is appropriate (see Figures A.3 and A.4 for examples). The letter should not exceed one page. Under no circumstances should you prepare and photocopy a generic form letter to be sent to numerous physicians. The applicant lacking the time and courtesy to write a personal letter will most probably not receive careful consideration.

Plan your cover letter in detail. If you are responding to an advertisement, mention in the first paragraph the specific position for which you are applying and the date and source of the advertisement. If the letter is unsolicited (that is, you are applying on your own initiative), say so in the first paragraph and indicate why you are interested in working for that particular practice.

Next, focus on and develop your best assets. A concise statement of your technical skills may be given along with mention of any more specialized skills. A sentence expanding on some aspect of your education or on your previous employment experience not already developed fully in the résumé can be included in the letter. Be straightforward yet modest and sincere.

Proofread the draft and the completed copy so that there are no grammatical, spelling, or typographical errors. Keep a copy of this letter for your records. (See Figure A.3 for a sample cover letter.)

Sources for Jobs

Newspaper Ads

The most available source of job listings are newspaper ads. Every day of the week, available positions in the medical office are listed in newspapers. Larger

Fig. A.3   Cover Letter, in Block Format

1216 Philadelphia St., S.E.
Grand Rapids, MI 49506

June 1, 1996

Ms. Anne Jones Peters
Office Manager
Falmouth Surgical Associates
56 Main St.
Hadley, MI 49708

Dear Ms. Peters:

I am sending my résumé in response to your ad for a medical assistant that appeared in the *Union News* on May 25.

I am a Certified Medical Assistant and have been working in a busy internal medicine practice for the past three years. I have experience in the full range of office and clinical duties, from handling reception and check-out to performing lab tests. In addition I assist in processing insurance claims.

I would like to expand my experience by working in a specialist's practice, and I value the excellent reputation of Falmouth Surgical Associates. I believe my experience would be useful in your medical office, and I look forward to meeting with you to learn more about this position. I will call you next week to follow up.

Sincerely,

Joan B. Connor

metropolitan areas will have new opportunities daily. The Sunday want ads tend to have the greatest number of advertisements. The serious applicant, however, should study the early edition of the paper each day to identify the best possible positions as they open.

The ads may vary as to whether or not the applicant should telephone the office to learn more about the job or submit a résumé. Other ads may ask prospective applicants to come to the office for an application form. The

Fig. A.4   Follow-up Letter, in Semiblock Format

1216 Philadelphia St., S.E.
Grand Rapids, MI 49506

June 12, 1996

Ms. Anne Jones Peters
Office Manager
Falmouth Surgical Associates
56 Main St.
Hadley, MI 49708

Dear Ms. Peters:

   It was a pleasure talking with you yesterday about the medical assistant's position at Falmouth Surgical Associates. I was very impressed with the job as you described it and with the professionalism of the staff.

   I hope you will give me the opportunity to put my skills and enthusiasm to work for your office. I believe my range of medical assisting skills would serve the practice well. The interview confirmed my interest in working with you, and I certainly hope to hear from you.

Sincerely yours,

Joan B. Connor

---

most common ads tend to ask the candidate to call the office, listing a name and phone number.

Answering an ad by telephone   When responding to a newspaper ad by telephone, the intent should be to sell yourself in order to obtain an interview. You want to make yourself appear to be a desirable candidate to the prospective employer, which will optimize your chances of obtaining maximum salary and benefits.

   Your inquiries about the job should center around the medical practice itself and the specific job opening. Take good notes on everything you are told about the practice, as well as what duties you will be expected to perform.

Always be honest, but be honest in a positive way. For example, if you are not familiar with one of the duties described by the prospective employer, rather than saying you are inexperienced, respond that although you have not had previous experience in that area, you have been known to be a fast learner. Explain that from what you have heard, the new task is something you would be very interested in learning to do, and are confident you would be able to perform it well within a short period of time.

Your positive characteristics   Most employers try to minimize the number of people who will actually receive interviews, hoping to limit the pool to the top candidates. In addition to determining your technical ability to perform the job, employers will try to identify prospective employees with certain positive characteristics. Some characteristics you should try to convey include loyalty, stability, enthusiasm, judgment, and intelligence. Try to make sure these positive characteristics come through on the phone, as the proper attitude will outweigh most other shortcomings of an employee. In other words, an employee with the proper attitude and a shortcoming in a particular technical area will generally be able to overcome the technical weakness within a matter of time.

In order to successfully sell yourself, be prepared for certain common questions that a prospective employer will ask before granting you an interview. Develop some positive answers, and if you are not having success after speaking with a few prospective employers, go over your answers with someone who may be able to coach you, such as a friend at the management level in the health care field, an executive in another field, or a career adviser.

Screening process   Questions that might be asked during the telephone screening process could include the following:
- Why does this job appeal to you?
- Why did you answer our ad?
- What work experience do you have that would be helpful in completing the duties with this position?
- If our office hours run over and you need to stay late, will that be a problem?
- What type of salary range are you interested in?

Be careful not to get trapped by the question on salary. Respond that you are hoping to receive a competitive salary for the job, but that the future opportunities within the practice are more important to you than the initial salary. Explain that you are looking for the opportunity to grow professionally with the practice.

Placement Agencies

Another way candidates are brought together with prospective employers is through placement agencies. Placement agencies can be expensive; however, the fee is normally paid by the employer. When dealing with a placement agency, be careful what you sign; agency commissions range from 10 to 20 percent of the first year's salary. Be cautious if the agency expects you to pay that fee rather than the employer.

A good placement agency can work as a buffer between the candidate and the employer, identifying and matching the needs and skill of the employer and employee. If the agency identifies you as a good candidate, it can help your chances of getting a job by preselling you to the employer before your interview. The agency may also be able to coach you on the specific attributes the prospective employer is looking for.

Approach the placement agency in the same way you would approach a prospective employer. A good employment agency will send its best prospects to its best clients. As such, it is to your benefit to be perceived by the agency as a top candidate. The rules explained above regarding the screening process will apply to your first contact with the employment agency.

State Employment Agencies

Government-supported employment agencies, such as state unemployment offices, will typically post job requirements for interested candidates. Many prospective employers, however, will not use public agencies, so your search should not be limited to them. Leads from public agencies should be followed up in the same manner as cold leads from the newspaper.

Networking

Networking always has been a method for matching prospective employees with employers. Finding a job through a network contact is generally to your advantage, since the employer is meeting a candidate with at least some sort of pre-interview reference check. Therefore, call everyone you know to see who they know in the medical field, or who they might know who know people in the medical field. This network could include parents, grandparents, siblings, aunts, uncles, neighbors, teachers, old friends, and new friends. People like to do other people favors and you never know where a lead might come from. In many cases, a job may be filled through a network contact before it ever is advertised in the newspaper or placed with an employment agency.

Interviewing

Prepare for the Interview

Once you have been scheduled for an interview, regardless of how you obtained it, you should begin some research and become as well-prepared as possible for that interview. First of all, identify the specialty or niche of the medical practice. If it is otolaryngology, for example, become as familiar with that specialty as possible. Know what type of procedures are performed, what type of patients are seen there, what type of ancillary services are likely to be performed, and what type of medical staff is likely to be on hand. Study a variety of reference sources, including the CPT-4 (Current Procedural Terminology), which lists all the different procedures performed by different specialties.

Research the specialty   If you have a friend or contact working in an office of this specialty, contact them to ask questions about the specialty and perhaps even get an office tour. In the absence of knowing someone, do not be afraid to contact the office manager of another office and see if you can arrange a tour and question-and-answer session. Simply introduce yourself as a recent graduate in the medical field and ask if you could spend 15 minutes to learn more about their specialty. This will not only give you an inside glimpse of the particular specialty, but it could lead to another inside network source.

Research the specific practice   After learning as much as you can about the specialty, try to find out about the specific practice. For example, study the names and pronunciations of each of the doctors working at the practice. Try to learn if any of the doctors has an outstanding reputation in a particular area. See if you know any patients of the practice; it will be in your favor. For example, it would be impressive for you to be able to say, "I have heard about Dr. Jones and have been impressed with his reputation. I know a patient of his, Jane Smith, who thinks he's the best doctor in the field. I would be honored to be associated with this type of practice."

If the prospective employer is a hospital, for example, do a little research to see how many beds the hospital is licensed for and how many are staffed. If you are in a metropolitan area, compare this with the other hospitals in the area. If you are in a rural area, compare this with some of the other hospitals in other towns. Find out if the hospital is known for any particular specialty and what level of care they are able to give. You may have the opportunity to request a tour of the hospital before your interview, or to at least go over and walk through the campus yourself. Having information on the prospective employer available will demonstrate a true interest on your part.

The Interview

You are now ready for the actual interview with the prospective employer. Following are some of the most important points to remember as you go through the interview.

Dress   An interview is not the place to make a fashion statement, so avoid trendy outfits. There are regional preferences as to what type of clothing is acceptable. A woman applying to a thoracic surgery group practice in a metropolitan area like Atlanta, Philadelphia, or St. Louis might wear a stylish suit; in a small rural community, a skirt and blouse and low heels would be considered appropriate dress. A man might wear freshly pressed slacks, shirt, and tie with dark shoes.

The interviewer will notice the overall impression you make; neat and clean appearance is important. Avoid wearing lots of jewelry and too much makeup. When you are speaking with the interviewer to set up the appointment, there is nothing improper in asking if they would like you to wear a uniform. By bringing the topic up, you might be given a hint of the employer's expectations. If the interview is held on a Saturday morning, for example, you may be told to dress casually (this does not mean blue jeans). A woman might choose a slacks outfit; a man might forgo a tie.

Punctuality Be on time for your interview. If you do not know exactly where the office is located, get directions beforehand. Give yourself plenty of time to get there with time to spare. The longer you wait in the office, the more you can observe about the office personality. You may want to make a dry run the day before the interview in case there is road construction along the route.

Arrival Identify yourself to the receptionist and state your business. "I'm Patty Perfect and I'm here to see Dr. Smith at 5 P.M. about a job." Be cheerful and polite.

Waiting If you have to wait before seeing the interviewer, sit quietly and observe the office routines. This process may provide you with additional questions to ask later in the interview.

Introductions When introduced to the physician or the office manager, repeat their names ("How do you do, Dr. Smith," or "It's nice to meet you, Ms. Jones"), and appear enthusiastic but not gushy.

Posture When sitting, do not sprawl, but do not sit rigidly like a stone. Try to relax.

Behavior No smoking and no gum chewing. If refreshment such as coffee is offered, decline the offer, unless you have a steady hand and a place to put the cup and saucer or mug.

Questions to ask Be prepared for certain questions during the interview, and also be prepared to ask questions. Avoid answering questions with a yes or no, but also avoid talking too much. Questions you could be prepared to ask could include the following:

- What things about the practice do employees appreciate the most?
- What things about the practice do employees seem to dislike the most?
- Do the employees tend to get along and work as a team?
- Does the practice provide time off for continuing education?
- How does the practice keep up with complex issues such as OSHA regulations and training, CLIA and Medicare rules and regulations?

Questions to answer Questions you should be prepared to answer could include the following:

- Why are you interested in our job; what is making you consider a change now?
- What attracted you to our position?
- What do you like best about your current job (or career choice) and what do you dislike the most?
- What do you like best about your current employer (teachers, school, etc.)?
- What attributes of our job do you like best?
- Where do you plan to be, in your career five years from now? (Watch out for this question; in answering, you want to show an enthusiasm for your selected career and an expectation that you will be well advanced in five years. It is better to project overambition than to have few expectations for yourself.)

Testing Many employers may have candidates take a test, particularly for business or clerical positions. These tests should be relatively simple, such as a typing test for a secretary or a day-sheet-balancing test for a bookkeeper. Psychologically, be prepared to take a test and don't be intimidated if you are requested to do so. In most cases, it is appropriate to put accuracy ahead of speed, since a quality product is essential in the medical field.

Termination of the interview Let the physician or the office manager terminate the interview. When he or she stands up, you may do the same. Shake hands, thank the interviewer for the time spent with you, say that it has been an interesting or enjoyable experience or whatever seems the most appropriate, and then say good-bye. Do not forget to say good-bye to the assistant or receptionist on the way out.

Follow-up letter When you get home, immediately send a letter (handwritten on personal stationery is acceptable) thanking the interviewer for the time spent with you. It is most effective to use statements such as "The interview confirmed my interest in working with you. I certainly hope to hear from you soon." (See Figure A.4 for a sample follow-up letter.)

Second Interview

Successful interviews will usually result in a second interview. Generally one or two candidates will be selected for a second interview, so if you are one, it means you performed well on your first interview. You are coming close to being offered the job; therefore, be prepared to accept an offer and negotiate a starting date. During your second interview, you will probably meet the same person you met in the first interview, as well as additional people. Remain calm, you are almost there.

General Pointers

Some additional tips can help during an interview. Make eye contact with the interviewer. Avoid the annoying verbal tics such as "ah" or "um" and the repetition of "you know" or "OK" throughout the conversation. Follow the interviewer's lead. Do not try to lead the conversation. You may interject questions when appropriate during lulls in the conversation or you may save them to ask at the end of the interview.

Salary

When wages are discussed, have a clear idea of what you expect. However, it is unwise to argue with a prospective employer about a salary you think is too low. If you can see that the interview is about to end and the employer has not yet brought up the subject of salary, you might say, "Oh, by the way, Dr. Smith, what do you feel is a reasonable salary based on your expectations and my qualifications?" Or you might say, "May I ask what the salary will be?"

You can also convey your knowledge of the usual and customary salary ranges in your particular geographical area by mentioning those ranges in round numbers; for example, "When I spoke with the medical society, it was suggested that the going salary for this type of position is currently $." You should not be insistent; just state the facts objectively.

Reducing Stress

The interview process is normally quite stressful and tension-filled for applicants. Do your best to reduce your stress by participating in some friendly chat before getting into the nitty-gritty of the interview. Comment on such superficial matters as the weather or perhaps compliment the employer on the appearance of the office, location, etc.

One way to control stress is to tell yourself that the worst thing that could happen is that you will not get the job. Since you did not have the job before the interview, you will not end up in a worse situation. Continue to tell yourself that you can only improve your situation by going to the interview. If you are not offered the job, you will be no worse off than when you started, but you will have gained some experience in interviewing. Like anything else, the more you do, the better you will become.

On the Job

After you have successfully obtained the position, it is a good idea to review the job description of your expected duties and to read the personnel policies manual.

Job Description

Smaller offices may not have formal job descriptions, because the doctor-owner may feel that they hinder flexibility and that people should be versatile enough to handle all different types of jobs. In reality, formal job descriptions do not hinder flexibility, but rather help employees identify the most important aspects of their job and prioritize. In the absence of job descriptions, it may take employees a while to identify what is most important to the organization.

Larger organizations will undoubtedly have formal job descriptions. Because of the ongoing changes in the health care field, job descriptions may become outdated unless they are frequently updated. If your employer does not take the initiative to review and update your job description at the time of your periodic review, take the initiative yourself. You can use the job description to evaluate yourself and point out your strengths to the employer. You can also use any changes in the job description to point out what expanded areas of responsibility you might have taken on since the previous job review.

Personnel Policies Manual

Small offices may not have written personnel policies, although this is becoming rare in all offices. It is difficult for any employer to be fair and consistent without having written guidelines, and the failure to have a written policy can lead to inconsistencies and potential personnel problems.

Therefore, you should generally expect to receive upon hiring, or at least on the first day, a personnel policies manual outlining the office's policy on various personnel issues. You should recognize that normally these are policies subject to change by the employer and are not employment contracts or guarantees. They should, however, be a dependable guide to personnel procedures. You should be notified in writing of any changes in personnel policy through the issuance of a new policy or an updated section to the manual.

When you receive the personnel policies manual, it may seem large and overwhelming and you may file it away without reading it. However, a good employee will read the manual and become familiar with it. A well-drafted policies manual should answer many questions you have now or questions that come up. If you are unable to read the whole manual at once, read it section by section over your first few weeks at the office and then keep it on hand to answer questions as they arise. (For details on information in a personnel policies manual, see Chapter 7, "Personnel Policies.")

Appendix B

Supplementary Information

Health Promotion and Disease Prevention 446
Schedules of Controlled Substances 449
Glossary of Managed Care Terms 451
National Practitioner Data Bank 453
Immunization Schedule 454
Poison Control Centers 454
Selected References 461

The following supplementary information includes material that further describes issues discussed in the various chapters.

Health Promotion and Disease Prevention

As the federal government became more and more involved in the financing of health care (through Medicare, Medicaid, the Veterans Administration, etc.), research (through the National Institutes of Health), and data collection, it began to realize that the prevention of illness offered an important avenue for not only controlling costs but also improving the quality of life of its citizens.

The year 1979 marked the first major federal effort to address this issue with the publication by the U.S. Public Health Service (PHS) of the report *Healthy People: The Surgeon General's Report on Health Promotion and Disease Prevention.* In 1980 a second publication by the PHS followed, *Promoting Health/ Preventing Disease: Objectives for the Nation.*

Adopting a "management by objectives" approach, the PHS set out objectives addressing improvements in health status expressed in measurable terms with clear targets to be accomplished by 1990. Midcourse reviews of progress were reported at intervals, and in 1987 a steering committee was formed within the PHS to oversee the process of revising the objectives to target the year 2000.

One of the committee's first efforts was to broaden the participation and involvement of a number of private and public entities with interests in health promotion and disease prevention.

With help from the Institute of Medicine, the National Academy of Sciences, and leading agencies of the PHS, a number of regional hearings were jointly convened to help explore and increase the participation of interested persons and organizations. New objectives were developed, which included targeting selected populations for specific attention as well as adding new areas such as HIV infection and cancer.

The result of months of intensive activity directed by the Office of Disease Prevention and Health Promotion, the PHS produced, among other substantial gains, the 1990 publication, *Healthy People 2000: National Health Promotion and Disease Prevention Objectives,*. This document presented three broad goals for the nation:

1. To increase the span of healthy life for Americans
2. To reduce health disparities among Americans
3. To achieve access to preventive services for all Americans

Healthy People 2000 identified 22 areas of priority comprising over 300 measurable objectives to be reached by the year 2000. Examples from the 22 areas include the following:

Health Promotion

1. Physical Activity and Fitness
- Increase to at least 30 percent the proportion of people aged 6 and older who engage regularly, preferably daily, in light to moderate physical activity for at least 30 minutes per day.

2. Nutrition
- Reduce overweight to a prevalence of no more than 20 percent among people aged 20 and older and no more than 15 percent among adolescents aged 12-19

3. Tobacco
- Reduce cigarette smoking to a prevalence of no more than 15 percent among people aged 20 and older

4. Alcohol and Other Drugs
- Reduce deaths caused by alcohol-related motor vehicle crashes to no more than 8.5 per 100,000 people

5. Family Planning
- Reduce pregnancies among girls aged 17 and younger to no more than 50 per 1,000 adolescents

6. Mental Health and Mental Disorders
- Reduce suicides to no more than 10.5 per 100,000 people

7. Violent and Abusive Behavior
- Reduce homicides to no more than 7.2 per 100,000 people

8. Educational and Community-Based Programs
- Increase to at least 50 percent the proportion of postsecondary institutions with institution-wide health promotion programs for students, faculty, and staff

Health Protection

9. Unintentional Injuries
- Reduce deaths caused by unintentional injuries to no more than 29.3 per 100,000 people

10. Occupational Safety and Health
- Reduce deaths from work-related injuries to no more than 4 per 100,000 full-time workers

11. Environmental Health
- Reduce outbreaks of waterborne disease from infectious agents and chemical poisoning to no more than 11 per year

12. Food and Drug Safety
- Reduce outbreaks of infections due to *S. enteritidis* to fewer than 25 per year

13. Oral Health
- Reduce to no more than 20 percent the proportion of people aged 65 and older who have lost all of their natural teeth

Preventive Services

14. Maternal and Infant Health
- Reduce the infant mortality rate to no more than 7 per 1,000 live births

15. Heart Disease and Stroke
- Reduce coronary heart disease deaths to no more than 100 per 100,000 people

16. Cancer
- Reverse the rise in cancer deaths to achieve a rate of no more than 130 per 100,000 people

17. Diabetes and Chronic Disabling Conditions
- Increase years of healthy life to at least 65 years

18. HIV Infection
- Confine annual incidence of diagnosed AIDS cases to no more than 98,000 cases

19. Sexually Transmitted Diseases (STD)
- Reduce gonorrhea to an incidence of no more than 225 cases per 100,000 people

20. Immunization and Infectious Diseases

- Improve the financing and delivery of immunizations for children and adults so that virtually no American has a financial barrier to receiving recommended immunizations

21. Clinical Preventive Services

- Increase to at least 95 percent the proportion of people who have a specific source of ongoing primary care for the coordination of their preventive and episodic health care

22. Surveillance and Data Systems

- Identify, and create where necessary, national data sources to measure progress toward each of the year 2000 national health objectives

The Office of Health Promotion and Disease Prevention has succeeded in enlisting the help of a number of national, state and local agencies, and has encouraged and supported the participation of all groups with interest in any or all of these goals and objectives. Periodic updates to the original *Healthy People 2000* are published, the most recent being *Healthy People 2000 Review, 1994,* and *1995 Healthy People 2000 Midcourse Review.* Copies of these publications are available from the Superintendent of Documents, U.S. Government Printing Office, Washington, D.C. 20402.

Schedules of Controlled Substances

As mentioned in Chapter 2, "Health Law," the enactment of the Controlled Substances Act in 1970 classified drugs into five schedules, according to their potential for abuse and user dependence. The schedules range from I (most restricted) to V (least regulated). Some examples of the drugs and the five schedules are shown below:

Schedule I

These substances may not be used for any purposes except medical research. Included are:

Narcotics: Heroin and many nonmarketed synthetic narcotics
Hallucinogens:
  LSD
  MDA, STP, DMT, DET,
    mescaline, peyote,
    bufotenine, ibogaine,
    psilocybin, phencyclidine
    (PCP) (veterinary drug only)

Marijuana, tetrahydrocannabinols
Methaqualone

Schedule II

These are substances available by written prescription only, without refills. Included are:

Narcotics:
Opium
Opium alkaloids and derived
phenanthrene alkaloids:
Morphine, codeine,
hydromorphone (Dilaudid),
oxymorphone (Numorphan),
oxycodone (dihydrohydroxy-
codeinone, a component of
Percodan, Percocet, Tylox)
Designated synthetic drugs:
Meperidine (Demerol),
methadone, levorphanol (Levo-
Dromoran), fentanyl
(Sublimaze), alphaprodine
(Nisentil), sufentanil (Sufenta)

Stimulants:
Coca leaves and cocaine
Amphetamine (Benzedrine)
Amphetamine complex
(Biphetamine)
Dextroamphetamine
(Dexedrine)
Methamphetamine (Desoxyn)
Phenmetrazine (Preludin)
Methylphenidate (Ritalin)
Above in mixtures iwth other
controlled or uncontrolled
drugs
Depressants:
Amobarbital (Amytal)
Pentobarbital (Nembutal)
Secobarbital (Seconal)
Mixtures of above (e.g., Tuinal)

Schedule III

Substances in this class require new prescriptions after six months or five refills. They include:

Narcotics: The following opiates in
combination with one or more
active nonnarcotic ingredients,
provided the amount does not
exceed that shown:
Codeine and dihydrocodeine:
Not to exceed 1800 mg/dL or
90 mg/tablet or other dose
unit
Dihydrocodeinone
(hydrocodone and in
Hycodan): Not to exceed 300
mg/dL or 15 mg/tablet
Opium: 500 mg/dL or 25 mg/
5 mL or other dosage unit
(paregoric)

Stimulants:
Benzphetamine (Didrex)
Phendimetrazine (Plegine)
Depressants:
Schedule II barbiturates in
mixtures with noncontrolled
drugs or in suppository dose
form
Aprobarbital (Alurate)
Butabarbital (Butisol)
Glutethimide (Doriden)
Talbutal (Lotusate)
Thiamylal (Surital)
Thiopental (Pentothal)

Schedule IV

Prescriptions for drugs in this group must also be rewritten after six months or five refills; the penalties for illegal possession differ from those under Schedule III. Drugs in this group include:

Narcotics:
Pentazocine (Talwin)
Propoxyphene (Darvon)
Stimulants:
Diethylpropion (Tenuate)
Mazindol (Sanorex)
Phentermine (Ionamin)
Fenfluramine (Pondimin)
Pemoline (Cylert)
Depressants:
Benzodiazepines:
Alprazolam (Xanax)
Chlordiazepoxide (Librium)
Clonazepam (Clonopin)
Clorazepate (Tranxene)
Diazepam (Valium)
Flurazepam (Dalmane)

Depressants: (cont)
Halazepam (Paxipam)
Lorazepam (Ativan)
Oxazepam (Serax)
Prazepam (Centrax)
Temazepam (Restoril)
Triazolam (Halcion)
Chloral hydrate
Ethchlorvynol (Placidyl)
Ethinamate (Valmid)
Meprobamate (Equanil,
Miltown, etc)
Mephobarbital (Mebaral)
Methohexital (Brevital)
Methyprylon (Noludar)
Paraldehyde
Phenobarbital

Schedule V

This class is the least restrictive and includes any other nonnarcotic prescription drug, as well as drugs that may be dispensed without prescription (unless prohibited by state regulations.)

Narcotics:
Diphenoxylate (not more than 2.5 mg and not less than 0.025 mg of atropine per dosage unit, as in Lomotil)
Loperamide (Imodium)

The following drugs in combination with other active, nonnarcotic ingredients and provided the amount per 100 mL or 100 g does not exceed that shown:
Codeine: 200 mg
Dihydrocodeine: 100 mg

Glossary of Managed Care Terms

This glossary of managed care terms applies to their use in Chapter 4, "Managed Care." Abbreviations or acronyms used in discussing managed care can also be found in Appendix C.

benefit package health services that an insurer, government agency, or health plan offers to a group or individual under the terms of a contract

capitation a stipulated amount of money paid out per member to cover the cost of health care per member

carve out to obtain separately a service that is usually part of an indemnity or HMO plan

case management a process in coordinating the care of a person with specific health care needs in order to achieve the ideal patient outcome in the most cost-effective manner

clinic without walls a group of physicians who have formed a single legal entity but maintain their individual practices

closed panel a managed health care plan that contracts with physicians for their services and requires these physicians to not see patients from other health care organizations

co-insurance the portion of covered health care costs for which the member has a financial responsibility to pay, usually a fixed percentage

community rating a process used to set premium rates based on a total community's or region's actuarial estimates of utilization

co-payment a fixed dollar amount that the member must pay for specified services at the time the health care is rendered

deductible the amount of health care expenses a covered person must pay each year before the plan will make any payments for eligible benefits

exclusive provider organization (EPO) a health care plan that provides coverage for the members if they utilize only contracted physicians

experience rating the process of setting premium rates based upon previous claims experience and projected required revenues for a specific group

fee-for-service (FFS) reimbursement the process under which physicians and other providers receive a payment that does not exceed their total expenses for each unit of service provided

gatekeeper a primary care case-management model where the primary care physician, or gatekeeper, serves as the patient's initial contact for medical care and referrals

group-model HMO an HMO that contracts with a physician group, reimbursing services rendered at a negotiated rate

health maintenance organization (HMO) an organization that provides coverage and health services needed by members for a fixed, prepaid premium

indemnity plan an insurance plan in which the insured person is reimbursed for covered expenses

independent practice association (IPA) an organization that contracts with a health care plan, which in turn contracts with physicians, to provide health care services in return for a negotiated fee

integrated service network a network of providers and payers which would provide care and compete with other systems for enrollees in their region

management services organization (MSO) an organization that provides practice management, administrative, and support services to individual physicians or group practices

network-model HMO an HMO plan that contracts with more than one physician group, and may contract with single- and multispecialty groups

physician-hospital organization (PHO/HPO) a health care plan formed and owned by one or more hospitals and physician groups in order to obtain payer contracts and further mutual interests

point-of-service (POS) plan a health plan that allows the member to choose which provider, participating or nonparticipating, to receive services from; reimbursement is based upon various benefit levels and the type of provider chosen

preadmission authorization a review to determine the need for inpatient hospital care, done before actual admission

preferred provider organization (PPO) a health care plan that contracts with medical care providers; the plan offers better benefits if members use these "preferred" providers

primary care physician (PCP) a physician whose practice is devoted to internal medicine, family/general practice, and pediatrics

staff-model HMO an HMO that employs providers and requires these providers to use the HMO's own facilities

utilization review (UR) a formal analysis of the medical necessity, efficiency, and/or appropriateness of health care services and treatment plans

National Practitioner Data Bank

The National Practitioner Data Bank is a resource available to state licensing boards, hospitals and other health care entities, professional societies, and federal agencies to identify problematic or incompetent performance or unprofessional conduct by physicians, dentists, and other health care providers. The Data Bank collects and releases to eligible entities information as it relates to the professional competence and conduct of physicians, dentists, and, in some cases, other licensed health care practitioners. Examples of such information include:

- Medical malpractice payments
- Adverse licensure actions
- Adverse actions on clinical privileges
- Adverse actions on professional society memberships.

All Title IV requirements for reporting to and requesting information from the Data Bank are applicable to physicians and dentists. Some elements of Title IV, such as reporting medical malpractice payments, also apply to other health care practitioners who are licensed or otherwise authorized by an individual state to provide health care services The Data Bank helpline is available at (800) 767-6732.

Immunization Schedule

The following list details the government's recommended schedule for childhood vaccinations:

Birth to 2 months:	hepatitis B
2 months:	polio; diphtheria, pertussis, tetanus (DPT); *Haemophilus influenzae* type B (Hib)
2 to 4 months:	hepatitis B
4 months:	polio; DPT; Hib
6 months:	DPT; Hib
6 to 18 months:	hepatitis B; polio
12 to 15 months:	DPT; Hib; measles, mumps, rubella (MMR)
12 to 18 months:	chicken pox
4 to 6 years:	polio; DPT; MMR

Poison Control Centers

The following list is compiled by the American Association of Poison Control Centers and includes names, addresses, and phone numbers of poison control centers as of April 1995; they are listed alphabetically by state.

Alabama

Alabama Poison Center, Tuscaloosa
408-A Paul Bryant Drive
Tuscaloosa, AL 35401
Emergency Phone: (800) 462-0800 (AL only) or (205) 345-0600

Regional Poison Control Center
The Children's Hospital of Alabama
1600 - 7th Ave. South
Birmingham, AL 35233-1711
Emergency Phone: (205) 939-9201, (800) 292-6678 (AL only), or (205) 933-4050

Arizona

Arizona Poison and Drug Information Center
Arizona Health Sciences Center; Rm. #3204-K
1501 N. Campbell Ave.
Tucson, AZ 85724
Emergency Phone: (800) 362-0101 (AZ only), (602) 626-6016

Samaritan Regional Poison Center
Good Samaritan Regional Medical Center
Ancillary-1
1111 E. McDowell Road
Phoenix, AZ 85006
Emergency Phone: (602) 253-3334

California

Central California Regional Poison Control Center

Valley Children's Hospital
3151 N. Millbrook, IN31
Fresno, CA 93703
Emergency Phone: (800) 346-5922 (Central CA only) or (209) 445-1222

San Diego Regional Poison Center

UCSD Medical Center
200 West Arbor Drive
San Diego, CA 92103-8925
Emergency Phone: (619) 543-6000, (800) 876-4766 (in 619 area code only)

San Francisco Bay Area Regional Poison Control Center

San Francisco General Hospital
1001 Potrero Ave., Building 80, Room 230
San Francisco, CA 94110
Emergency Phone: (800) 523-2222

Santa Clara Valley Regional Poison Center

Valley Health Center - Suite 310
750 South Bascom Ave.
San Jose, CA 95128
Emergency Phone: (408) 885-6000, (800) 662-9886 (CA only)

University of California, Davis, Medical Center Regional Poison Control Center

2315 Stockton Blvd
Sacramento, CA 95817
Emergency Phone: (916) 734-3692; (800) 342-9293 (Northern California only)

Colorado

Rocky Mountain Poison and Drug Center

645 Bannock St.
Denver, CO 80204
Emergency Phone: (303) 629-1123

District of Columbia

National Capital Poison Center

3201 New Mexico Avenue, NW, Suite 310
Washington, DC 20016
Emergency Numbers: (202) 625-3333; (202) 362-8563 (TTY)

Florida

Florida Poison Information Center—Jacksonville

University Medical Center
University of Florida Health Science Center—Jacksonville
655 West 8th Street
Jacksonville, FL 32209
Emergency Numbers: (904) 549-4480; (800) 282-3171 (FL only)

Florida Poison Information Center and Toxicology Resource Center

Tampa General Hospital
P.O. Box 1289
Tampa, FL 33601
Emergency Phone: (813) 253-4444 (Tampa) (800) 282-3171 (Florida)

Georgia

Georgia Poison Center

Grady Memorial Hospital
80 Butler Street S.E.
P.O. Box 26066
Atlanta, GA 30335-3801
Emergency Phone: (800) 282-5846 GA only; (404) 616-9000

Indiana

Indiana Poison Center

Methodist Hospital of Indiana
1701 N. Senate Boulevard
P.O. Box 1367
Indianapolis, IN 46206-1367
Emergency Phone: (800) 382-9097 (IN only), (317) 929-2323

Kentucky

Kentucky Regional Poison Center of Kosair Children's Hospital

P.O. Box 35070
Louisville, KY 40232-5070
Emergency Phone: (502) 629-7275 or (800) 722-5725 (KY only)

Maryland

Maryland Poison Center

20 N. Pine St.
Baltimore, MD 21201
Emergency Phone: (410) 528-7701, (800) 492-2414 (MD only)

National Capital Poison Center (D.C. suburbs only)

3201 New Mexico Avenue, NW, Suite 310
Washington, DC 20016
Emergency Numbers: (202) 625-3333; (202) 362-8563 (TTY)

Massachusetts

Massachusetts Poison Control System

300 Longwood Ave.
Boston, MA 02115
Emergency Phone: (617) 232-2120, (800) 682-9211

Michigan

Poison Control Center

Children's Hospital of Michigan
3901 Beaubien Blvd.
Detroit, MI 48201
Emergency Phone: (313) 745-5711

Minnesota

Hennepin Regional Poison Center

Hennepin County Medical Center
701 Park Ave.
Minneapolis, MN 55415
Emergency Phone: (612) 347-3141, Petline: (612) 337-7387, TDD (612) 337-7474

Minnesota Regional Poison Center

St. Paul-Ramsey Medical Center
640 Jackson Street
St. Paul, MN 55101
Emergency Phone: (612) 221-2113

Missouri

Cardinal Glennon Children's Hospital Regional Poison Center

1465 S. Grand Blvd.
St. Louis, MO 63104
Emergency Phone: (314) 772-5200, (800) 366-8888

Montana

Rocky Mountain Poison and Drug Center

645 Bannock St.
Denver, CO 80204
Emergency Phone: (303) 629-1123

Nebraska

The Poison Center

8301 Dodge St.
Omaha, NE 68114
Emergency Phone: (402) 390-5555 (Omaha), (800) 955-9119 (NE & WY)

New Jersey

New Jersey Poison Information and Education System

201 Lyons Ave.
Newark, NJ 07112
Emergency Phone: (800) 962-1253

New Mexico

New Mexico Poison and Drug Information Center

University of New Mexico
Albuquerque, NM 87131-1076
Emergency Phone: (505) 843-2551, (800) 432-6866 (NM only)

New York

Hudson Valley Regional Poison Center

Phelps Memorial Hospital Center
701 North Broadway
North Tarrytown, NY 10591
Emergency Phone: (800) 336-6997, (914) 366-3030

Long Island Regional Poison Control Center

Winthrop University Hospital
259 First Street
Mineola, NY 11501
Emergency Phone: (516) 542-2323, 2324, 2325, 3813

New York City Poison Control Center

N.Y.C. Department of Health
455 First Ave., Room 123
New York, NY 10016
Emergency Phone: (212) 340-4494, (212) P-O-I-S-O-N-S, TDD (212) 689-9014

North Carolina

Carolinas Poison Center

1000 Blythe Boulevard
P.O. Box 32861
Charlotte, NC 28232-2861
Emergency Phone: (704) 355-4000, (800) 84-TOXIN (1-800-848-6946)

Ohio

Central Ohio Poison Center

700 Children's Drive
Columbus, OH 43205-2696
Emergency Phone: (614) 228-1323, (800) 682-7625, (614) 228-2272 (TTY),
(614) 461-2012

Cincinnati Drug & Poison Information Center and Regional Poison Control System

231 Bethesda Avenue, M.L. 144
Cincinnati, OH 45267-0144
Emergency Phone: (513) 558-5111, 800-872-5111 (OH only)

Oregon

Oregon Poison Center

Oregon Health Sciences University
3181 S.W. Sam Jackson Park Road
Portland, OR 97201
Emergency Phone: (503) 494-8968, (800) 452-7165 (OR only)

Pennsylvania

Central Pennsylvania Poison Center

University Hospital
Milton S. Hershey Medical Center
Hershey, PA 17033
Emergency Phone: (800) 521-6110

The Poison Control Center, serving the greater Philadelphia metropolitan area

One Children's Center
Philadelphia, PA 19104-4303
Emergency Phone: (215) 386-2100

Pittsburgh Poison Center

3705 Fifth Avenue
Pittsburgh, PA 15213
Emergency Phone: (412) 681-6669

Rhode Island

Rhode Island Poison Center

593 Eddy St.
Providence, RI 02903
Emergency Phone: (401) 277-5727

Texas

North Texas Poison Center

5201 Harry Hines Blvd.
P.O. Box 35926
Dallas, TX 75235
Emergency Phone: (214) 590-5000, Texas Watts (800) 441-0040

Southeast Texas Poison Center

The University of Texas Medical Branch
Galveston, TX 77550-2780
Emergency Phone: (409) 765-1420 (Galveston), (713) 654-1701 (Houston)

Utah

Utah Poison Control Center

410 Chipeta Way, Suite 230
Salt Lake City, UT 84108
Emergency Phone: (801) 581-2151, (800) 456-7707 (UT only)

Virginia

Blue Ridge Poison Center

Box 67
Blue Ridge Hospital
Charlottesville, VA 22901
Emergency Phone: (804) 924-5543, (800) 451-1428

National Capital Poison Center (Northern VA only)

3201 New Mexico Avenue, NW, Suite 310
Washington, DC 20016
Emergency Numbers: (202) 625-3333; (202) 362-8563 (TTY)

West Virginia

West Virginia Poison Center

3110 MacCorkle Ave. S.E.
Charleston, WV 25304
Emergency Phone: (800) 642-3625 (WV only), (304) 348-4211

Wyoming

The Poison Center

8301 Dodge St.
Omaha, NE 68114
Emergency Phone: (402) 390-5555 (Omaha), (800) 955-9119 (NE & WY)

Selected References

The following selected references apply to information presented in the chapters of this book.

Health Information Management

American Health Information Management Association. 1994a. *Health information management*. 10th ed. Berwyn, Ill.: Physician Record Company.

———. 1994b. *Guidelines for faxing patient health information*. Chicago: AHIMA.

———. 1994c. Managing health information in facility mergers and acquisitions. *Journal of American Health Information Management* 65, no. 4 (April).

———. 1994d. Protecting patient information after a closure. *Journal of American Health Information Management* 65, no. 4 (April).

American Medical Association. 1995. *Medicare RBRVS: The physicians' guide*. Chicago: AMA.

Bonewit-West, K. 1993. *Computer concepts and applications for the medical office*. Philadelphia: W.B. Saunders Co.

Borglum, K.C., and D.M. Cate. 1995. *Medical practice forms: Every form you need to succeed*. New York: McGraw-Hill.

Brandt, M.D. 1993. *Maintenance, disclosure, and redisclosure of health information*. Chicago: AHIMA.

Fordney, M.T. 1995. *Insurance handbook for the medical office*. 4th ed. Philadelphia: W.B. Saunders Co.

Insurance Career Development Center. 1995. *Guide to medical billing*. St. Louis, Mo.: Mosby Lifeline.

Kinn, M.E. 1993. *The administrative medical assistant*. 3d ed. Philadelphia: W.B. Saunders Co.

Kotoski, G.M., and M.S. Stegman. 1994. *Physician documentation for reimbursement*. Gaithersburg, Md.: Aspen Publishers.

Roach, W.H., Jr. 1994. *Medical records and the law*. 2d ed. Gaithersburg, Md.: Aspen Publishers.

Rowell, J.C. 1994. *Understanding medical insurance: A step-by-step guide*. 2d ed. Albany, N.Y.: Delmar Publishers.

Tomes, J.P. 1993. *Healthcare records management: Disclosure and retention*. Chicago: Healthcare Financial Management Association/Probus Publishing Co.

Managed Care

Berkowitz, E.D., and Wolff, W. 1988. *Group Health Association: A portrait of a health maintenance organization*. Philadelphia: Temple University Press.

Kongstvedt, P.R. 1995. *Essentials of managed health care*. Gaithersburg, Md.: Aspen Publishers.

Luft, H.S. 1981. *Health maintenance organizations: Dimensions of performance*. New York: John Wiley & Sons.

Mayer, T.R., and Mayer, G.G. 1985. HMOs: Origins and developments. *The New England Journal of Medicine* 312, no. 9:591.

Nelson, J.A. 1987. The history and spirit of the HMO movement. *HMO Practice* 1, no. 2:75.

PACE (Program of All-Inclusive Care for the Elderly). 1994. *A description of an integrated model of medical and long-term care services.* San Francisco: PACE.

Soper, M.R., et al. 1990. *Balancing the triad: Cost containment, quality of service and quality of care in managed care systems.* Kansas City, Mo.: National Center for Managed Health Care Administration.

Starr, P. 1982. *The social transformation of American medicine: The rise of a sovereign profession and the making of a vast industry.* New York: Basic Books.

Zander, K. 1992. Critical pathways. *Total quality management: The health care pioneers.* Eds. M.M. Melum and M.K. Siniori. Chicago: American Hospital Publishing.

Medical Dictionaries

Dorland's illustrated medical dictionary. 1994. 28th ed. Philadelphia: W.B. Saunders Co.

Merriam-Webster's medical desk dictionary. 1996. Springfield, Mass.: Merriam-Webster.

Physician's desk reference. 1994. 48th ed. Montvale, N.J.: Medical Economics Data Production Co.

Quick look drug book. 1995. Hudson, Ohio: Lexi-Comp.

Stedman's medical dictionary. 1995. 26th ed. Baltimore: Williams and Wilkins.

Medical Ethics

Beauchamp, T.L., and J.F. Childress. 1994. *Principles of biomedical ethics.* New York: Oxford University Press.

Beauchamp, T.L., and L. Walters. 1994. *Contemporary issues in bioethics.* Belmont, Calif.: Wadsworth Publishing Co.

Bishop, A.H., and J.R. Scudder, Jr., eds. 1985. *Caring, curing, coping: Nurse, physician, patient relationships.* Birmingham: University of Alabama Press.

Brody, H. 1992. *The healer's power.* New Haven, Conn.: Yale University Press.

Council of Ethical and Judicial Affairs, American Medical Association. 1995. Ethical issues in managed care. *Journal of the American Medical Association* 273, no. 4:330-35.

Fletcher, J.C., and R. Boyle. 1995. *Introduction to clinical ethics.* Frederick, Md.: University Publishing Group.

Graber, G.C., A.D. Beasley, and J.A. Eaddy. 1985. *Ethical analysis of clinical medicine.* Baltimore: Urban & Schwarzenberg.

Jecker, N.S., J.A. Carrese, and R.A. Pearlman. 1995. Caring for patients in cross-cultural settings. *Hastings Center Report* 25, no. 1:6-14.

Murray, T.H., and E. Livny. 1995. The human genome project: Ethical and social implications. *Bulletin of the Medical Library Association* 83, no. 1:14-21.

Pellegrino, E.D. 1994. Words can hurt you: Some reflections on the metaphors of managed care. *Journal of the American Board of Family Practice* 7, no. 6:505-10.

Purtillo, R.B., and A.M. Haddad. 1996. *Health professional and patient interaction.* Philadelphia: W.B. Saunders Co.

Reich, W.T., ed. 1995. *Encyclopedia of bioethics.* New York: Macmillan.

Thomasma, D.C., P.A. Marshall, and D. Kondratowicz. 1995. *Clinical medical ethics: Cases and readings.* Lanham, Md: University Press of America.

Watson, James D. 1990. The human genome project: Past, present, and future. *Science* 248 (April 6):44-49.

Medical Office Design

Farber, L. 1987. *Encyclopedia of practice and financial management.* 2d. ed. Oradell, N.J.: Medical Economics Books.

Haines, R.C., Jr. 1994. Patient per hour: The pulse of your practice. *Administrative Ophthalmology.* 3, no. 1 (Winter):28-29.

———. 1988. Goal setting for facility development. *Medicenter Management* 3, no. 7 (July):21.

Haines, R.C., Jr., and T.C. Quirk. 1992. Successful medical office design. *Administrative Ophthalmology* 1, no. 1 (Spring):37-40.

Wold, C.R. 1995. *Managing your medical practice.* White Plains, N.Y.: AHAB Press.

Quality of Care

Agency for Health Care Policy and Research. 1995. *Using clinical practice guidelines to evaluate quality of care.* Vol. 1, no. 95-0045. Rockville, Md.: AHCPR..

Anderson, C., and P.A. Rivenburgh. 1995. Benchmarking. *Quality in health care: Theory, application, and evolution.* Ed. N.O. Graham. Gaithersburg, Md.: Aspen Publishers.

Benjamin, K. 1995. Outcomes research and the allied health professional. *Journal of Allied Health* 24, no, 1 (Winter):3-17.

Benson, D.S. 1992. *Measuring outcomes in ambulatory care.* Chicago: American Hospital Publishing.

Berwick, D.M. 1995. Continuous improvement as an ideal in health care. *Quality in health care.* Ed. N.O. Graham. Gaithersburg, Md.: Aspen Publishers.

Berwick, D.M., A.B. Godfrey, and J. Roessner. 1990. *Curing health care: New strategies for quality improvement.* New York: Jossey-Bass.

Brassard, M., and D. Ritter. 1994. *The memory jogger II: A pocket guide of tools for continuous improvement and effective planning.* Methuen, Mass.: GOAL/QPC.

Coffey, R.S., et al. 1995. Introduction to clinical paths. *Quality in health care.* Ed. N.O. Graham. Gaithersburg, Md.: Aspen Publishers.

Donabedian, A. 1993. Quality in health care: Whose responsibility is it? *American Journal of Medical Quality* 18, no. 2 (Summer):32-36.

———. 1985. *Explorations in quality assessment and monitoring.* 3 vols. Ann Arbor, Mich.: Health Administration Press.

————. 1969. *Medical care administration.* Vol. 2. *Medical care appraisal: Quality and utilization.* New York: American Public Health Association.

Epstein, A. 1995a. The outcomes movement: Will it get us where we want to go? *Quality in health care.* Ed. N.O. Graham. Gaithersburg, Md.: Aspen Publishers.

————. 1995b. Performance reports on quality: Prototypes, problems, and prospects. *New England Journal of Medicine.* 333, no. 1 (July):57-61.

Graham, N.O., ed. 1995. *Quality in health care: Theory, applications, and evolution.* Gaithersburg, Md.: Aspen Publishers.

Hospital and Health Services Administration 40, no. 1 (Spring 1995). Special issue on CQI.

Journal of Allied Health 24, no. 1 (Winter 1995). Special issue on outcomes asessment.

Leebov, W. 1991. *The quality quest.* Chicago: American Hospital Publishing.

Leininger, L.S., et al. 1994. CQI in primary care. *Continuous quality improvement in health care.* Eds. C.P. McLaughlin and A.D. Kaluzny. Gaithersburg, Md.: Aspen Publishers.

Lohr, K.. ed. 1990. *Medicare: A strategy for quality assurance.* Vol. 1. Washington, D.C.: National Academy Press.

McLaughlin, C.P., and A.D. Kaluzny, eds. 1994. *Continuous quality improvement in health care: Theory, implementation, and applications.* Gaithersburg, Md.: Aspen Publishers.

National Committee for Quality Assurance. *Reviewer guidelines for the standards for accreditation.* Washington, D.C.: NCQA.

————. *Health plan employer data and information set.* Washington, D.C.: NCQA.

————. *Report card pilot project.* Washington, D.C.: NCQA.

Pathek, D.S., and Z. Hakim. 1993. An overview of total quality management: Applications for health care systems. *Topics in Hospital Pharmacy Management* 12, no. 4 (January):1-13.

Plsek, P.S. 1995a. Tutorial: Quality improvement project models. *Quality in health care.* Ed. N.O. Graham. Gaithersburg, Md.: Aspen Publishers.

————. 1995b. Techniques for managing quality. *Hospital and Health Services Administration* 40, no. 1 (Spring):50-79.

Roberts, J.S. 1987. A history of the Joint Commission on Accreditation of Hospitals. *Journal of the American Medical Association* 258, no. 7.

Wakefield, D., and B.J. Wakefield. 1995. Overcoming the barriers to implementation of TQM/CQI in hospitals: Myths and realities. *Quality in health care.* Ed. N.O. Graham. Gaithersburg, Md.: Aspen Publishers.

Walton, M. 1986. *The Deming management method.* New York: Perigree Books.

Whetsell, G.W. 1995. Total quality management. *Quality in health care.* Ed. N.O. Graham. Gaithersburg, Md.: Aspen Publishers.

Young, M., S. Rallison, and P. Eckman. 1995. Patients, physicians, and professional knowledge: Implications. *Hospital and Health Services Administration* 40, no. 1 (Spring):40-49.

Style Manuals

American Medical Association manual of style. 1989. 8th ed. Baltimore: Williams and Wilkins.

The Chicago manual of style. 1993. 14th ed. Chicago: University of Chicago Press.

Sabin, W.A. 1992. *The Gregg reference manual.* 7th ed. Lake Forest, Ill.: Glencoe div. Macmillan/McGraw-Hill.

Transcription

Blake, R.S. 1993. *The medical transcriptionist's handbook.* Albany, N.Y.: Delmar Publishers.

Davis, N.M. 1994. *Medical abbreviations: 10,000 conveniences at the expense of communications and safety.* 7th ed. Huntingdon Valley, Pa.: Neil M. Davis.

Davis, N.M., M.R. Cohen, and B.S. Teplitsky. 1992. Look-alike and sound-alike drug names: The problem and the solution. *Hospital Pharmacology* 27:95-110.

Novak, N.N., and P.A. Ireland. 1995. *Hillcrest Medical Center: Beginning medical transcription course.* 4th ed. Albany, N.Y.: Delmar Publishers.

Pyle, V. 1994. *Current medical terminology.* 5th ed. Modesto, Calif.: Health Professions Institute.

Appendix C

Medical Abbreviations and Vocabulary

| Abbreviations 466
| Frequently Confused and Misused Words 486

The following section includes abbreviations that are often used in medical offices, as well as words and phrases that are frequently misused or easily confused.

Abbreviations

The following list of abbreviations contains many of the most commonly used medical abbreviations. Most of these appear without periods, in keeping with standard medical style; however, some abbreviations may be regularly used with periods—either form is acceptable in standard use.

a about; absent; absolute; absorbency; absorbent; accommodation; acetum; acid, acidity; actin; active, activity; allergist, allergy; alpha; anode; answer; ante; anterior; aqua; area; artery; asymmetric, asymmetry

A adenine; ampere

Å angstrom

a̅a̅ *also* **aa** [Latin *ana*] of each — used at the end of a list of two or more substances in a prescription to indicate that equal quantities of each are to be taken

AA achievement age; Alcoholics Anonymous

AAF ascorbic acid factor

AAL anterior axillary line

AAMA American Association of Medical Assistants

AAMT American Association for Medical Transcription

A&P anterior and posterior; auscultation and percussion

A&W alive and well

AAPCC adjusted average per capita cost

ab abort, abortion; about

AB aid to blind; [Latin *artium baccalaureus*] bachelor of arts

ABC atomic, biological, and chemical

abd abdomen, abdominal

abdom abdomen, abdominal

ABFP American Board of Family Practice

abs absent; absolute

abt about

ac acute; [Latin *ante cibum*] before

meals — used in writing prescriptions

Ac actinium

AC alternating current

acc acceleration; according

ACE angiotensin converting enzyme

AcG accelerator globulin (*syn* factor V)

ACh acetylcholine

AChE acetylcholinesterase

ACLS advanced cardiac life support

ACNM American College of Nurse-Midwives

ACS antireticular cytotoxic serum

ACSW Academy of Certified Social Workers

act active

ACTH adrenocorticotropic hormone

AD Alzheimer's disease; average deviation

ADA adenosine deaminase; American Dietetic Association

ADC aid to dependent children

add adduction, adductor

ADD attention deficit disorder

ADH antidiuretic hormone

ADHD attention-deficit hyperactivity disorder

adj adjunct

ADL activities of daily living

adm administration, administrator; admission, admit

ADP adenosine diphosphate

ae *or* **aet** *or* **aetat** [Latin *aetatis*] of age, aged

AF atrial fibrillation; audio frequency

AFB acid-fast bacillus

AFP alpha-fetoprotein

Ag [Latin *argentum*] silver

agglut agglutination

agt agent

AHA American Hospital Association

AHCPR Agency for Health Care Policy and Research

AHF antihemophilic factor (*syn* factor VIII)

AHG antihemophilic globulin

AHIMA American Health Information Management Association

AI artificial insemination

AICD automatic implantable cardioverter defibrillator

AID artificial insemination by donor

AIDS acquired immune deficiency syndrome

AIH artificial insemination by husband

AJ ankle jerk

AK above knee

Al aluminum

ALA aminolevulinic acid

alb albumin

alc alcohol

ALD adrenoleukodystrophy

ALG antilymphocyte globulin, antilymphocytic globulin

alk alkaline

alky alkalinity

ALL acute lymphoblastic leukemia

ALS amyotrophic lateral sclerosis; antilymphocyte serum, antilymphocytic serum

alt alternate; altitude

ALT alanine aminotransferase

alv alveolar

Am americium

AM [Latin *ante meridiem*] before noon; [Medieval Latin *Artium Magister*] master of arts

AMA against medical advice; American Medical Association

amb ambulance; ambulatory

AMI acute myocardial infarction

AML acute myeloblastic leukemia, acute myelocytic leukemia, acute myelogenous leukemia, acute myeloid leukemia

amp amperage; ampere; ampule; amputation

AMP adenosine monophosphate

amt amount

ANA American Nurses Association; antinuclear antibodies, antinuclear antibody

anal analysis; analytic; analyze
anat anatomic, anatomical, anatomy
ANF atrial naturetic factor
anhyd anhydrous
ANP atrial natriuretic peptide
ans answer
ANS autonomic nervous system
AOB alcohol on breath
AOTA American Occupational Therapy Association
ap apothecaries
AP action potential; alkaline phosphatase; anterior pituitary; anteroposterior; aortic pressure
APC aspirin, phenacetin, and caffeine
APF animal protein factor
app appendix
appl applied
approx approximate, approximately
appt appointment
APSAC anisoylated plasminogen-streptokinase activator complex (*syn* anistreplase)
aq aqua, aqueous
AQ accomplishment quotient, achievement quotient
Ar argon
ARC AIDS-related complex; American Red Cross
ARD acute respiratory disease
ARDS acute respiratory distress syndrome, adult respiratory distress syndrome
ARRT American registered respiratory therapist; American Registry of Radiologic Technologists
ART accredited record technician
as astigmatism
As arsenic
AS aortic stenosis; arteriosclerosis
ASA acetylsalicylic acid (*syn* aspirin)
ASAP as soon as possible
ASCP American Society of Clinical Pathologists
ASCVD arteriosclerotic cardiovascular disease
ASHD arteriosclerotic heart disease

assn association
asst assistant
AST aspartate transaminase
as tol as tolerated
at airtight
At astatine
ATLS advanced trauma life support
atm atmosphere, atmospheric
ATP adenosine triphosphate
at wt atomic weight
au angstrom unit; antitoxin unit
Au [Latin *aurum*] gold
aux auxiliary
av average; avoirdupois
AV arteriovenous; atrioventricular
avdp avoirdupois
AVP arginine vasopressin
ax axis
Az [French *azote*] nitrogen
AZT azidothymidine
b bacillus; barometric; bath; Baumé scale; behavior; bel; bicuspid; born; brother
B boron
Ba barium
BA bronchial asthma
bact bacteria, bacterial; bacteriological, bacteriology; bacterium
BaE *or* **BAE** barium enema
bal balance
BAL British anti-lewisite (*syn* dimercaprol)
bar barometer, barometric
baso basophil
BBB blood-brain barrier; bundle branch block
BBT basal body temperature
BC board-certified
BCG bacillus Calmette-Guérin; ballistocardiogram; bromocresol green
BCLS basic cardiac life support
bd [Latin *bis die*] twice a day — used in writing prescriptions
Bé Baumé
Be beryllium
BE barium enema; below elbow; board-eligible

BFP biologic false-positive
BH bill of health
BHA butylated hydroxyanisole
BHT butylated hydroxytoluene
Bi bismuth
bid [Latin *bis in die*] twice a day — used in writing prescriptions
bili bilirubin
biol biologic, biological, biologist, biology
BJ biceps jerk
Bk berkelium
BK below knee
bld blood
BLS basic life support
BM Bachelor of Medicine; basal metabolism; bowel movement
BMI body mass index
BMR basal metabolic rate
BMT bone marrow transplantation
BNA Basle Nomina Anatomica
BO body odor
BOD biochemical oxygen demand, biological oxygen demand
bot botanical, botanist, botany; bottle
bp base pair
BP blood pressure; boiling point; British Pharmacopoeia
BPH benign prostatic hyperplasia, benign prostatic hypertrophy
Br bromine
BRP bathroom privileges
BS bowel sounds; breath sounds
BSE bovine spongiform encephalopathy
BSN bachelor of science in nursing
BST blood serological test
BT bedtime; brain tumor
Btu British thermal unit
BUdR bromodeoxyuridine
BUN blood urea nitrogen
BW blood Wassermann; body weight
Bx [by analogy with *Rx*] biopsy
c calorie; canine; cathode; centimeter; clonus; closure; cobalt; coefficient; contact; contraction; coulomb; curie; cylinder; *or* c̄ [Latin

cum] with — used in writing prescriptions
C carbon; Celsius; centigrade; cervical — used esp. with a number from 1 to 7 to indicate a vertebra or segment of the spinal cord; cocaine; [Latin *congius*] gallon; cytosine
Ca calcium
CA cancer; carcinoma; cardiac arrest; chronological age
CABG coronary artery bypass graft
CAC cardiac accelerator center
CAD coronary artery disease
CAI confused artificial insemination
cal small calorie
Cal large calorie
cAMP cyclic adenosine monophosphate
canc canceled
cap capacity; capsule
CAT computed axial tomography, computerized axial tomography
cath cathartic; catheter, catherization; cathode
cav cavity
cb centibar
Cb columbium
CB [Latin *Chirurgiae Baccalaureus*] bachelor of surgery
CBC complete blood count
CBD closed bladder drainage; common bile duct
CBF cerebral blood flow
CBR chemical, bacteriological, and radiological; chemical, biological, and radiological
CBW chemical and biological warfare
cc cubic centimeter
CC chief complaint; commission certified; critical condition; current complaint
CCI chronic coronary insufficiency
CCK cholecystokinin
CCT chocolate-coated tablet
CCU cardiac care unit; coronary care unit; critical care unit
cd candela

Cd cadmium

CD cluster of differentiation — used with a number to denote any of numerous antigenic proteins; communicable disease; constant drainage; contagious disease; convulsive disorder; curative dose

CDC calculated date of confinement; Centers for Disease Control

cDNA complementary deoxyribonucleic acid

Ce cerium

CE cardiac enlargement

CEA carcinoembryonic antigen

Cel Celsius

cen central

CER conditioned emotional response

cert certificate, certification, certified, certify

cerv cervical

CES central excitatory state

cf [Latin *confer*] compare

Cf californium

CF complement fixation; cystic fibrosis

CFS chronic fatigue syndrome

CFT complement fixation test

CG chorionic gonadotropin

ch child; chronic

ChB [Latin *Chirugiae Baccalaureus*] Bachelor of Surgery

CHD childhood disease; coronary heart disease

ChE cholinesterase

chem chemical, chemist, chemistry

CHF congestive heart failure

chg change

chl chloroform

CHO carbohydrate

chol cholesterol

chr chronic

CI chemotherapeutic index

CICU coronary intensive care unit

CIS carcinoma in situ

CK creatine kinase

cl centiliter; clavicle; clinic; closure

Cl chloride; chlorine

CL chest and left arm; corpus luteum; critical list

CLA certified laboratory assistant

CLIA Clinical Laboratory Improvement Act

clin clinical

CLL chronic lymphocytic leukemia

cm centimeter

Cm curium

CM [Latin *Chirurgiae Magister*] Master of Surgery; circular muscle

CMA certified medical assistant

CMHC Community Mental Health Center

CML chronic myelocytic leukemia, chronic myelogenous leukemia, chronic myeloid leukemia

CMV cytomegalovirus

CN chloroacetophenone

CNA certified nurse's aide

CNM certified nurse-midwife

CNP continuous negative pressure

CNS central nervous system

Co cobalt; coenzyme

CO carbon monoxide; cardiac output

c/o complains of

coag coagulation

COC cathodal opening contraction

COCl cathodal opening clonus

coeff *or* **coef** coefficient

COH carbohydrate

col colony; color

COLD chronic obstructive lung disease

coll collect, collection; colloidal; collyrium

comp comparative, compare; composition; compound

conc concentrated, concentration

cond condition

cond ref conditioned reflex

cond resp conditioned response

conf conference

cong congenital; [Latin *congius*] gallon

const constant

cont containing; contents; continue, continued

conv convalescent

coord coordination

COPD chronic obstructive pulmonary disease

COPE chronic obstructive pulmonary emphysema

cor corrected

CoR Congo red

cort cortex, cortical

COTA certified occupational therapy assistant

CP capillary pressure; cerebral palsy; chemically pure; compare; constant pressure; cor pulmonale

CPAP continuous positive airway pressure

CPB competitive protein binding

CPC chronic passive congestion

cpd compound

CPE cytopathogenic effects

CPI constitutional psychopathic inferiority

CPK creatine phosphokinase

CPM counts per minute

CPR cardiopulmonary resuscitation

CPT Current Procedural Terminology

CPZ chlorpromazine

CQI continuous quality improvement

Cr chromium; creatinine

CR cardiorespiratory; chest and right arm; clot retraction; conditioned reflex, conditioned response

CRD chronic respiratory disease

CRF corticotropin-releasing factor

CRH corticotropin-releasing hormone

crit critical

CRNA certified registered nurse anesthetist

CRO cathode-ray oscilloscope

CrP creatine phosphate

CRP C-reactive protein

CRT cathode-ray tube; complex reaction time

CRTT certified respiratory therapy technician

cryst crystalline, crystallized

cs case; cesarean section; conditioned stimulus; consciousness; corticosteroid; current strength

Cs cesium

CSF cerebrospinal fluid; colony-stimulating factor

CSM cerebrospinal meningitis

CT circulation time; coated tablet; compressed tablet; computed tomography, computerized tomography

CTa catamenia

CTC chlortetracycline

ctr center

cu cubic

Cu copper

CU clinical unit

CUC chronic ulcerative colitis

cult culture

cur curative; current

CV cardiovascular

CVA cerebrovascular accident

CVD cardiovascular disease

CVP central venous pressure

CVR cardiovascular renal; cardiovascular respiratory; cerebrovascular resistance

CVS chorionic villus sampling

CW crutch walking

Cy cyanogen

cyl cylinder, cylindrical

cytol cytological, cytology

d date; daughter; day; dead; deceased; deciduous; degree; density; developed; deviation; dexter; diameter; died; diopter; disease; divorced; dorsal; dose; duration

D deuterium

da daughter; day

DA delayed action

DAH disordered action of the heart

dam dekameter

D&C dilation and curettage

D&E dilation and evacuation
DAT delayed action tablet
dau daughter
dbl double
DBP diastolic blood pressure
DC Dental Corps; diagnostic center; direct current; doctor of chiropractic
DCc double concave
DCR direct critical response
DD developmentally disabled
DDC dideoxycytidine
DDI dideoxyinosine
DDS doctor of dental science, doctor of dental surgery
DDT dichlorodiphenyltrichloroethane
dec deceased
decd deceased
def defecation; deficient; definite
deg degeneration; degree
del delusion
dent dental, dentist, dentistry
depr depression
derm dermatologist, dermatology
DES diethylstilbestrol
detn detention
devel development
DFP diisopropyl fluorophosphate (*syn* isoflurophate)
dg decigram
DHA dehydroepiandrosterone; dihydroxyacetone
DHEA dehydroepiandrosterone
DHPG 1,3 - dihydroxy - 2 - propoxymethyl guanine (*syn* ganciclovir)
DHT dihydrotestosterone
DI diabetes insipidus
dia diameter; diathermy
diam diameter
dil dilute
dilat dilatation
dim diminished
DIP distal interphalangeal
diph diphtheria
dis disabled; disease
disch discharge, discharged
disp dispensary

dissd dissolved
div divide, division; divorced
DJD degenerative joint disease
dkg dekagram
dkl dekaliter
dkm dekameter
dl deciliter
DL danger list
DLE disseminated lupus erythematosus
dm decimeter
DM diabetes mellitus
DMBA dimethylbenzanthracene
DMD [Latin *dentariae medicinae doctor*] doctor of dental medicine
DMF decayed, missing, and filled teeth
DMSO dimethyl sulfoxide
DMT dimethyltryptamine
DNA deoxyribonucleic acid
DNase *also* **DNAase** deoxyribonuclease
DNOC dinitro-o-cresol
DNR do not resuscitate
DO doctor of optometry; doctor of osteopathy
DOA dead on arrival
DOB date of birth
doc document
DOE dyspnea on exertion
DOM 2,5-dimethoxy-4-methylamphetamine (*syn* STP)
dos dosage
doz dozen
DP doctor of pharmacy; doctor of podiatry
DPA diphenylamine
DPH department of public health; doctor of public health
DPM doctor of podiatric medicine
DPT diphtheria-pertussis-tetanus (vaccine)
DQ developmental quotient
dr dram; dressing
Dr doctor
DR delivery room
DRG diagnosis-related group

DrPH doctor of public health
DSC doctor of surgical chiropody
DSD dry sterile dressing
DT delirium tremens; distance test; duration of tetany
DTN diphtheria toxin normal
DTP diphtheria, tetanus, pertussis (vaccine)
dt's delirium tremens
DU diagnosis undetermined
dup duplicate
DV dilute volume
DVM doctor of veterinary medicine
DW distilled water
dwt [Latin *denarius* + *weight*] pennyweight
Dx diagnosis
Dy dysprosium
E emmetropia; enema; enzyme; experimenter; eye
ea each
EA educational age
EAE experimental allergic encephalomyelitis, experimental autoimmune encephalomyelitis
EBV Epstein-Barr virus
ECF extracellular fluid
ECG electrocardiogram
ECT electroconvulsive therapy
ED effective dose; emergency department; erythema dose
EDB ethylene dibromide
EDR electrodermal response
EDTA ethylenediaminetetraacetic acid
EEE eastern equine encephalomyelitis
EEG electroencephalogram; electroencephalograph
EENT eye, ear, nose, and throat
EGF epidermal growth factor
Eh standard oxidation-reduction potential
EHBF extrahepatic blood flow
EIA enzyme immunoassay; equine infectious anemia; exercise-induced asthma

EKG electrocardiogram; electrocardiograph
elec electric, electrical, electricity
ELISA enzyme-linked immunosorbent assay
EM electromagnetic; electron microscope, electron microscopy; emergency medicine
emb embryo, embryology
embryol embryology
EMF electromotive force; electromagnetic field
EMG electromyogram, electromyograph, electromyography
EMS emergency medical service, emergency medical services; eosinophilia-myalgia syndrome
EMT emergency medical technician
emul emulsion
enl enlarged
ENT ear, nose, and throat
EOG electrooculogram
eos *or* **eosin** eosinophil
epil epilepsy, epileptic
epith epithelial, epithelium
EPO erythropoietin; exclusive provider organization
eq equal; equivalent
Er erbium
ER emergency room
ERG electroretinogram
ERPF effective renal plasma flow
ERT estrogen-replacement therapy
Es einsteinium
ESB electrical stimulation of the brain
ESF erythropoietic stimulating factor
ESP extrasensory perception
ESR erythrocyte sedimentation rate
ESRD end-stage renal disease
EST electroshock therapy
esu electrostatic unit
Eu europium
ex examined; example; exercise
exc except, exception
exp experiment, experimental; expired

expt experiment
exptl experimental
ext external; extract; extremity
f farad; faraday; father; female; focal length; formula; function
F Fahrenheit; filial generation — usu. used with a subscript F_1 for the first, F_2 for the second, etc.; fluorine
FA fatty acid
FACC Fellow of the American College of Cardiology
FACD Fellow of the American College of Dentists
FACOG Fellow of the American College of Obstetricians and Gynecologists
FACP Fellow of the American College of Physicians
FACR Fellow of the American College of Radiology
FACS Fellow of the American College of Surgeons
FAD flavin adenine dinucleotide
Fah *or* **Fahr** Fahrenheit
fam family
FAMA Fellow of the American Medical Association
FAP familial adenomatous polyposis
FAPA Fellow of the American Psychological Association
FAS fetal alcohol syndrome
fasc fasciculus
FD focal distance
FDA Food and Drug Administration
Fe iron
FeLV feline leukemia virus
fem female; feminine; femur
FF fat free; filtration fraction
FFA free fatty acids
FGF fibroblast growth factor
FHS fetal heart sounds
FHT fetal heart tone
fib fibrillation
FICS Fellow of the International College of Surgeons
FID free induction decay
fig figure
fl fluid

FL focal length
fl oz fluid ounce
Fm fermium
FMN flavin mononuculeotide
FNA fine needle aspiration
fp freezing point
FP family physician, family practitioner; family practice
FPC fish protein concentrate
fpm feet per minute
fps foot-pound-second
Fr francium
FR flocculation reaction
FRCP Fellow of the Royal College of Physicians
FRCS Fellow of the Royal College of Surgeons
freq frequency
FRSC Fellow of the Royal Society of Canada
FSH follicle-stimulating hormone
ft feet, foot
FUO fever of undetermined origin
g gauge; gender; gingival; glucose; grain; gram; gravity, acceleration of gravity
G guanine
Ga gallium
GABA gamma-aminobutyric acid
gal galactose; gallon
galv galvanic, galvanism, galvanized
GAS general adaptation syndrome
GB gallbladder
GC gas chromatograph, gas chromatography; gonococcus
G-CSF granulocyte colony-stimulating factor
Gd gadolinium
Ge germanium
GE gastroenterology
gen general; genus
GFR glomerular filtration rate
GG gamma globulin
GH growth hormone
GI gastrointestinal
GL greatest length
GLC gas-liquid chromatography
gm gram

GM and S General Medicine and Surgery

GM-CSF granulocyte-macrophage colony-stimulating factor

GN graduate nurse

GnRH gonadotropin-releasing hormone

gp group

GP general paresis; general practitioner

gr grain; gram; gravity

GRAS generally recognized as safe

grav gravida

GRE gradient echo, gradient-recalled echo

GSH glutathione (reduced form)

G6PD glucose-6-phosphate dehydrogenase

GSR galvanic skin response

GSSG glutathione (oxidized form)

GSW gunshot wound

GTH gonadotropic hormone

GTP guanosine triphosphate

GU genitourinary

GVH graft-versus-host

GVHD graft-versus-host disease

Gy gray

gyn gynecologic, gynecologist, gynecology

h height; [Latin *hora*] hour — used in writing prescriptions

H heroin; hydrogen

Hb hemoglobin

HBsAg hepatitis B surface antigen

HBV hepatitis B virus

HCFA Health Care Financing Administration

HCG human chorionic gonadotropin

HCPCS Health Care Financing Administration Common Procedural Coding System

HCT hematocrit

HCV hepatitis C virus

HD Hansen's disease; hearing distance

HDL high-density lipoprotein

He helium

HEDIS Health Plan Employer Data and Information Set

HELLP hemolysis, elevated liver enzymes, and low platelet count (syndrome)

HEW Department of Health, Education, and Welfare

hex hexosaminidase

Hf hafnium

hg hectogram

Hg [New Latin *hydrargyrum*] mercury

Hgb hemoglobin

HGH human growth hormone

HHS Department of Health and Human Services

HHV human herpesvirus

HI hemagglutination inhibition

5-HIAA 5-hydroxyindoleacetic acid

Hib *Haemophilus influenzae,* serotype B

HIPC health insurance purchasing cooperative

HIV human immunodeficiency virus

hl hectoliter

HLA *also* **HL-A** human leukocyte antigen — often used with one or more identifying letters or with letters and a number

HMD hyaline membrane disease

HMO health maintenance organization

HNPCC hereditary nonpolyposis colon cancer, hereditary nonpolyposis colorectal cancer

Ho holmium

HOP high oxygen pressure

hosp hospital

HPI history of present illness

HPLC high-performance liquid chromatography

HPV human papillomavirus

hr [Latin *hora*] hour — used in writing prescriptions

HRT hormone replacement therapy

hs [Latin *hora somni*] at bedtime — used esp. in writing prescriptions

HS house surgeon

HSA human serum albumin

HSV herpes simplex virus
ht height
5-HT 5-hydroxytryptamine (*syn* serotonin)
HTLV human T-cell leukemia virus
HUS hemolytic uremic syndrome
HVL half-value layer
Hz hertz
i incisor; optically inactive
I iodine
IAA indoleacetic acid
ib *or* **ibid** [Latin *ibidem*] in the same place
IBS irritable bowel syndrome
ICD International Classification of Diseases — usu. used with a number indicating the revision
ICN International Council of Nurses
ICSH interstitial-cell stimulating hormone
ICSS intracranial self-stimulation
ICT inflammation of connective tissue; insulin coma therapy
ICU intensive care unit
id [Latin *idem*] the same
ID identification; inside diameter, internal diameter; intradermal
IDDM insulin-dependent diabetes mellitus
ID$_{50}$ median infective dose
IDU idoxuridine
IF interferon
IFN interferon
Ig immunoglobulin — often used with an identifying letter
IGF insulin-like growth factor
IH infectious hepatitis
Il illinium
IL interleukin — often used with an identifying number
IM internal medicine; intramuscular, intramuscularly
IMP inosine 5'-monophosphate (*syn* inosinic acid)
in inch
In indium
IND investigational new drug
INH isoniazid

inj injection
Io ionium
IP intraperitoneal, intraperitoneally
IPA independent practice association
IPPB intermittent positive pressure breathing
IPSP inhibitory postsynaptic potential
IPT interpersonal psychotherapy, interpersonal therapy
Ir iridium
IR infrared
ITP idiopathic thrombocytopenic purpura
IU immunizing unit; international unit
IUCD intrauterine device
IUD intrauterine device
IUDR idoxuridine
IV intravenous, intravenously; intraventricular
IVF in vitro fertilization
IVP intravenous pyelogram
J mechanical equivalent of heat
JAMA Journal of the American Medical Association
JCAH Joint Commission on Accreditation of Hospitals
JCAHO Joint Commission on Accreditation of Healthcare Organizations
JND just noticeable difference
K dissociation constant, ionization constant; [New Latin *kalium*] potassium; kelvin
ka [German *kathode*] cathode
kb kilobase
kc kilocycle
kcal kilocalorie, kilogram calorie
kc/s kilocycles per second
kg kilogram
kgm kilogram-meter
KJ knee jerk
kl kiloliter
km kilometer
Kr krypton
KS Kaposi's sarcoma

KUB kidney, ureter, and bladder

L left; levorotatory; light; liquid; liter; lithium; lumbar — used esp. with a number from 1 to 5 to indicate a vertebra or segment of the spinal cord in the lumbar region

La lanthanum

LAK lymphokine-activated killer cell

lap laparotomy

laryngol laryngological

LATS long-acting thyroid stimulator

lb pound

LC liquid chromatography

LCMV lymphocytic choriomeningitis virus

LD learning disabled, learning disability; lethal dose

LD$_{50}$ median lethal dose

LDH lactate dehydrogenase, lactic dehydrogenase

LDL low-density lipoprotein

LE lupus erythematosus

Leu leucine

LFA lymphocyte function-associated antigen

LFD least fatal dose

LH luteinizing hormone

LHRH luteinizing hormone-releasing hormone

Li lithium

liq liquid; liquor

LLQ left lower quadrant (abdomen)

L-PAM levorotatory-phenylalanine mustard (*syn* melphalan)

LPN licensed practical nurse

LPS lipopolysaccharide

Lr lawrencium

LRCP Licentiate of the Royal College of Physicians

LRCS Licentiate of the Royal College of Surgeons

LRF luteinizing hormone-releasing factor

LSD lysergic acid diethylamide

LTH luteotropic hormone

LTP long-term potentiation

LTR long terminal repeat

Lu lutetium

LUQ left upper quadrant (abdomen)

LV left ventricle

LVN licensed vocational nurse

m Mach; male; married; masculine; mass; meter; [Latin *mille*] thousand; million; minim; minute; molal; molality; molar; molarity; mole; mucoid; muscle

M [Latin *misce*] mix — used in writing prescriptions; mitosis

ma milliampere

MA mental age

mac macerate

MAC maximum allowable concentration

MAO monoamine oxidase

MAOI monoamine oxidase inhibitor

masc masculine

MASH mobile army surgical hospital

MAST military antishock trousers

max maximum

MB [New Latin *medicinae baccalaureus*] bachelor of medicine

mbar millibar

MBC minimal bactericidal concentration, minimum bactericidal concentration

MBD minimal brain dysfunction

MBP major basic protein; myelin basic protein

mc megacycle; millicurie

MC medical corps; [New Latin *magister chirurgiae*] master of surgery

MCAT Medical College Admissions Test

mcg microgram

MCh [New Latin *magister chirurgiae*] master of surgery

MCH maternal and child health; mean corpuscular hemoglobin (concentration)

MCHC mean corpuscular hemoglobin concentration

mCi millicurie

MCO managed care organization

M-CSF macrophage colony-stimulating factor

MCV mean corpuscular volume
Md mendelevium
MD medical department; [Latin *medicinae doctor*] Doctor of Medicine; muscular dystrophy
MDMA 3,4-methylenedioxymethamphetamine (*syn* ecstasy)
MDR minimum daily requirement
MDS master of dental surgery
Me methyl
ME medical examiner
meg megacycle
mEq milliequivalent
Met methionine
mg milligram
Mg magnesium
mgm milligram
MHC major histocompatibility complex
MHPG 3-methoxy-4-hydroxyphenylglycol
MHz megahertz
MI mitral incompetence, mitral insufficiency; myocardial infarction
MIC methylisocyanate; minimal inhibitory concentration, minimum inhibitory concentration
MID minimal infective dose
min minim; minimum; minute
mixt mixture
ml milliliter
mL millilambert
MLD median lethal dose; minimum lethal dose
MLT medical laboratory technician
mm millimeter
mmole *also* **mmol** millimole
MMPI Minnesota Multiphasic Personality Inventory
MMR measles-mumps-rubella (vaccine)
Mn manganese
MN master of nursing
mo month
Mo molybdenum
MO medical officer
MODY maturity-onset diabetes of the young
MOH medical officer of health
mol molecular, molecule
MOPP mechlorethamine, vincristine, procarbazine, and prednisone
morph morphological, morphology
mOsm milliosmol
mp melting point
MPC maximum permissible concentration
MPD multiple personality disorder
MPF maturation promoting factor
MPH master of public health
MPTP 1-methyl-4-phenyl-1,2,3,6-tetrahyropyridine
mR milliroentgen
MR magnetic resonance
mrad millirad
Mrad megarad
mrem millirem
Mrem megarem
MRI magnetic resonance imaging
mRNA messenger ribonucleic acid
MRS magentic resonance spectroscopy
ms millisecond
MS mass spectrometry; master of science; multiple sclerosis
MSc master of science
msec millisecond
MSG monosodium glutamate
MSH melanocyte-stimulating hormone
MSN master of science in nursing
MSO management services organization
MsTh mesothorium
MSW master of social work
MT medical technologist
MTD maximum tolerated dose
mtDNA mitochondrial deoxyribonucleic acid
mV millivolt
MVP mitral valve prolapse
mW milliwatt
MW megawatt
N nasal; newton; nitrogen — usu ital when used as a prefix; normal —

used of solutions; index of refraction

Na sodium

NA Nomina Anatomica; numerical aperture; nurse's aide

NAD nicotinamide adenine dinucleotide; no appreciable disease

NADH nicotinamide adenine dinucleotide (reduced form)

NADP nicotinamide adenine dinucleotide phosphate

NADPH nicotinamide adenine dinucleotide phosphate (reduced form)

nanosec nanosecond

Nb niobium

NB newborn

NBRT National Board for Respiratory Therapy

NCA neurocirculatory asthenia

nCi nanocurie

NCI National Cancer Institute

NCQA National Committee for Quality Assurance

Nd neodymium

NDT neurodevelopmental treatment

Ne neon

neurol neurological; neurology

NF National Formulary; neurofibromatosis

ng nanogram

NG nasogastric

NGF nerve growth factor

NGU nongonococcal urethritis

NHS National Health Service

Ni nickel

NICU neonatal intensive care unit

NIDDM non-insulin-dependent diabetes mellitus

NIH National Institutes of Health

NIMH National Institute of Mental Health

NIOSH National Institute of Occupational Safety and Health

NK natural killer (cell)

nl nanoliter

nm nanometer

NMDA *N*-methyl-D-aspartate

nmol *also* **nmole** nanomole

NMR nuclear magnetic resonance

no number

No nobelium

NOPHN National Organization for Public Health Nursing

Np neptunium

NP neuropsychiatric, neuropsychiatry; nurse practitioner

NPN nonprotein nitrogen

NPO [Latin *nil per os*] nothing by mouth

NPT normal pressure and temperature

nr near

NR no refill

NREM nonrapid eye movement (sleep)

ns nanosecond

NSAID nonsteroidal anti-inflammatory drug

nsec nanosecond

NSU nonspecific urethritis

nT nanotesla

NTD neural tube defect

NTP normal temperature and pressure

O opening; [Latin *octarius*] pint — used in writing prescriptions; oxygen

OB obstetric; obstetrician; obstetrics

OB-GYN obstetrician-gynecologist; obstetrics-gynecology

OBS obstetrician; obstetrics

obstet obstetric; obstetrics

OCD obsessive-compulsive disorder

od [Latin *omnes dies*] every day — used in writing prescriptions

OD doctor of optometry; [Latin *oculus dexter*] right eye — used in writing prescriptions; overdose

OI opportunistic infection

ol oleum

OL [Latin *oculus laevus*] left eye — used in writing prescriptions

OMPA octamethylpyrophosphoramide

OPD outpatient department

opt optician
OPV oral polio vaccine
OR operating room
ORF open reading frame
org organic
ORS oral rehydration salts, oral rehydration solution
Os osmium
OS [Latin *oculus sinister*] left eye — used in writing prescriptions
OSHA Occupational Safety and Health Administration
Osm osmol
ost osteopathic
OT occupational therapist, occupational therapy; old tuberculin
OTC over-the-counter
OTR registered occupational therapist
oz ounce, ounces
P parental; parental generation — usu. used with a numerical subscript; part; percentile; pharmacopeia; phosphorus; pint; pole; population; position; positive; posterior; pressure; pulse; pupil
Pa protactinium
PA pernicious anemia; physician assistant
PABA para-aminobenzoic acid
PACU postanesthesia care unit
PAF platelet-activating factor
PAH para-aminohippurate; para-aminohippuric acid; polycyclic aromatic hydrocarbon, polynuclear aromatic hydrocarbon
2-PAM 2-pyridine aldoxime methyl (*syn* pralidoxime)
P&A percussion and auscultation
Pap Papanicolaou (smear, test)
PAS para-aminosalicylic acid; periodic acid-Schiff
PASA para-aminosalicylic acid
PAT paroxysmal atrial tachycardia
path pathological, pathology
pathol pathological, pathologist, pathology
Pb lead

PBB polybrominated biphenyl
PBI protein-bound iodine
PC percent, percentage; [Latin *post cibos*] after meals — used in writing prescriptions; professional corporation; purified concentrate
PCB polychlorinated biphenyl
pCi picocurie
PCP pentachlorophenol; phencyclidine; Pneumocystis carinii pneumonia; primary care physician
PCR polymerase chain reaction
Pcs preconscious
PCV packed cell volume
PCWP pulmonary capillary wedge pressure
Pd palladium
PD interpupillary distance
PDGF platelet-derived growth factor
PDR *Physicians' Desk Reference*
PE physical examination
PEEP positive end-expiratory pressure
PEP phosphoenolpyruvate
per period, periodic; person
perf perforated, perforation
PET positron-emission tomography
pf picofarad
pg picogram
PG prostaglandin
PGA pteroylglutamic acid
PGR psychogalvanic reaction, psychogalvanic reflex, psychogalvanic response
PGY postgraduate year
ph pharmacopoeia; phosphor; phot
PHA phytohemagglutinin
Phar D doctor of pharmacy
pharm pharmaceutical, pharmacist, pharmacy
Pharm D doctor of pharmacy
PhD [Latin *philosophiae doctor*] doctor of philosophy
PhG graduate in pharmacy
PHN public health nurse
PHO physician-hospital organization
PHS Public Health Service

phys physical; physician; physiological

PID pelvic inflammatory disease

pil [Latin *pilula*] pill — used in writing prescriptions

PK psychokinesis

PKU phenylketonuria

PLSS portable life-support system

pm premolar

Pm promethium

PM [Latin *post meridiem*] after noon; postmortem

PMA Pharmaceutical Manufacturers Association

PMN polymorphonuclear neutrophilic leukocyte

pmol *or* **pmole** picomole

PMS premenstrual syndrome

PN psychoneurotic

PNH paroxysmal nocturnal hemoglobinuria

po [Latin *per os*] by mouth — used esp. in writing prescriptions

Po polonium

POD postoperative day

poly(A) polyadenylate, polyadenylic acid

poly(C) polycytidylic acid

poly I:C *also* **poly I·C** polyinosinic and polycytidylic acids

POMR problem-oriented medical record

POS point-of-service (plan)

pp parts per

PP pellagra preventive

PPA phenylpropanolamine

ppb parts per billion

PPD purified protein derivative

PPLO pleuropneumonia-like organism (*syn* mycoplasma)

ppm parts per million

PPO preferred provider organization

ppt parts per thousand; parts per trillion; precipitate

Pr praseodymium

prn [Latin *pro re nata*] as needed; as

the circumstances require — used in writing prescriptions

PRO Peer Review Organization

PrP prion protein

ps picosecond

PSA prostate-specific antigen

PSRO professional standards review organization

PSVT paroxysmal supraventricular tachycardia

psych psychology

psychol psychologist, psychology

pt patient; pint

Pt platinum

PT physical therapist; physical therapy

PTA plasma thromboplastin antecedent

PTC phenylthiocarbamide; plasma thromboplastin component

PTFE polytetrafluoroethylene

PTH parathyroid hormone

PTSD post-traumatic stress disorder

Pu plutonium

PUFA polyunsaturated fatty acid

pulv [Latin *pulvis*] powder — used in writing prescriptions

PUO pyrexia of unknown origin

PUVA psoralen ultraviolet A

PVD peripheral vascular disease

PVE prosthetic valve endocarditis

PVP polyvinylpyrrolidone

pvt private

PWA person with AIDS

Px pneumothorax; prognosis

PZI protamine zinc insulin

q [Latin *quaque*] every — used in writing prescriptions

QA quality assurance

qd [Latin *quaque die*] every day — used in writing prescriptions

qh *or* **qhr** [Latin *quaque hora*] every hour — used in writing prescriptions often with a number indicating the hours between doses

qid [Latin *quater in die*] four times a day — used in writing prescriptions

ql [Latin *quantum libet*] as much as you please — used in writing prescriptions

qn [Latin *quaque nocte*] every night — used in writing prescriptions

qp [Latin *quantum placet*] as much as you please — used in writing prescriptions

qt quart

qv [Latin *quantum vis*] as much as you will

r roentgen

R Reaumur; rough — used in bacteriology

Ra radium

rad [Latin *radix*] root — used in writing prescriptions

RAST radioallergosorbent test

Rb rubidium

RBC red blood cells; red blood count

RBE relative biological effectiveness

RBRVS resource-based relative value scale

RCT randomized clinical trial; randomized controlled trial

rd rutherford

RD reaction of degeneration; registered dietitian

RDA Recommended Daily Allowance

RDMS registered diagnostic medical sonographer

RDS respiratory distress syndrome

Re rhenium

redox oxidation-reduction

REM rapid eye movement

rep [Latin *repetatur*] let it be repeated — used in writing prescriptions

RES reticuloendothelial system

RF rheumatic fever

RFLP restriction fragment length polymorphism

Rh rhesus (factor); rhodium

RH relative humidity

RIA radioimmunoassay

RICE rest, ice, compression, elevation

RK radial keratotomy

RLF retrolental fibroplasia

RLQ right lower quadrant (abdomen)

Rn radon

RN registered nurse

RNA ribonucleic acid

RNase *or* **RNAase** ribonuclease

ROP retinopathy of prematurity

RPh registered pharmacist

rpm revolutions per minute

RPR rapid plasma reagin (test)

RPT registered physical therapist

RQ respiratory quotient

RR recovery room

RRA registered records administrator

RRL registered records librarian

rRNA ribosomal ribonucleic acid

RRT registered respiratory therapist

RSD reflex sympathetic dystrophy

RSV respiratory syncytial virus; Rous sarcoma virus

RT reaction time; recreational therapy; respiratory therapist

Ru ruthenium

RU rat unit

RUQ right upper quadrant (abdomen)

S sacral — used esp. with a number from 1 to 5 to indicate a vertebra or segment of the spinal cord in the sacral region; signa — used to introduce the signature in writing a prescription; smooth — used of bacterial colonies; subject; sulfur; svedberg

sa [Latin *secundum artem*] according to art — used in writing prescriptions

S-A sinoatrial

SAD seasonal affective disorder

sat saturated

Sb [Latin *stibium*] antimony

SBS sick building syndrome

Sc scandium

ScD doctor of science

SCID severe combined immunodeficiency

ScM master of science

SCM state certified midwife

SCN suprachiasmatic nucleus

SDA specific dynamic action

Se selenium

SED skin erythema dose

SEM scanning electron microscope, scanning electron microscopy

sg specific gravity

SGOT serum glutamic-oxaloacetic transaminase

SGPT serum glutamic pyruvic transaminase

SH serum hepatitis

Si silicon

SI [French *Système International d'Unités*] International System of Units

SIDS sudden infant death syndrome

Sig signa — used to introduce the signature in writing a prescription

SIV simian immunodeficiency virus

SK streptokinase

SLE systemic lupus erythematosus

Sm samarium

Sn tin

SNF skilled nursing facility

SOAP subjective, objective, assessment, and plan

SOB short of breath

SOS [Latin *si opus sit*] if occasion require; if necessary — used in writing prescriptions

sp species (singular)

SPCA serum prothrombin conversion accelerator; Society for the Prevention of Cruelty to Animals

SPECT single photon emission computed tomography

SPF sun protection factor

sp gr specific gravity

sp nov [Latin *species nova*] new species — used following a taxonomic binomial proposed as new

spp species (plural)

Sr strontium

S-R stimulus-response

sRNA soluble ribonucleic acid (*syn* transfer ribonucleic acid)

SRS-A slow-reacting substance of anaphylaxis

ss [Latin *semis*] one half — used in writing prescriptions

SSPE subacute sclerosing panencephalitis

SSRI selective serotonin reuptake inhibitor

SSSS staphylococcal scalded skin syndrome

STD sexually transmitted disease

STH somatotropic hormone

STM short-term memory

STP standard temperature and pressure

STS serologic test for syphilis

surg surgeon; surgery; surgical

SV simian virus

SVT supraventricular tachycardia

T absolute temperature; tesla; thoracic — used with a number from 1 to 12 to indicate a vertebra or segment of the spinal cord; thymine; tritium

Ta tantalum

TA transactional analysis

T and A tonsillectomy and adenoidectomy

TAT thematic apperception test

Tb terbium

TB tubercle bacillus; tuberculosis

TBG thyroid-binding globulin, thyroxine-binding globulin

TBI traumatic brain injury

Tc technetium

TCA tricyclic antidepressant

TCDD 2,3,7,8-tetrachlorodibenzo-para-dioxin, 2,3,7,8-tetrachlorodibenzo-p-dioxin

TCE trichloroethylene

TCR T cell (antigen) receptor

Td tetanus diphtheria (toxoids)

TD tardive dyskinesia

tds [Latin *ter die sumendum*] to be

taken three times a day — used in writing prescriptions

Te tellurium

TEA tetraethylammonium

tech technician

TEM transmission electron microscope, transmission electron microscopy; triethylenemelamine

TENS transcutaneous electrical nerve stimulation

TEPP tetraethyl pyrophosphate

TGF transforming growth factor

Th thorium

THA 1,2,3,4 - tetrahydro - 9 - acridinamine (*syn* tacrine)

THC tetrahydrocannabinol

Ti titanium

TIA transient ischemic attack

tid [Latin *ter in die*] three times a day — used in writing prescriptions

TIL tumor-infiltrating lymphocyte

tinct tincture

Tl thallium

TLC tender loving care; thin-layer chromatography

TLE temporal lobe epilepsy

Tm thulium

TM transcendental meditation

TMD temporomandibular disorder

TMJ temporomandibular joint, temporomandibular joint syndrome

TNF tumor necrosis factor

TOF time-of-flight

TORCH toxoplasmosis, other, rubella, cytomegalovirus, and herpes simplex virus

TPA tissue plasminogen activator

TPI Treponema pallidum immobilization (test)

TPN triphosphopyridine nucleotide (*syn* NADP)

TPP thiamine pyrophosphate

TPR temperature, pulse, respiration

TQM total quality management

TRF thyrotropin-releasing factor

TRH thyrotropin-releasing hormone

tRNA transfer ribonucleic acid

Try tryptophan

TSH thyroid-stimulating hormone (*syn* thyrotropin)

TSS toxic shock syndrome

U uracil; uranium

UDP uridine diphosphate

UMP uridine 5'-monophosphate (*syn* uridylic acid)

ung [Latin *unguentum*] ointment — used in writing prescriptions

Unh unnilhexium

Unp unnilpentium

Unq unnilquadium

URI upper respiratory infection

USAN United States Adopted Names — used to designate officially recognized nonproprietary names of drugs as established by a joint committee of medical and pharmaceutical professionals

USP United States Pharmacopeia

ut dict [Latin *ut dictum*] as directed — used in writing prescriptions

UTI urinary tract infection

UTP uridine triphosphate

UV ultraviolet

V vanadium; volt

VAD ventricular assist device

VCG vectorcardiogram

VD venereal disease

VDRL venereal disease research laboratory

VF ventricular fibrillation

Vi virulent

VIP vasoactive intestinal peptide, vasoactive intestinal polypeptide

VLDL very low-density lipoprotein

VMA vanillylmandelic acid

VMD doctor of veterinary medicine

VNA Visiting Nurse Association

VOC volatile organic compound

vol volume

VS vesicular stomatitis

VSD ventricular septal defect

VT ventricular tachycardia

v/v volume per volume

W [German *wolfram*] tungsten
WAIS Wechsler Adult Intelligence Scale
WBC white blood cell
WDHA watery diarrhea, hypokalemia, and achlorhyria (syndrome)
WEE western equine encephalomyelitis
WHO World Health Organization
WPW Wolff-Parkinson-White (syndrome)
ws water-soluble

wt weight
w/v weight in volume
w/w weight in weight
x power of magnification
Xe xenon
XP xeroderma pigmentosum
Y yttrium
Yb ytterbium
Z atomic number; impedance
Zn zinc
ZPG zero population growth
Zr zirconium

Frequently Confused and Misused Words

The following list includes nonmedical words that are often confused in general usage. A list of easily confused medical words and phrases is included in Chapter 11, "Medical Transcription and Correspondence."

abjure to reject solemnly
adjure to command

abrogate to nullify
arrogate to claim

abstruse hard to understand
obtuse dull, slow

accede to agree
exceed to go beyond

accent to emphasize
ascent climb
assent to agree to something

access right or ability to enter
excess intemperance

ad advertisement
add to join to something; to find a sum

adapt to adjust to something
adept highly skilled
adopt to take as one's child; to take up

addenda additional items
agenda list of things to be done

addition part added
edition publication

adjoin to be next to
adjourn to suspend a session
adjure to command

adverse unfavorable
averse disinclined

advert to refer
avert to avoid
overt unconcealed

advice counsel or information
advise to give advice

affect to act upon or influence
effect result; to bring about

agenda *see* ADDENDA

alimentary relating to nourishment
elementary simple or basic

allude to refer indirectly
elude to evade

allusion indirect reference
illusion misleading image

amenable accountable, agreeable
amendable modifiable

amend to alter in writing
emend to correct

anymore any longer, now
any more more

appraise to set a value on
apprise to give notice of
apprize to appreciate or value

arraign to bring before a court
arrange to come to an agreement

arrogate *see* ABROGATE

ascent *see* ACCENT

assay to test for valuable content
essay to try tentatively

assent *see* ACCENT

assure to give confidence to
ensure to make certain
insure to guarantee against loss

aural relating to the ear or hearing
oral relating to the mouth, spoken

averse *see* ADVERSE

avert *see* ADVERT

bail security given
bale bundle of goods

base bottom
bass fish; deep voice

biannual usu. twice a year; sometimes every two years
biennial every two years

bloc group working together
block tract of land

born produced by birth
borne carried

breadth width
breath breathed air
breathe to draw in air

canvas strong cloth; oil painting
canvass to solicit votes or opinions

capital city that is the seat of government
capitol state legislature building
Capitol U.S. Congress building

casual not planned
causal relating to or being a cause

casually by chance or accident
casualty one injured or killed

censor to examine for improper content
censure to express disapproval of

cession a yielding
session meeting

cite to summon; to quote
sight payable on presentation
site piece of land

collaborate to work or act jointly
corroborate to confirm

collision act of colliding
collusion secret cooperation for deceit

complacent self-satisfied
complaisant amiable

complement remainder
compliment admiring remark

concert to act in harmony or conjunction
consort to keep company

consul diplomatic official
council administrative body

counsel legal representative; to give advice

corespondent joint respondent
correspondent one who communicates

corroborate *see* COLLABORATE

council *see* CONSUL

councilor member of a council
counselor lawyer

counsel *see* COUNCIL

credible worthy of being believed
creditable worthy of praise
credulous gullible

currant raisinlike fruit
current stream; belonging to the present

cynosure one that attracts
sinecure easy job

decent good or satisfactory
descent downward movement
dissent difference of opinion

decree official order
degree extent or scope

defuse to make less harmful
diffuse to pour out or spread widely

deluded misled or confused
diluted weakened in consistency

demur to protest
demure shy

deposition testimony
disposition personality; outcome

depraved corrupted
deprived divested or stripped

deprecate to disapprove of
depreciate to lower the worth of

descent *see* DECENT

desperate having lost hope
disparate distinct

detract to disparage or reduce
distract to draw attention away

device piece of equipment or tool
devise to invent, to plot

diffuse *see* DEFUSE

diluted *see* DELUDED

disassemble to take apart
dissemble to disguise feelings or intentions

disburse to pay out
disperse to scatter

discreet capable of keeping a secret
discrete individually distinct

disparate *see* DESPERATE

disperse *see* DISBURSE

disposition *see* DEPOSITION

dissemble *see* DISASSEMBLE

dissent *see* DECENT

distract *see* DETRACT

edition *see* ADDITION

effect *see* AFFECT

e.g. for example
i.e. that is

elementary *see* ALIMENTARY

elicit to draw or bring out
illicit not lawful

eligible qualified to have
illegible not readable

elude *see* ALLUDE

emanate to come out from a source
eminent standing above others
immanent inherent
imminent ready to take place

emend *see* AMEND

emigrate to leave a country
immigrate to come into a place

eminence prominence or superiority
immanence restriction to one domain
imminence state of being imminent

ensure *see* ASSURE

envelop to surround
envelope letter container

equable free from unpleasant extremes
equitable fair

erasable removable by erasing
irascible hot-tempered

essay *see* ASSAY

every day each day
everyday ordinary

exceed *see* ACCEDE

excess *see* ACCESS

extant currently existing
extent size, degree, or measure

flaunt to display ostentatiously
flout to scorn

flounder to struggle
founder to sink

forego to precede
forgo to give up

formally in a formal manner
formerly at an earlier time

forth forward, out of
fourth 4th

gage security deposit
gauge to measure

gait manner of walking
gate opening in a wall or fence

generic general
genetic relating to the genes

gibe to tease or mock
jibe to agree
jive foollish talk

guarantee to promise to be responsible for
guaranty something given as a security

hail to greet
hale to compel to go; healthy

hearsay rumor
heresy dissent from a dominant theory

i.e. *see* E.G.

illegible *see* ELIGIBLE

illicit *see* ELICIT

illusion *see* ALLUSION

immanence *see* EMINENCE

immanent *see* EMANATE

immigrate *see* EMIGRATE

imminence *see* EMINENCE

imminent *see* EMANATE

imply hint, indicate
infer conclude, deduce

impracticable not feasible
impractical not practical

inapt not suitable
inept unfit or foolish

incite to urge on
insight discernment

incredible unbelievable
incredulous disbelieving, astonished

incurable not curable
incurrable capable of being incurred

inept *see* INAPT

inequity lack of equity
iniquity wickedness

infer *see* IMPLY

ingenious very clever
ingenuous innocent and candid

inherent intrinsic
inherit to receive from an ancestor

iniquity *see* INEQUITY

insight *see* INCITE

install to set up for use
instill to impart gradually

insure *see* ASSURE

interment burial
internment confinement   or   impounding

interstate involving more than one state
intestate leaving no valid will
intrastate existing within a state

irascible *see* ERASABLE

it's it is
its belonging to it

jibe *see* GIBE

jive *see* GIBE

lead to guide; heavy metal
led guided

lean to rely on for support
lien legal claim on property

lesser smaller
lessor grantor of a lease

levee embankment   to   prevent flooding
levy imposition or collection of a tax

liable obligated by law
libel to make libelous statements; false publication

lien *see* LEAN

material having relevance or importance; matter
matériel equipment and supplies

median middle value in a range
medium intermediate; means of communication

meet to come into contact with
mete to allot

meretricious falsely attractive
meritorious deserving   reward   or honor

meticulous extremely careful about details

militate to have effect
mitigate to make less severe

miner mine worker
minor one of less than legal age; not important or serious

moot having   no   practical   significance

mute a person unable to speak; to tone down or muffle

naval relating to a navy
navel belly button

obtuse *see* ABSTRUSE

oral *see* AURAL

ordinance law, rule, or decree
ordnance military supplies
ordonnance compilation of laws

overt *see* ADVERT

parlay to bet again a stake and its winnings

parley discussion of disputed points

peer one of equal standing
pier bridge support

peremptory ending a right of action, debate or delay
preemptory preemptive

perpetrate to be guilty of
perpetuate to make perpetual

perquisite a right or privilege
prerequisite a necessary preliminary

persecute to harass injuriously
prosecute to proceed against at law

personal relating to a particular person
personnel body of employees

perspective view of things
prospective relating to the future
prospectus introductory description of an enterprise

perspicacious very discerning
perspicuous easily understood

pier *see* PEER

plain ordinary
plane airplane; surface

plaintiff complaining party in litigation

plaintive sorrowful

plat plan of a piece of land
plot small piece of land

pole long slender piece of wood or metal

poll sampling of opinion

pore to read attentively
pour to dispense from a container

practicable feasible
practical capable of being put to use

precede to go or come before
proceed to go to law

precedence priority
precedents previous examples to follow

preemptory *see* PEREMPTORY

preposition part of speech
proposition proposal

prerequisite *see* PERQUISITE

prescribe to direct to use; to assert a prescriptive right
proscribe to forbid

preview advance view
purview part or scope of a statute

principal main body of an estate; chief person or matter
principle basic rule or assumption

proceed *see* PRECEDE

proposition *see* PREPOSITION

proscribe *see* PRESCRIBE

prosecute *see* PERSECUTE

prospective *see* PERSPECTIVE

prospectus *see* PERSPECTIVE

purview *see* PREVIEW

raise to lift, to increase
raze to destroy or tear down

reality the quality or state of being real
realty real property

rebound to spring back or recover
redound to have an effect

recession ceding back
recision cancellation
rescission act of rescinding or abrogating

respectfully with respect
respectively in order

resume to take up again
résumé summary

role part, function
roll turn

session *see* CESSION

shear to cut off
sheer very thin or transparent

sight *see* CITE

sinecure *see* CYNOSURE

site *see* CITE

stationary still
stationery writing material

statue piece of sculpture
stature natural height or achieved status
statute law enacted by a legislature

tack course of action
tact sense of propriety

tenant one who occupies a rental dwelling
tenet principle

therefor for that
therefore thus

tortuous lacking in straightforwardness
torturous very painful or distressing

track path or course
tract stretch of land; system of body organs

trustee one entrusted with something
trusty convict allowed special privileges

venal open to bribery
venial excusable

waive to give up voluntarily
wave to motion with the hands

waiver act of waiving a right
waver to be irresolute

who's who is
whose of whom

your belonging to you
you're you are

Index

A

A, an, 404
AAAHC. *See* Accreditation Association for Ambulatory Health Care
AAMA. *See* American Association of Medical Assistants
AAMT. *See* American Association for Medical Transcription
Abbreviations, 400–410
  a or *an* with, 404
  and contractions, 401
  at beginning of sentences, 402
  capitalization of, 362, 402
  division of, 400
  drug names, 322
  in addresses, 406
  in compound words, 402–403
  in dates, 405–406
  inflected forms of, 326, 346
  medical, 466–485
  of academic degrees, 338, 406
  of Bible books, 405
  of Latin words and phrases, 407
  of proper nouns and adjectives, 362, 401
  of scientific terms, 409
  plural forms, 380, 402–403
  possessive forms, 387, 402–403
  punctuation of, 400–401
  units of measurement, 403, 410
  variation in styling of, 400
  with ampersand, 404–405
  with apostrophe, 326
  with hyphen, 346, 403
  with names, 408
  with period, 349–350, 400–401
  with slash, 359, 401
  within parentheses, 347
Abdominal ultrasound report, 308 (illus.)
ABMS. *See* American Board of Medical Specialties
Abstracting health information, 228
Abstractions, 362
Abuse, substance
  confidentiality and, 37
  consent to release health information and, 27
  managed care and, 81–82
Academic degrees
  abbreviation of, 338, 406
  capitalization of, 362
Accented English, transcribing, 313
Access to care, 46
Access to specialists, in health maintenance organizations, 83
Accessibility, for people with disabilities, 29, 139, 140, 145
Accounting computer software, 119
Accounts receivable. *See also* Financial management
  billing cycle, 271–272
  data entry, 272
  patient services, 272
  receipt processing, 272
Accounts receivable verification, 278
Accreditation. *See* Certification and accreditation
Accreditation Association for Ambulatory Health Care, 52
Accuracy, when entering computer data, 109
Act phase of TQM, 62–63
Activation sequence, computer, 107–108

Active patient files, retention of, 249
Acute vs. chronic conditions, 225
A.D., 404, 419–420
ADA. *See* Americans with Disabilities Act
Addresses, street
abbreviations in, 406
numbers in, 417–418
punctuation of, 338
ADEA. *See* Age Discrimination in Employment Act
Adjectives
compound, 392–395
in compound words, 390
nouns used as, 392
Administration, 365–366
Administrator, 147–148
Administrator's office design, 129 (illus.)
Adolescents
autonomy of, 9–10
confidentiality and, 11
consent and, 27
Adverbial clauses and phrases, 331–332
Adverbs
as modifiers of compounds, 395
compound, 396
conjunctive, 357
Advocating autonomy for patients, 8
Age, numbers for, 426–427
Age Discrimination in Employment Act, 170
Agency for Health Care Policy and Research, 66, 84
A.H., 419
AHA. *See* American Hospital Association
AHCPR. *See* Agency for Health Care Policy and Research
AHIMA. *See* American Health Information Management Association
Alcohol use, health promotion and, 447
Allergy procedure room design, 135
Alphabet. *See* Letters of the alphabet
Alphabetical filing, 239
Alphabetical index for numerical files, 241
a.m., 409, 425
AMA. *See* American Medical Association
America Online, 120
American Association for Medical Transcription, 288
American Association of Medical Assistants, 3–4, 19, 144
code of ethics, 4 (illus.)
American Association of Poison Control Centers, 454

American Board of Medical Specialties, 34
American Health Information Management Association, 226, 231, 233, 293
health record retention schedules, 248, 251–252
American Hospital Association
health record retention schedules, 248
patient rights and, 6
American Medical Association, 19, 293
CPT-4 and, 234
position on computer security, 101 (illus.)
principles of medical ethics, 3–4 (illus.)
American Medical Association Manual of Style, 428, 465
American Medical Association Principles of Medical Ethics, 3, 179
American Medical Technologists, 144
American Nurses' Association, 3–4, 19
code of ethics, 5 (illus.)
Americans with Disabilities Act, 28, 29, 140, 145, 170
Ampersand, 404–405
An, a, 404
ANA. *See* American Nurses' Association
And, replaced by slash, 358
And/or, 358
Animal names, 362, 380–381
Apostrophe
and plurals, 326, 380
and possessives, 325, 385–388
in compound words, 396
in numbers, 326, 418, 419
to show omission, 326
Appearance, appropriate job interview, 441–442
Appointment book, 207–208
Appointment scheduler, 146
Appointment system, computerized, 253
Appointments, 206–210
failed, 210
reminders, 209–210
scheduling, 206–207
scheduling guidelines, 208–209
Appositives, 333, 328
Archives, health record, 252–253
Art, works of, 375
Article titles. *See under* Titles of works
capitalization, 428
Articles
in titles of works, 375
documentation of, 428–429
indefinite, 404

Assault, defined, 43
Assessing risk, 96–97
Assignment of benefits form, 213 (illus.)
Association names. *See* Organizations, names of
Astronomy, 374
Asynchronous Transfer Mode, 118
ATM. *See* Asynchronous Transfer Mode
Attentiveness, as patient service indicator, 180–181
Attorneys, as users of health information, 206
Attribution of sources within text, with dash, 341
Attributive position of compounds, 392
At-will employee, 152
Audiocassette tapes, 292
Authorization, to release health information, 227
Authors, documentation of, in references, 428
Autonomy, 8–10
   advocating, 8
   determining capacity for, 9
   of children and adolescent patients, 9–10
   of patient, 7–10
   protecting elderly patients, 8
   providing health information to patient, 8
Awards, 362

B

Backing up computer data, 109–111
Backup cycle, 110
Bad-debt ceiling, 267
Bank memos, 276
Bank statements and reconciliations, 276
Bankers, relationships with, 274
Banking, 273–276
   checking accounts, 274–276
   location and services, 273–274
   relationships with banker, 274
Bar chart, 60–61 (illus.)
Basic four, 293, 295–299 (illus.)
Batch, 272
Bathroom designs for clinical office, 139, 140
Battery, defined, 43
b.c., 404, 419–420
b.c.e., 419–420

Beginning of sentences and phrases, 359–361
   abbreviations, 402
   numerals, 411
Behavior, fostering healthy, 97
Behavioral health managed care, 81–82
   limitation of benefits, 85
Beneficence, 12–14
   dilemmas of, 13–14
   limitations to, 12–13
   paternalism, 13
   to do no harm, 13–14
Benefit package, 451
Benefits, 174–176. *See also* Employee insurance
   health, life, and disability insurance, 175
   intangible, 176
   limitation of, 85–86
   personal days, 174–175
   wages in lieu of, 176
Between, used to indicate range, 416
Bible and biblical books, 373, 405
   citations to, 329
Biblical names, 373, 386
Bibliographic format, 329
Bibliographies, 461–465. *See also* References
   health information management, 461
   managed care, 461–462
   medical dictionaries, 462
   medical ethics, 462–463
   medical office design, 463
   medical transcription, 465
   quality of care, 463–464
   style manuals, 465
Billing and collection, 36, 263–273. *See also* Insurance billing
   cycle of reimbursement, 263–266 (illus.)
   Guide to Medical Billing, 461
   health record and, 204
   managing accounts receivable, 271–272
   managing collection, 266–271 (illus.)
   outside services, 273
Billing cycle, 271–272
Billion, 412
Binomial nomenclature, 373
Block quotation, 354
Blue Cross, 51
Board certification, 34
Boldface type, use of, 379–380
Book titles, 375
   capitalization, 428

Bookkeeper, 146–147
Books
  documentation of, 428
  reference number to parts of, 427
  titles of, 375
B.P., 419–420
Brackets, 326–328
  with comma, 339
  with other punctuation, 328
  with parentheses, 327
  with period, 350
Brainstorming, 58–60
Brand names, 376. *See also* Trademarks
Breach of duty, 39
Breast ultrasound report, 307 (illus.)
Budgeting, 279–280
  physician salaries and, 280
Building permits, 30
Bulleted list, 422
Business office design, 124–129. *See also*
    Clinical office design; Medical office
    design
  administrator's office, 129 (illus.)
  credit-counseling area, 128
  financial areas, 129
  medical records storage, 126, 128
  medical transcription workstation, 129,
    289–290
  office management area, 128–129
  payment and reappointment, 125–126
    (illus.)
  photocopy area, 126
  reception area, 124–125, 127 (illus.)
Business personnel, 145–148. *See also* Per-
    sonnel policies; Personnel policies
    manual
  administrator, 147–148
  appointment scheduler, 146
  bookkeeper or financial manager,
    146–147
  medical assistant, 145
  medical transcriptionist, 147, 287–290
  office manager, 147
  receptionist, 145–146
  telephone staff, 187–189
Byte, 117

C

Cables, computers and, 113
Canceled checks, 276
Cancer, prevention of, 448

Capitalization, 359–380
  abbreviations, 362, 402
  abstractions, 362
  academic degrees, 362
  animal names, 362
  awards and prizes, 362–363
  beginnings of sentences and phrases,
    359–361
  computer software titles, 374
  derivatives of proper names, 363
  for emphasis, 378
  geographical terms, 363
  governmental and political bodies, 365
  historical periods and events, 366–367,
    419
  in compound words, 367–368
  in hyphenated compounds, 367–368,
    393–394
  in lists, 421–423
  in quotations, 327, 360
  in reference entries, 428–429
  Internet, 374
  labels, 379
  legal material, 368
  letters representing shapes, 377
  medical terms, 368
  military terms, 368–369
  modes of transportation, 376–377
  musical compositions, 376
  numerical designations, 369–370
  of governmental titles, 371–372
  of professional titles, 371
  of salutation, 361
  on-line services, 374
  organization names, 370
  outline heading, 361
  parenthetical elements, 348–349,
    359–360
  people, 370–371
  plant names, 362
  poetry, 360
  prayers, 373
  proper nouns and adjectives, 361–377
  religious terms, 372–373
  scientific terms, 373–374
  signs, 379
  time periods and dates, 374
  titles of works, 375–376
  trademarks, 376
  U.S. Supreme Court, 365
  word following colon, 360–361
Capitation, 35–36, 71, 451
  managing health benefits, 85

physician fees and, 257–258
primary care, 262
provider system models and, 86
Carbon-copy notations, 330
Cardiology procedure room design, 134
Carve out, 451
Case management, 452
Cases in law, 368
Causation, 39
Cause-and-effect diagram, 56, 58 (illus.)
CD-ROM programs, 119–120
C.E., 419–420
Celestial objects, 374
Central dictation systems, 291
Central processing unit. *See* CPU
Cents, 423
Centuries, 419
Certification and accreditation, 32–34
    board certification, 34
    managed care organizations and, 33–34
    of hospital medical staff, 33
Certified Medical Transcriptionist, 288
Chapter titles, 375
Chart notes, transcription of, 302,
    312–313 (illus.)
Check endorsements, 275–276
Check phase of TQM, 60–62
Checkbooks, 275
Checking accounts, 274–276
    check endorsements, 275–276
    checkbooks, 275
    deposit slips, 275
    overdrafts, 275
    stop payment, 275
Checks, 276
Check-writing procedures, 278
Chemical elements and compounds, 394,
    409
Chemical formulas, 327
Chest X-ray report, 310 (illus.)
Chief complaint, 217
Children. *See also* Adolescents
    autonomy of, 9–10
    consent and, 27
Chronic care solutions, 91
Chronic vs. acute conditions, 225
Church, 373
Church names, 424
Citations, legal, 368
Civil liability, 42–43
Civil Rights Act of 1964, 29
Claims, internal control of, 278
Clauses
    adverbial, 332

and parentheses, 347, 349
elliptical, 357
main (independent), 330–331,
    356–357
restrictive and nonrestrictive, 332
subordinate (dependent), 332
with colon, 328–329, 330
with conjunctive adverbs, 357
CLIA. *See* Clinical Laboratory Improve-
    ment Act
Clinic without walls, 92–93, 452
Clinical encounter, 87–91
    managing, 88–89
    managing in facilities, 89–91
Clinical guidelines
    hospital-based, 90
    in clinical encounters, 89
Clinical Laboratory Improvement Act, 32,
    139
Clinical office design, 130–141. *See also*
    Business office design; Medical office
    design
    doctor's office, 133–134
    doctor's station, 133
    exam modules, 130 (illus.)
    exam rooms, 131–133
    laboratory department, 139
    nurse's station, 138–139 (illus.)
    primary care exam room, 132 (illus.)
    procedure rooms, 134–138
    X-ray department, 139–140
Clinical personnel, 141–145. *See also* Per-
    sonnel policies; Personnel policies
    manual
    licensed practical nurse, 143
    medical assistant, 143–144
    medical technician, 144
    nurse practitioner, 143
    physical/occupational therapists, 145
    physician assistant, 143
    physician, 141
    registered nurse, 143
Clinical preventive services, 449
Clinical process. *See* Clinical encounter
Closed panel, 75, 452
Closed patient files, retention of, 249
COBRA, 169, 170, 283
Coded mailboxes, 231
Codes, 233–235. *See also* Insurance billing
    confidentiality of, 235
    diagnosis, 233–234
    procedure, 234
    resource-based relative value scale,
        234–235

Coding, 36, 266
Co-insurance, 452
Collaborative relationship, between pro-
    vider and patient, 10
Collection, 36, 266–271 (illus.). *See also*
    Billing and collection
  bookkeeper and, 147
  goals, 267
  letters requesting payment, 268–270
    (illus.)
  schedule, 267
  telephone calls, 268–271
Colon, 328–330
  and dash compared, 339–340
  as an introductory mark, 328
  capitalization of word following,
    360–361
  ellipsis points and, 343
  in biblical references, 329
  in bibliographies, 329
  in ratios, 329, 425
  in reference entries, 428–429
  in salutation of letter, 329
  in time expressions, 329, 425–426
  in titles, 329
  spacing of, 329
  with appositives, 328
  with clauses, 328–329
  with comma, 329
  with parentheses, 330
  with phrases, 328–329
  with quotation marks, 330, 354
  with quotations, 329
Color names, 395
Color-coding, of files, 246
Columbia Registry of Clinical Trials, 88
Combined profit sharing and money pur-
    chase pension plans, 285–286
Combining forms, 397, 399–400
Comma, 330–339
  and dash compared, 334, 339
  and inverted order, 339
  and semicolon, 331, 339, 354–356
  as clause connector, 330
  in questions, 337
  in quotations, 336–337
  omission of, 332, 333, 335, 414–415
  serial, 335
  to avoid ambiguity, 339
  with addresses, 338
  with appositives, 333, 337
  with colon, 336, 339
  with compound predicates, 331

  with contrasting expressions, 334–335
  with coordinate modifiers, 335–336
  with dash, 334, 339, 341
  with dates, 338
  with degrees and titles, 338–339
  with exclamation point, 336, 339
  with introductory and interrupting ele-
    ments, 333–334
  with items in a series, 335
  with names, 338
  with nonrestrictive clauses, 332
  with numbers, 338, 414–415
  with omitted words, 337
  with other punctuation, 339
  with parenthetical elements, 333
  with question mark, 337, 339
  with quotation marks, 337, 355
  with restrictive clauses, 333, 337
  with salutation, 339
  with sentence within a sentence, 337,
    355
  with subordinate clauses and phrases,
    331–332
Comma fault, 331
Comma splice, 331
Common values, among health profession-
    als, 18
Communications computer software, 120,
    255
Community rating, 452
Company, Co., 404
Company names, 339, 370, 404
Compass points, 363, 405
Complaints and incidents
  responding to, 39–40
  resolving on telephone, 190–192
  sample script for irate callers, 192–195
Complimentary close, 339, 361
Compound adjectives, 392–395
Compound adverbs, 396
Compound names, filing, 242
Compound nouns, 389–392
Compound predicates, 331
Compound terms
  permanent, 388
  plural, 381–382
  open, 388
  slash and, 358
  solid, 388
  temporary, 388
Compound verbs, 390–391, 396–397
Compound words, 388–400
  abbreviated, 403

capitalization of, 367–368
hyphenated, 367–368, 389, 400, 403, 411
CompuServe, 120
Computer
Computer Concepts and Applications for the Medical Office, 461
future trends in managed care and, 120–121
in medical office, 99–100, 102–103, 105–107
paperless office and, 121–122
security passwords, 101–102
support services, 101
Computer activation sequence, 107–108
Computer backup, lockbox service and, 274
Computer data, 109–111
accuracy, 109
backing up, 109–111
Computer disconnection sequence, 108
Computer environment, 113–114
Computer hardware
cables, 113
chairs, 114
keyboard, 107, 114
modem, 118
monitor, 114
mouse, 118
printers, 113
server, 113
terminals, 114
Computer networks, 111–112
Computer operating distance, 107
Computer operating systems, 111–112
Computer security, 101–102
American Medical Association position on, 102–103 (illus.)
health information and, 237
Computer software
accounting programs, 119
billing and collection, 273
communications programs, 120, 255
for health information management, 253–255
for medical office, 100
multimedia programs, 120
word processing and desktop publishing programs, 119
Computer software titles, capitalization of, 374
Computer terms, 114–119, 374, 409
Computer-related work habits, 107–111

backing up data, 109–110
basic rules, 107–109
saving your work, 110–111
Concurrent review, 84
Conference room design, 140
Confidentiality, 10–12
breaching, 12
computerized records and, 10
defined, 226
fax transmission of health information and, 231
for adolescents, 11
of health information, 37, 226
third-party requests for information and, 11
threats to, 10–11
waiving right to, 11
Confidentiality of codes, insurance billing and, 235
Conjunctions
and semicolon, 356–358
capitalization of, in titles, 375
coordinating, 332, 357
correlative, 334–335
Conjunctive adverbs, 334
Consent forms, 224
insurance forms and, 212
Consent, 26–27
release of health information and, 227, 229–230 (illus.), 235
Consolidated Omnibus Budget Reconciliation Act. *See* COBRA
Constitution, citing Articles, 414
Consultation report, 224
transcription of, 294, 298 (illus.)
Continuing education, license renewal requirements and, 29–30
Continuity of medical care, 202
Continuous Quality Improvement, 51
TQM and, 54
Contraception
confidentiality and, 11
consent and, 27
Contract numbers, 427
Contractions, 326, 401
Contracts
employment, 38
with third-party payers, 34–35
Contrasting expressions, 334–335
Controlled substances, 31
schedules of, 449–451
Controlled Substances Act of 1970, 449
Conversion factor, 260

Coordinate modifiers, 335–336, 392
Co-payment, 86, 452
Corporate names, 339, 370, 404
Corporation, Corp., 404
Corrections to health records, making, 224–225
Correspondence, 329, 339, 361
  medical, 302, 305, 314–317 (illus.)
Council on Ethical and Judicial Affairs of the American Medical Association, 3
Country names, 407
Court cases, citations to, 368
Courtesy copies, punctuation, 330
Courtesy titles, 409
Courts
  as users of health information, 206
  capitalization of, 365
  names of, 365, 424
Cover letter, job application, 436–437 (illus.)
CPT. *See* Current Procedural Terminology
CPT-4, 146, 234, 261, 266
CPU, 112
CQI. *See* Continuous Quality Improvement
Credit-counseling area design, 128
Criminal liability, 43–44
Critical paths. *See* Critical pathways
Critical pathways, 66–67, 90–91
Current performance, measuring, 56
Current Procedural Terminology, 4th edition. *See* CPT-4
Current professional knowledge, quality of care and, 47–48
Cycle of reimbursement, 263 (illus.)
  coding, 266
  collection, 266
  documentation of services, 264–266
  insurance claims, 266
  patient registration, 263–264
  reimbursement, 266
Cytology report, transcription of, 301–302 (illus.)

D

Dash, 334, 339–343
  and colon compared, 341
  and comma compared, 339–340, 341
  and parentheses compared, 342, 347, 349
  and question mark, 342, 351

  and semicolon, 341–342
  em, 340
  en, 340, 342
  spacing of, 340
  three–em, 340, 343
  two–em, 340, 344
  with comma, 334, 339, 341
  with exclamation point, 342
  with period, 342
  with quotation marks, 355
Data collection sheet, 57, 59 (illus.)
Data entry
  accounts receivable, 272
  computer, 109–110
Data systems, 449
Database
  capitalization of, 374
  problem-oriented medical record, 214
Database management, 255
Dates, 418–420
  abbreviations in, 405–406
  A.D. and B.C., 404, 419–420
  and apostrophe, 418
  elided, 419
  geological, 419
  in military correspondence, 406, 418
  in reference entries, 428–429
  inverted styling of, 418
  punctuation of, 338
Days of the week, 374
dBase, 255
de
  capitalization, 370
  filing, 242
DEA. *See* Drug Enforcement Agency
Death, of physician, 176–177
Decades, 419
Decimal fractions, 421
  in monetary units, 423
Decision-making capacity, autonomy and, 9
Decorations, military, 369
Deductible, 86, 452
Defamation, defined, 43
Degrees, academic, 338, 362, 406
Degrees, of arc, 420
Degrees, of temperature, 420
Deming, W. Edwards, 51
Department of Labor, 168, 170, 284
Dependent clauses. *See* Clauses, subordinate
Deposit slips, 275
Depositions, 40

Deposits-in-transit, 276
Depressants, 449–451
Dermatology procedure room design, 135
Design. *See* Business office design; Clinical office design; Medical office design
Desktop dictation machines, 291
Desktop publishing computer software, 119
Destruction methods, for health records, 251
Determining capacity for autonomy, 9
Diabetes, prevention of, 448
Diagnosis codes, insurance billing and, 233–234
Diagnosis-related group, 51, 205, 206
Diagnostic procedure reports, 223
Diagonal. *See* Slash
Dialogue
   capitalization of, 360
   punctuation of, 352–356
Dictation equipment, 290–291. *See also* Medical transcription equipment.
Dictionaries, medical, 462
Diminished capacity, waiving right to confidentiality and, 11
Direct access, to health information, 228
Direct address, 334
Direct question, 337, 350–352
Direct quotation, 336, 352
Directions. *See* Compass points
Directory, computer, 116
Disabilities, ensuring access for people with. *See* Americans with Disabilities Act; Accessibility
Disability, of physician, 176–177
Disability insurance, as employee benefit, 175–176
Discharge summary, transcription of, 300–302 (illus.)
Disclosures, 37
Disconnection sequence, computer, 108
Disease prevention, 448–449. *See also* Health promotion; Health protection
   managed care and, 97–98
Disease terminology, 368
Diskettes, computer, 116
Disks, computer, 116
Dissatisfied patients
   resolving complaints, 190–192
   sample script for irate callers, 192–195
Division of responsibility, financial control and, 277
Do phase of TQM, 60

Docking pay, 173
Doctor, Dr., 409
   filing, 242
Doctor-assisted suicide, medical ethics and, 14
Doctor's office design, 133–134
Doctor's station design, 130 (illus.), 133
Documentation
   employee termination and, 168
   of articles, 428–429
   of books, 428
   of newspapers, 429
   of periodicals, 428–429
Documentation and coding, insurance billing and, 235
Documentation guidelines for health records, 225–226
Documentation of services, 264–266
   encounter form, 264–265 (illus.)
   out-of-office journal, 264, 266
Dollar amounts, 423
Donabedian, Avedis, 48, 50
DOS, 111–112, 115
Dot-matrix printer, 108
Dots. *See* Ellipsis points
Dr. See Doctor, Dr.
Drawer, 275
Dress, for job interview, 441–442
Dressing rooms, in X-ray department design, 140
DRG. *See* Diagnosis-related group
Drive, computer, 115–116
Drug addiction
   confidentiality and, 11, 37
   consent to release health information and, 27
   managed care and, 81–82
Drug and sample storage area design, 140
Drug Enforcement Agency, 31
Drug names, 368, 449–451
   abbreviated, 322
Drugs
   health promotion and, 447
   regulation of, 31–32
   schedules of, 449–451
Dust problems, computers and, 113
Duty, medical malpractice and, 38–39

E

E&M codes. *See* Evaluation and management codes
Earth, 374

Editing, 306–308, 310, 313
frequently confused words, 318–321
health care vocabulary standards,
321–324
of accented English, 313
problems, 308, 310
Editorial insertions, 326–328
Education, continuing and license renewal requirements, 29–30
Education needs, health record retention
and, 248
Educational and community-based health
promotion programs, 447
EEOC. *See* Equal Employment Opportunity Commission
EIN. *See* Employee identification number
Elderly patients
managing risk of, 97
protecting autonomy of, 8
Electroencephalographic report, 316
(illus.)
Electromagnetic fields, computer monitors and, 114
Electronic remittance, 106
Elements, chemical, 394, 409
Elision of numbers, 416–417
Ellipsis points, 343–345
and comma, 339
and extracts, 343–344
and period, 344
and poetry, 344
omission of, 343–344
spacing of, 343
with other punctuation, 344
Elliptical clauses, 357
ELSI. *See* Human Genome Project
Em dash, 340
three-em, 340, 343
two-em, 340, 343
E-mail, 120
Emergency room report, 311 (illus.)
transcription of, 302, 311 (illus.)
Emergi-centers, 207
Emotional distress, intentional infliction
of, 43
Empathy, for patients, 196–197
Emphasis, styling for, 378
Employee confidentiality agreement, 238
(illus.)
Employee identification number, 280
Employee insurance. *See also* Benefits
COBRA, 283
Family and Medical Leave Act, 284
Employee performance evaluation, tele-
phone service, 195

Employee Polygraph Protection Act of
1988, 170
Employee Retirement Income Security
Act, 170
Employees. *See also* Personnel policies; Personnel policies manual
hiring, 156–161
obligations to by employer, 19
recruiting, 153–156
replacing, 167
terminating, 165–169
Employer, obligations of employee, 18–19
Employers' rights, 167–168
Employment
application for, 432–436
interviewing, 440–444
search for, 431–432
sources of, 436–440
Employment contracts, 38
Employment statement, 152
En dash, 340, 342
with inclusive numbers, 416
Encounter form, 264–265 (illus.)
End-of-line division, 346, 400
English, accented, 313
Enumerations, 421–423
capitalization in, 421–423
punctuation of, 348, 351, 421–423
Environmental health, health protection
and, 448
Epigraph, 341, 355
Epithet, personal, 370–372
EPOs. *See* Exclusive provider organiza-
tions
Equal Employment Opportunity Commis-
sion, 168
Equal Pay Act, 170
Equipment
dictation, 290–291
medical transcription, 291–292
Equipment leases, 38
Equity ownership models, 95–96
Era designations, 416, 419–420
Ergonomics, 290
ERISA. *See* Employee Retirement Income
Security Act
Errors, correcting in health records,
224–225
Esquire, Esq., 409
Essay titles, 375
et al., 428
Ethical obligations, 18–20
to other health professionals, 18–19
to society, 19–20
Ethical practice, ensuring, 17

Ethical rights of patients, vs. legal, 2
Ethics, defined, 5. *See also* Medical ethics
Etiquette
  job interview, 441–443
  patient relations, 197–199
  telephone, 179–181, 189–190, 192–195
Evaluation and management codes, 264
Ex- compounds, 398
Exam modules, 130 (illus.)
  placement of nurse's station, 138
    (illus.)
Exam rooms, 131–133
  attributes, 131–133
  design, 131–132 (illus.)
Excel, 254
Exclamation point, 345–346
  with brackets, 345
  with comma, 339, 345–346
  with dash, 345
  with parentheses, 345, 348
  with period, 345
  with question mark, 345
  with quotation marks, 345, 355
Exclamations, 345–346
Exclusive provider organizations, 78, 452
Experience rating, 452
External commands, 115
External controls, health maintenance or-
    ganizations and, 82–83
Extracts, quotation marks and, 354–355
Eyeglasses, computer working distance
    and, 114

F

Facilities, scheduling appointments and,
    209
Failed appointments, 210
Fair Credit Reporting Act, 36
Fair Debt Collection Practices Act, 36
Fair Labor Standards Act, 170, 171, 173
False imprisonment, defined, 43
Family and Medical Leave Act, 169–170,
    284
Family history, 217
Family planning, health promotion and,
    447
Family relationship terms, 371
Fax cover sheet, 232 (illus.)
Fax transmission
  *Guidelines for Faxing Patient Health Infor-
    mation, 461*
  of health information, 228, 231

FDA. *See* U.S. Food and Drug Administra-
    tion
Federal Insurance Contributions Act. *See*
    FICA
Federal regulations
  confidentiality of health information,
    226
  governing working relationships,
    169–171
  health record and, 203
  health record disposition, 251
  health record retention, 247–248
Federal taxes, 280
Federal unemployment tax, 281
Federal Unemployment Tax Return, 281
Federal, capitalization of, 365–366
Fee analysis, 259–261
Fee schedule, 258–259
Fee-for-service reimbursement, 452
FFS. *See* Fee-for-service reimbursement
FICA, 280–281
Figures (numerals), 410–414, 418. *See also*
    Numbers
-fold (suffix), use with numbers, 399
File
  folders, 244–245
  labels, 245
Files, color-coding, 246
Filing systems, 239–246
  alphabetical, 239
  equipment, 243
  laboratory reports, 223
  numeric, 240–241
  preventing misfiles, 246
  procedures, 245–246
  rules of filing, 241–243
  storage needs, 243–244
  supplies, 244–245
FIN. *See* Employee identification number
Financial area design, 129
Financial counselor, 256–257
  collection and, 266–267
  role in patient registration, 264
Financial management, 256
  banking, 273–276
  billing and collection, 263–273
  budgeting, 279–280
  financial counselor, 256–257
  insurance, 281–284
  internal controls, 277–279
  physician fees, 257–262
  retirement plans, 284–286
  taxes, 280–281

Financial manager, 146–147
Financing health care. *See* Health insurance
Flexible office hours, 207
Floppies, 116
Flowchart, 56, 57 (illus.)
  medical office management structure, 148 (illus.)
Flowcharting, 56, 60
FLSA. *See* Fair Labor Standards Act
FMLA. *See* Family and Medical Leave Act
Folders, 244–245
Follow-up letter, 438 (illus.), 443
Follow-up notes in SOAP format, transcription of, 294, 297 (illus.)
Food and drug safety, health protection and, 448
For deposit only, 276
Foreign language interpreters, 145
Foreign words and phrases, 353, 377, 382, 393
Fort, Ft., 407
401(k), 286
Fractions
  common, 420–421
  decimal. *See* Decimal fractions
  mixed, 420–421
  spelled-out form, 415, 420
Freedom of Information Act, 152
Frequently confused words, 318–321, 486–491
From, used to indicate range, 416
-ful words, plurals of, 384
Future trends
  for medical secretaries, 122–123
  in health promotion and disease prevention, 446–449
  in managed care, 97–98, 120–121
  in medical ethics, 20–22

G

G.P.M.S., 273
Gantt charts, 60
Gastroenterology procedure room design, 137
Gatekeeper, 452
Gatekeeper structures, 83–84
General liability insurance, 282
General surgery exam room attributes, 132
Genetics, Human Genome Project, 20–22
Genus names, 373
Geographical terms, 363–364, 406–407

Geological dates, 419
Geological terms, 374
Global physician compensation, 262
Government, as users of health information, 206
Government programs, measuring quality of care, 51
Government regulation of health care professionals, 29–32. *See also* Federal regulations; State regulations
  building permits, 30
  individual licenses, 29–30
  narcotic and drug regulation, 31–32
  office laboratories, 32
  organizational licenses, 30
  X-ray and health care equipment permits, 31
Governmental bodies, 365–366, 424
Gross conversion, 259
Gross conversion factor worksheet, 259–260 (illus.)
Group, in physician-patient relationship, 24–25
Group managed care models, 74–75
Grouping procedures, 209
Group-model health maintenance organization, 452

H

H&P. *See* History and physical examination
Hardware, computer. *See* Computer hardware
HCFA. *See* Health Care Financing Administration
HCFA-1500. *See* HCFA Health Insurance Claim Form
HCFA Health Insurance Claim Form, 235–236 (illus.)
HCPCS, 234
Headings, memorandum, 330, 361
Health benefits, managing, 85–86
Health Care Financing Administration, 46, 80, 206, 234, 260
Health Care Financing Administration Common Procedural Coding System. *See* HCPCS
Health care provider-patient relationship, terminating, 16
Health care providers, as user of health information, 204
Health care team, 1

Health care vocabulary standards, 321–324
Health information, appointments, 206–210
  appointment book, 207–208
  appointment reminders, 209–210
  scheduling appointments, 206–207
  scheduling guidelines, 208–209
  time management, 209
Health information, insurance billing, 233–236
Health information, releasing, 226–233
  confidentiality and, 226
  consent to release, 227
  fax transmission, 228, 231
  methods of, 228
  patient access, 8, 231–233
  policies and procedures, 227–228
Health information management, 237–239
  bibliography, 461
  defined, 201
Health information management, computers and, 253–255
  business applications, 254–255
  specialized medical-office systems, 253–254
Health information management components, 201–206
  health record, 202–204
  users, 204–206
Health information manager, 201–202
Health information users, 204–206
  attorneys and courts, 206
  government, 206
  hospitals, 204–205
  managed care organizations, 205
  physician's business office, 204
  providers, 204
  third-party payers, 205
Health insurance. *See also* COBRA
  as employee benefit, 175
  private, 70–71
Health insurance reform, 70–71
Health maintenance organizations, 25, 82–85, 452. *See also* Integrated health systems; Managed care organizations
  as third-party payers, 34–35
  capitation and, 71
  changing physician behavior, 82
  external controls, 82–83
  gatekeeper structures, 83–84
  measuring quality of care and, 51

  termination of physician-patient relationship and, 26
  utilization review, 84–85
Health of populations, managing, 96–98
  assessing risk, 96–97
  fostering healthy behavior, 97
  future challenges, 97–98
Health Plan Employer Data and Information Set, 67, 84, 181
Health professionals, ethical obligations among, 18–19
Health promotion, 446–447. *See also* Disease prevention; Health protection
  managed care and, 97–98
Health protection, 448
Health records, 202–204, 212–226. *See also* Health information *entries*
  as insurance documents, 203–204
  as legal documents, 203
  consent forms, 224
  consultation reports, 224
  diagnostic procedures, 223
  documentation guidelines, 225–226
  format, 212–216
  laboratory reports, 222–223
  making corrections, 224–225
  medical history, 217–221 (illus.)
  medication sheet, 223–224
  microfilming, 249–250
  patient access, 231, 233
  physical examinations, 217, 222
  physician orders, 222
  progress notes, 222
  radiology reports, 223
  storage, 249
  transcription of, 292–293
  transfer to archives, 252–253
Health records disposition, 250–253
  during practice mergers or closings, 251–253
  one-time destruction, 250–251
Health records format, 212–216
  integrated, 216
  problem-oriented, 214, 216
  source-oriented, 212–213
Health records retention, 246–250
  active, inactive, and closed files, 249
  continuity of patient care, 247
  evidence in future litigation, 247–248
  microfilming health records, 249–250
  research and education needs, 248
  retention schedule, 248–249
  statutory regulatory requirements, 247
  storage, 249

Healthy behavior, fostering, 97
Healthy People: The Surgeon General's Report on Health Promotion and Disease Prevention, 446
Healthy People 2000: National Health Promotion and Disease Prevention Objectives, 447, 449
Healthy People 2000 Review, 1994, 449
Heart disease, prevention of, 448
HEDIS. *See* Health Plan Employer Data and Information Set
Highway numbers, 418
Hippocrates, 2, 12
Hippocratic oath, 2 (illus.), 12, 13, 48, 179
Hiring process, 156–161
  checking references, 159–161
  interviewing, 157–159
  job application, 156–157
  making job offer, 161
Historical periods and events, 366–367, 416, 419–420
History and physical examination, transcription of, 293–296 (illus.)
History, physical, impression, plan. *See* HPIP
HIV, prevention of, 448
HIV status
  confidentiality and, 37
  nondiscrimination and, 29
HMO Act of 1973, 74, 78, 86
HMOs. *See* Health maintenance organizations
Holiday
  pay, 173
  pay for forgoing, 173
Holidays and holy days, 374
Honorable, Hon., 409
Hospital
  as user of health information, 204–205
  medical staff, 33
  recruiters, 154
Hospital-based clinical guidelines, 90
HPIP, 302
Human Genome Project, 20–22
  ethical implications, 21
Human relations, among medical staff and with patients, 195–199
  examples of patient service, 197–199
  practice limitations on patient services, 197
  respect among staff, 195–196
  sensitivity to the sick, 196–197

Human relations, in patient service, 178–184
  as choice or mandate, 181
  indicators of, 179–181
  measuring patient satisfaction, 181–183 (illus.)
  patient-service employees, 182, 184
Human relations, telephone and, 184–195
  importance, 184–186
  equipment, 186–187
  etiquette, 189–190
  evaluating service, 195
  quality assurance, 190
  resolving patient complaints, 190–195
  staffing and training, 187–189
Hundred, 411
Hyphen, 346
  in addresses, 417
  in compound names or words, 367–368, 389, 400, 403, 411
  in ratios, 425
  with abbreviations, 346, 403
  with numbers, 346, 415–416
  with prefixes and suffixes, 346, 397–399
  word division and, 346
Hyphenated names, filing, 242

I

ICD-9-CM, 146, 233, 266
Illustrations, labels for, 378
Immunization, 449
  forms, 223–224
  schedule, 454
Implied consent, 26
Inactive patient files, retention of, 249
Incapacitated patients, consent and refusal and, 27–28
Inclusive numbers, 416–417
  elided forms, 416
  with dash, 342
  with percentages, 424
Incorporated, Inc., 339, 404
Indefinite articles, 404
Indefinite pronouns, 404
Indemnity plan, 70, 452
Indention of extracts, 354
Independent clauses. *See* Clauses, main
Independent practice associations, 73, 76, 452
  and computer networks, 112
  as third-party payers, 34–35

Indirect discourse, 337
Indirect question, 337, 351
Indirect quotation, 337, 351, 352
Individual possession, 388
Infectious diseases, 449
Inflected forms of verbs, 326, 346
Information management. *See* Health information management
Informed consent, 26, 227
Initials
  in reference entries, 428
  of company names, 404
  of personal names, 350, 408
Injury, 39
In-person surveys of patient satisfaction, 182
Insertions, editorial, 326–328
Institute of Medicine, 47, 446
Institution, as integrated health system, 87–88
Insurance, 281–284
  employee, 283–284
  general, 282
  insurance management, 284
  professional liability, 40–41, 283
  workers' compensation, 282
Insurance billing, 203–204, 233–236. *See also* Billing and collection
  confidentiality of coding, 235–236 (illus.)
  diagnosis codes, 233–234
  documentation and coding, 235
  procedure codes, 234
  resource-based relative value scale, 234–235
Insurance billing system, computerized, 254
Insurance claims, 266
Insurance conference room, office design, 129
Insurance forms
  HCFA-1500 Insurance Form, 235–236 (illus.)
  patient information, 212
Insurance management, 284
Intangible benefits, 176
Integrated health record, 216
Integrated health systems, 91–96. *See also* Health maintenance organizations; Managed care organizations
  clinic without walls, 92–93
  management services organizations, 94–95

ownership models, 95–96
  physician-hospital organizations, 93–94
Integrated pathways, 91
Integrated progress notes, 216
Integrated service network, 452
Intentional infliction of emotional distress, 43
Intentional torts, 42–43
Interjections, 334, 345
Internal commands, 115
Internal control
  clinical encounters and, 89
  of claims, 278
  of reimbursement, 278–279
Internal financial controls, 277–279
  accounts receivable verification, 278
  check-writing procedures, 278
  division of responsibility, 277
  internal control of claims, 278
  internal control of reimbursement, 278–279
  internal monitoring, 277–278
Internal Revenue Service, 280, 284
International Classification of Diseases, 9th revision, Clinical Modification. *See* ICD-9-CM
Internet, 120, 374
Interpreters, for non-English speakers and deaf people, 145
Interrogative elements and sentences, 350–351
Interrupted speech, 340, 344
Interrupting elements, 333–334, 347–349
Interviewing (as employer), 157–159
  physicians, 157–158
  support staff, 158–159
Interviewing (as potential employee) 440–444
  discussing salary, 444
  interview, 441–443
  preparation, 440–441
  reducing stress, 444
  second interview, 443
Introductory elements in sentences, 333–334
Invasion of privacy, defined, 43
Investigational drug, 31–32
Investigational drug exemption, 31
IPAs. *See* Independent practice associations
IRS. *See* Internal Revenue Service
Italic type, 377–378

Italicization
  and plural forms, 383
  and possessive endings, 386
  for emphasis, 378
  in lists, 378
  in reference entries, 428–429
  of foreign words and phrases, 377
  of legal case titles, 368
  of letters of the alphabet, 377
  of medical terms, 368
  of musical compositions, 376
  of numerals, 378
  of scientific terms, 373
  of titles, 375–376
  of words referred to as words, 377
  of words suggesting sounds, 378
  punctuation following, 378

J

Jacket, 250
JCAH. *See* Joint Commission on Accreditation of Hospitals
JCAHO. *See* Joint Commission on Accreditation of Healthcare Organizations
Job application, 156–157, 432–437
  cover letter, 436–437 (illus.)
  references, 435–436
  résumé, 432–434 (illus.)
Job description, 444–445
  for telephone professional, 188 (illus.)
Job evaluations, 164
Job interview questions, 442–443
  for patient-service employees, 182, 184
Job offer, making, 161
Job search, 431–432
Job sources, 436–440
Joint Commission on Accreditation of Healthcare Organizations, 51–52
Joint Commission on Accreditation of Hospitals, 51
Joint possession, 388
Journal title. *See* Periodical titles
Judicial bodies. *See* Courts
Junior, Jr., 338, 408, 409
  filing, 242
Juran, Joseph, 51
Just-cause employment, 152
Justice, social, 16–17
Justice for patient, 14–16
  appropriate remuneration, 15
  patients' obligation, 15–16

professional standards, 15
termination of provider relationship, 16
undue advantage, 15

K

Kaiser Permanente Health Plan, 75, 141
Kaiser Permanente Medical Care Program, 72
Keogh plan, 286
Keyboards
  height, 107
  location, 114

L

La
  capitalization, 370
  filing, 242
Labels, file, 245
Labor unions, 424
Laboratory
  design, 139
  regulation of, 32
Laboratory reports, 222–223
Laboratory technician, 144
Languages, names of, 371
Laser treatment for emphysema, 317 (illus.)
Lateral files, 243
Latin abbreviations, 407
Latin names (biology), 373
Latitude, 407
Law, 23–24. *See also* Federal regulations; Liability; State regulations
  consent forms, 224
  health record and, 203
  health record retention and, 247–248
  working relationship requirements, 169–174
Lawful orders, 41
Layoff notice, 167
Layoffs, WARN Act and, 165–167
Leases, office equipment, 38
Lecture titles, 375
Legal case titles. *See* Case titles
Legal citations, 368
Legal documents
  capitalization and, 364, 368
  numbers in, 423
Legal obligations
  physician-patient, 24–29

of health providers to patients, 2
  vs. ethical and moral rights, 2
Legal review, of personnel policies manual, 153
Legislation, 367
Legislative bodies, 365
Letters of the alphabet
  in lists and outlines, 350, 422–423
  plurals of, 383
  referred to as letters, 353, 377
  representing shapes, 377–378
  within compound words, 391
Letters. *See* Correspondence
Liability, 38–44. *See also* Litigation
  civil, 42–43
  criminal, 43–44
  insurance, 40–41
  medical malpractice, 38–39
  office staff and, 41–42
  responding to complaints and incidents, 39–40
  responding to suits, 40
Libel, defined, 43
Library design, 140
Licensed practical nurse, 143
Licenses, 29–30
  individual, 29–30
  organizational, 30
Life insurance, as employee benefit, 175
Life support, medical ethics and, 14
Lighting, 289–290
Lightning storms, computers and, 108
Limitations to beneficence, 12–13
Line breaks
  and abbreviations, 400
  and numbers, 416
Lists, 421–423
  bulleted, 422
  run-in, 421
  vertical, 422–423
Lists of references, 461–465
  health information management, 461
  managed care, 461–462
  medical dictionaries, 462
  medical ethics, 462–463
  medical office design, 463
  medical transcription, 465
  quality of care, 463–464
  style manuals, 465
Litigation. *See also* Liability
  employee termination and, 168
  health record retention and, 247–248

Lockbox service, 274
Long dash. *See* Em dash; En dash
Longitude, 407
Losses, 348
Lotus 1–2–3, 254
LPN. *See* Licensed practical nurse
Lumbar spine X-ray report, 306 (illus.)

M

M.D., 409
Mac
  capitalization, 370
  filing, 242
Magazine titles, 375
Main clauses. *See* Clauses, main
Maintenance, of files, 245
Malpractice. *See* Medical malpractice liability
Malpractice insurance. *See* Professional liability insurance
Managed care, 67–78. *See also* Health maintenance organizations; Integrated health systems; Managed care organizations
  bibliography, 461–462
  defined, 67–70
  development of plans, 72–73
  early models, 73
  exclusive provider organizations, 78
  future trends, 120–121
  group models, 74–75
  health care financing system reform and, 70–71
  historical background, 71–72
  independent practice associations, 76
  managed indemnity plans, 77
  medical ethics and, 16–17
  mixed models, 79
  network models, 75–76
  patient service and, 181
  physician reimbursement, 262
  point-of-service plans, 78–79
  preferred provider organizations, 77–78
  prototype, 72
  staff models, 73–74
Managed care, specialized models, 79–82
  behavioral health, 81–82
  Medicaid, 80–81
  Medicare, 79–80

Managed care organizations, 33–35. *See also* Health maintenance organizations; Integrated health systems
  accreditation and, 33–34
  as third-party payers, 34–35
  as users of health information, 205
  financial counselor and, 257
  referrals and, 28
Managed care terms, 451–453
Managed care tracking sheet, 258 (illus.)
Managed indemnity plans, 77
Management services organizations, 94–95, 452
Management structure, medical office, 148–149 (illus.)
Managing for motivation, 162, 164–165
Maps, CD-ROMs and, 120
Marine, capitalization of, 369
Maternal and infant health, disease prevention and, 448
Mathematical copy, 327
Maxims. *See* Mottoes and maxims
Mayo, Charles, 72
Mayo, William, 72
Mayo Clinic, 141
MCOs. *See* Managed care organizations
Meal periods, 173
Measurement, units of, 426
  abbreviated, 410
  with slash, 358
Measuring patient satisfaction, 181–182
Measuring quality of care, 48–53
  outcomes, 50
  process, 49
  programs, 51
  structure, 48–49
  three aspects, 50 (illus.)
  TQM and, 51–53
Medic Software, 273
Medicaid, 24, 29, 46, 48, 80–81, 97, 146, 206, 212, 259, 446
  HCFA Health Insurance Claim Form and, 235
  HCPCS and, 234
  investigational drugs and, 31
  measuring quality of care and, 51
Medical abbreviations and vocabulary, 466–491
Medical assistant, 143–144, 145
Medical care, continuity of, 202
Medical care quality. *See* Quality of care
Medical confidentiality, defined, 226

Medical correspondence, 302, 305, 314–317 (illus.)
Medical dictionaries, 462
Medical ethics, 2–22
  applied to medical practice, 6
  autonomy of patient, 7–10
  beneficence, 12–14
  bibliography, 462–463
  codes, 2–5 (illus.)
  defined, 6
  Human Genome Project, 20–22
  justice, 14–17
  maintaining privacy and confidentiality, 10–12
  need for, 5
  obligation to colleagues, 18–19
  obligation to society, 19–20
  respect for patient, 6–7
Medical Group Management Association, 286
Medical group practices, 72–76
Medical history, 217–221 (illus.)
Medical history update, 221 (illus.)
Medical information
  confidentiality, 37
  record keeping, 36–37
  required reports and disclosures, 37
Medical information technologist, 122–123
Medical language specialist. *See* Medical transcriptionist
Medical malpractice liability, 24, 38–39. *See also* Professional liability insurance
Medical Manager, 273
Medical office. *See also* TQM in the medical office
  as user of health information, 204
  computers and, 99–100, 102–103, 105–107
  management structure, 149–149, 148 (illus.)
  quality of care and, 46
  telephone etiquette, 179–181, 189–190, 192–195
Medical office design, 142 (illus.). *See also* Business office design; Clinical office design
  bibliography, 463
Medical office personnel, 141–149. *See also* Personnel policies
  business, 145–148
  clinical, 141–145

management structure, 148–149 (illus.)
recruiting, 153–156
Medical practice
guidelines, 66
insurance, 281–284
taxes, 280–281
Medical record. *See* Health records
Medical records administration. *See*
Health information management
Medical records storage area design, 126,
128
Medical resources, competing claims for,
16–17
Medical secretary, future trends, 122–123
Medical staff, replacing, 167
Medical technician, 144
Medical terms, 368, 394
drug names, 368, 449–451
Medical transcriber, 291–292
Medical transcription, 292–302
bibliography, 465
chart notes, 302, 312–313 (illus.)
consultation report, 294, 298 (illus.)
diagnostic reports, 302–311 (illus.)
discharge summary, 300–302 (illus.)
follow-up notes in SOAP format, 292,
297 (illus.)
health records, 292–293
history and physical examination,
293–296 (illus.)
operative report, 294, 299 (illus.)
Medical transcription area design, 129
Medical transcription equipment,
291–292. *See also* Dictation equipment
Medical transcriptionist, 147, 287–290
production standards, 288
workstation, 289–290
Medical Treatment Effectiveness Program, 66
Medicare, 29, 46, 48, 79–80, 97, 146, 212,
259, 446
HCFA Health Insurance Claim Form
and, 235
HCPCS and, 234
investigational drugs and, 31
measuring quality of care and, 51
resource-based relative value scale and,
234–235, 261
retrospective review and, 84
Medication sheet, 223–224
Medline, 120

Meeting minutes, capitalization in, 361
Meg, 117
Megahertz, 117
Memorandum heading, 330, 361
Memory-resident program, 118
Mental disorders, health promotion and,
447
Mental health
managed care and, 81–82
promotion of, 447
Menu, computer, 115
Merriam-Webster's Collegiate Dictionary, 377,
380
*Merriam-Webster's Standard American Style
Manual*, 428
Messrs., 409
Meteorological phenomena, 374
Metric units, abbreviated, 410, 426
MGMA. *See* Medical Group Management
Association
Microfiche, 250
Microfilming, of health records, 249–250
Microsoft Word, 254
Middle digit filing method, 240–241
Military terms, 368–369, 408
dates, 406, 418
decorations, 367
ranks, 369, 408
time, 426
Million, 411, 412, 423
Misfiles, preventing, 246
Miss, 409
Mixed managed care models, 79
Modem, 118
Modified fee-for-service compensation,
262
Modifiers
coordinate, 335–336, 392
punctuation of, 335–336
Monetary amounts, 423
in legal documents, 423
Money purchase pension plan, 285
Monitor, computer, 114
Months, names of, 374, 405–406
Moon, 374
Motivation, of personnel, 162, 164–165
Mottoes and maxims, 360, 377
punctuation of, 336–337, 353
Mount, Mt., 407
Mouse, 118
Movie titles, 375
Mr., Mrs., Ms., 409
filing, 242

MSOs. *See* Management services organizations

Multimedia computer software, 120

Musical compositions, 376

N

Names, personal. *See* Nicknames; Personal names

Names, proper. *See* Proper names

Narcotics, 449–451

National Academy of Sciences, 446

National Committee for Quality Assurance, 33, 52, 85
  patient service and, 178–179, 181
  report cards and, 67–68

National Committee for Quality Assurance standards, 65–66

National Institutes of Health, 446

National Practitioner Data Bank, 160, 453

National, capitalization of, 365–366

Naval, capitalization of, 369

NCQA. *See* National Committee for Quality Assurance

Network, computer, 111–112

Network managed care models, 75–76

Networking, 440

Network-model health maintenance organization, 452

New Latin names, 373

New patient registration form, 211 (illus.)

Newsletter, 119

Newspaper ads, as job source, 438–440

Newspapers
  capitalization, 375
  documentation of, 429

Nicknames, 371

1995 Healthy People 2000 Midcourse Review, 449

Nominal group technique, 59–60

Noncomputerized medical office, 103–105

Noncoordinate modifiers, 335–336

Nondiscrimination, 29

Nonrestrictive clauses and phrases, 332

Not sufficient funds. *See* NSF

Notes. *See* References

Nouns
  adjectival use, 393
  compound, 389–392
  plural forms, 380–385

possessive case, 385–386

proper. *See* Proper names; Proper nouns

Novellas, 375

NP. *See* Nurse practitioner

NSF, 275

Number, No., 408

Number-access register for numerical files, 241

Numbered reference, 427

Numbers, 410–427. *See also* Dates; Fractions
  adjacent or paired, 411, 416–417
  and comma, 338, 414–415
  as words or figures, 410–414
  at beginning of sentence, 411
  in addresses, 417–418
  in legal documents, 423
  in lists, 421–423
  in references, 427
  in series, 412
  inclusive. *See* Inclusive numbers
  omission of, 326
  ordinal. *See* Ordinal numbers
  plural forms of, 424–425
  possessive forms of, 387–388
  punctuation of, 414–415
  referred to as numerals, 378
  Roman numerals, 413–414, 422–423
  round, 412–413
  searching for misfiles, 246
  whole, 411
  with enumerations, 348, 351, 421
  with hyphen, 415–416
  with slash, 358–359
  with suffixes, 399
  with units of measurement, 426
  within compound words, 395, 398, 399

Numerical filing, 240–241

Nurse practitioner, 143

Nurse's station design, 138–139 (illus.)

Nurse's station with exam modules, 138 (illus.)

Nutrition, health promotion and, 447

O

Obstetrics and gynecology procedure room design, 134–135

Occupational safety and health, health protection and, 448

Occupational Safety and Health Act, 32, 139, 170
Occupational therapist, 145
O'clock, 425
Office computer systems, 113–114
  location, 113
  working conditions, 113–114
Office design. *See* Business office design; Clinical office design; Medical office design
Office hours
  flexible, 207
  open, 207
Office laboratories, 32
Office leases, 38
Office management area design, 128–129
Office manager, 147
Office of Disease Prevention and Health Promotion, 447, 449
Office staff. *See also* Business personnel; Clinical personnel; Personnel policies
  liability and, 41–42
  recruiting, 154–156
Office staff responsibilities, physician-patient relationship and, 25
Older Workers Benefit Protection Act, 169
Omission
  of words, and slash, 358, 359
  of comma in large numbers, 414–415
  of comma in sentence, 332, 333, 335
  of letters, 326
  of numerals, 326
  of words and phrases, 337
  within quotation, 343–344
Oncology procedure room design, 137
One (number), in addresses, 417
One-time destruction of health records, 250–251
On-line services, capitalization, 374
Open compounds, 388. *See also* Compound words
Open office hours, 207
Open shelf files, 243
Open-access policy, 152–153
Operating distance, from computer, 107
Operating systems, computer, 111–112
Operative report, transcription of, 294, 299 (illus.)
Ophthalmology exam room attributes, 133
Ophthalmology procedure room design, 136

Optical shop design, 136
Oral health, health protection and, 448
Oral release, of health information, 228, 230 (illus.)
Orders, lawful, 41
Ordinal numbers, 413
  in addresses, 417
  in dates, 418
  in spelled-out fractions, 420
  with personal names, 413
Organizations, names of, 370, 404, 424
Orientation, 161–163
  checklist, 162–163 (illus.)
Orthopedics exam room attributes, 132
Orthopedics procedure room design, 134
OSHA. *See* Occupational Safety and Health Act
Otolaryngology exam room attributes, 133
Otolaryngology procedure room design, 136–137
Outcomes analysis, computers and, 121
Outcomes of care, 47, 50
  measuring, 66
Outguides, 244
Outlines, 422–423
Out-of-office journal, 264, 266
Outside services, billing and collection, 273
Outstanding checks, 276
Overall physician compensation, 262
Overdrafts, 275
Overtime
  payment of, 173
  regulations, 171–172
Ownership models, 95–96
  equity, 95–96
  staff, 95

P

p.m., 409, 425
PA. *See* Physician assistant
Page numbers, 416
  as Roman numerals, 413
  colon with, 329
  elided, 416
  inclusive. *See* Inclusive numbers
Paperless office, 121–122
Paradox, 255
Parallel constructions, 335

Parentheses, 347–349
  and comma compared, 333, 347
  and dash compared, 347, 349
  and exclamation point, 345, 348
  and monetary amounts, 423
  and period, 348, 350
  and question mark, 348, 351
  and semicolon, 349, 358
  for explanatory material. *See* Parenthetical elements
  in mathematical copy, 327
  in references, 427
  with abbreviations, 347
  with colon, 330
  with dash, 342, 349
  with lists, 421
  with nicknames and epithets, 371
  with numbers, 347–348
  with quotations, 348
  within parentheses, 349
Parenthetical elements, 347–348
  capitalization of, 348
  punctuation of, 339, 341, 348–349
Parenthetical reference, 427
Pareto chart, 61–62 (illus.)
Participles, 390, 391, 392
Particles, 391, 396
  in personal names, 370
Parties, political, 366
Pass-through toilet area design, 139
Past medical history, 217
Paternalism, 13
Patient. *See also* Physician-patient relationship.
  as health care consumer, 200
  autonomy of, 7–10
  collaborative relationship with provider, 10
  incapacitated, 27–28
  privacy and confidentiality of, 10–12
  respect for, 6–7
  sensitivity to, 196–197
  terminating relationship with provider, 16
Patient access to health records, 231, 233
Patient billing system, computerized, 254
Patient care, continuity of and health record retention, 247
Patient information sheets, 119
Patient notification, of practice closing, 252
Patient obligations, in health care relationship, 15–16

Patient outcomes, 42
Patient Outcomes Research Teams, 66
Patient population, scheduling appointments and, 208
Patient registration, 263–264
Patient registration information, 210–212 (illus.)
Patient registration system, computerized, 253
Patient relations, 196–199
  examples of patient service, 197–199
  practice limitations on service, 197
  sensitivity to sick, 196–197
Patient release of information, 229 (illus.)
Patient rights, 6
  ethical vs. legal, 2
Patient satisfaction, measuring, 181–182
Patient satisfaction questionnaire, 183 (illus.)
Patient service, 178–195
  evaluating telephone performance, 195
  examples of, 197–199
  indicators of, 179–181
  managed care and, 181
  measuring patient satisfaction, 181–182
  practice limitations on, 197
  resolving complaints, 190–192
  sample script for irate callers, 192–195
  staff member attitudes and, 185–186
  words and phrases, 198–199
Patient services, accounts receivable and, 272
Patient's interest, health record and, 203
Patient-service employees, 182, 184
Pay. *See also* Wages
  docking, 173
  overtime, 173–174
  raises, 164–165
  vacation, 173
Payee, 275
Payment and reappointment area design, 125–126, 127 (illus.)
PCP. *See* Primary care physician
Pediatrics exam room attributes, 132–133
Peer review, 51
Peer Review Organization, 51
Peoples, words pertaining to, 371
Per, slash used for, 358
Percent, percentage, 424
Performance evaluation, of telephone service, 195
Period, 349–350
  and ellipsis points, 344

and semicolon compared, 354
in polite requests, 351
spacing of, 350
with abbreviations, 349–350, 400–401
with brackets, 350
with dash, 342
with exclamation point, 345–346
with names, spacing of, 350
with numerals, 350
with parentheses, 348, 350
with quotation marks, 350, 355
Periodical articles, 375–376
Periodical titles, 375
Periodicals, documentation of, 428–429
Permanent compounds, 388
Permanente Medical Groups, 75
Permits
building, 30
X-ray and health care equipment, 31
Personal asides, 348
Personal days, 174–175
Personal history, 217
Personal names, 338–339, 350, 370–371, 408
Personal secretary, 147
Personifications, 362
Personnel policies manual, 119, 150–153, 445
employee termination and, 168
legal review of, 153
writing, 151–153
Personnel policies
death or disability of physician, 176–177
fringe benefits, 172–174
hiring process, 156–161
legal requirements of working relationships, 169–174
recruiting physicians, 153–154
recruiting support staff, 154–156
terminating employees, 165–169
wages, 172–174
working relationships, 161–165
Personnel security, health information and, 237
Pew Health Professions Commission, 22
Phone nurse's area design, 139
Phonetic classification, in alphabetic filing, 239
PHOs. See Physician-hospital organizations
Photocopy work area design, 126
Photocopying health information, 228
Phrases
absolute, 333
adverbial, 332
introductory, 333–334
Latin, abbreviations of, 407
nonrestrictive, 332
plural forms, 381–382
possessive forms, 387
restrictive, 332
with colon, 328
with parentheses, 347–348
Physical activity and fitness, health promotion and, 447
Physical examination, 217, 222
Physical security, of health information, 237–238
Physical therapist, 145
Physician
changing behavior of and health maintenance organizations, 82
checking references of, 160
death or disability of, 176–177
interviewing for employment, 157–158
recruiting, 153–154
relation with staff, 195–196
time management, 209
Physician assistant, 143
Physician Fee Analyzer, 259
Physician fees, 257–262
fee analysis, 259–261
reimbursement under managed care, 262
resource-based relative value scale and, 261
Physician orders, 222
Physician salaries, budget planning and, 280
Physician's business office, as user of health information, 204
Physician's interest, health record and, 203
Physician's work habits, scheduling appointments and, 208
Physician-hospital organizations, 93–94, 205, 452–453
and computer networks, 112
as third-party payers, 35
Physician-patient relationship, 24–29
consent and referral, 26–28
initiation of, 24–25
nondiscrimination, 29
termination, 25–26
Placement agencies, 439–440

Planning phase of TQM, 54–60
  assemble team, 57–59
  develop and plan solutions, 59–60
  identify problem, 55–57
Plant names, 362
Plastic surgery procedure room design,
  135–136
Plays
  acts of, 414
  titles of, 375
Plurals, 380–385
  irregular, 382–383
  of abbreviations, 380, 402–403
  of animal names, 380–381
  of compounds and phrases, 381–382
  of foreign words, 382
  of italic elements, 383
  of letters, 383
  of nouns, 381–383
  of numbers, 326, 383, 425
  of proper nouns, 383–384
  of quoted elements, 384
  of symbols, 384
  of words ending in *-ay, -ey,* and *-oy,* 384
  of words ending in *-ful,* 384
  of words ending in *-o,* 384
  of words used as words, 384–385
  possessive forms, 385
  with apostrophe, 326, 380
Poetry
  and ellipsis points, 344
  and quotation marks, 354
  capitalization of, 360
  slash as line divider, 354–355, 359
  titles of, 375–376
Point, Pt., 407
Point-of-service plans, 78–79, 453
Poison control centers, 454–460
Polite requests, 351
Political organizations, 365
POMR. *See* Problem-oriented medical
  record
Pop-up menu, 115
Portable dictation units, 291
PORTs. *See* Patient Outcomes Research
  Teams
POSs. *See* Point-of-service plans
Possession, individual and joint, 388
Possessive, 385–388
  of abbreviations, 387, 402–403
  of common nouns, 385
  of numerals, 387–388

  of phrases, 387
  of plurals, 385
  of pronouns, 386–387
  of proper names, 385–386
  of words in quotation marks, 387
Possessive pronouns, 386–387
Posting transactions system, computer-
  ized, 253–254
Potential liability, office staff and, 42
PPOs. *See* Preferred provider organiza-
  tions
PPS. *See* Prospective payment system
Practice closings, disposition of health records and, 252
Practice limitations on patient service,
  197
Practice managers, patient service and,
  197
Practice merger, disposition of health rec-
  ords and, 251–252
Practice sale, disposition of health records
  and, 252
Prayers, 373
Preadmission authorization, 453
Predicate, compound, 331
Preferred provider organizations, 77–78,
  453
  and computer networks, 112
  as third-party payers, 34–35
Prefixes, 397–399
  capitalization of, 397
  with abbreviations, 403
  with hyphen, 397–399
Pregnancy, confidentiality and, 11
Pregnancy Discrimination Act, 170
Prepaid managed care prototype,
  72–73
Preparedness, as patient service indicator,
  180
Prepositions within compounds, 381,
  396
Present illness, 217
President, 372
Preventive disease services, 448. *See also*
  Health promotion; Health
  protection
Primary care capitation, 262
Primary care exam room attributes,
  131–132
Primary care exam room design, 132
  (illus.)

Primary care physician, 83, 453
Principles of medical ethics of the American Medical Association, 3 (illus).
Printers, computer, 113
Prior approvals, 35
Prior care, 42
Privacy, 10
  defined, 226
  invasion of, 43
Privacy Act of 1974, 152
Privacy of the body, 10
Private practice inducements, 154
Private programs, measuring quality of care, 51
PRO. *See* Peer Review Organization
Problem list, 214–215 (illus.)
Problem-oriented format, 302
Problem-oriented medical record, 214–216
  advantages and disadvantages, 216
  database, 214
  problem list, 214–215 (illus.)
  progress notes, 214, 216
  treatment plans, 214
Procedure codes, insurance billing and, 234
Procedure room design, 134–138. *See also individual specialties*
Procedures handbook, telephone, 189–190
Process of care, 49
Process outcomes, evaluating in clinical encounter, 88–89
Production standards, for medical transcription, 288
Professional codes of conduct, 2–5
Professional ethics. *See* Medical ethics, Professional codes of conduct
Professional liability insurance, 40–41, 283. *See also* Medical malpractice liability
Professional ratings, 406
Professional relationships, 1–6
  legal obligations, 2
Professional standards, 15
Professional Standards Review Organizations, 51
Profit sharing plan, 285
Progress notes, 214, 216, 222
  integrated, 216
Promed, 273
Promoting Health/Preventing Disease: Objectives for the Nation, 446

Pronouns
  indefinite, 404
  possessive, 386–387
Proof of destruction, of health records, 251
Proofreading, 305–306
  frequently confused words, 318–321, 486–491
  health care vocabulary standards, 321–324
Proper adjectives, 361–377
Proper names, 393. *See also* Personal names; Proper nouns
  derivatives of, 363–364
  possessive forms, 383–386
  with numbers, 413
Proper nouns
  capitalization of, 361–377, 402
  plural forms of, 383–384
Prospective payment system, 206
Prospective review, 84
Protecting children and adolescent patients, 9–10
Provider number, 280
Provider system models, 86–91
  managing clinical encounters, 88–89
  managing clinical processes, 89–91
  structure, 87–88
PSROs. *See* Professional Standards Review Organizations
Psychiatry procedure room design, 137
Psychosocial history, 217
Pull-down menu, 115
Punctuation, 325–359. *See also individual marks of punctuation*
  of abbreviations, 400–401
  of addresses, 338
  of biblical references, 329, 405
  of numbers, 326, 329, 338, 346, 414–417
  purposes of, 325
  to avoid ambiguity, 339

Q

QA
  compared to TQM, 52
  integrating with TQM, 65–68
  telephone and, 190
Quality, defined, 47–48
Quality assurance. *See* QA
Quality council, 56

Quality management, 202–203
Quality of care
  access to care, 47
  bibliography, 463–464
  current professional knowledge and,
    47–48
  measuring, 48–53
  medical office and, 46
  regional variations in, 46
  reimbursement and, 47
  TQM and QA and, 52, 65–68
  TQM and, 51–65
  uniform agreement on, 46–47
Quattro Pro, 254
Question mark, 350–352
  and parentheses, 351
  and period, 351
  with brackets, 351
  with comma, 339
  with dash, 342, 351
  with exclamation point, 345, 355
  with quotation marks, 351, 355
Questionnaires
  patient satisfaction, 181–183 (illus.)
  telephone quality assurance, 190
Questions, 337, 350–352. *See also* Question mark
  and quotation marks, 353
  direct, 337, 350–352
  indirect, 337, 351
Quotation marks, 352–356
  and italics, 352
  British usage, 355
  omission of , 353
  with colon, 329, 355
  with comma, 336–337, 355
  with dash, 355
  with exclamation point, 345, 355
  with extracts, 354–355
  with foreign terms, 353
  with parentheses, 347
  with period, 350, 355
  with possessive, 387
  with question mark, 351, 355
  with semicolon, 355, 358
  with single quotation marks, 355–356
Quotations, 352–356. *See also* Direct quotation; Indirect quotation
  and attribution of sources, 341
  and comma, 336–337
  capitalization of, 329, 344, 360
  colon introducing, 329
  direct, 336, 352

  editorial insertions in, 326–327
  in parentheses, 348
  in running text, 329
  indirect, 352
  of poetry. *See* Poetry
  omissions in, 343–344
  with brackets, 326–327
  within quotations, 355–356
Quoted elements
  compounds, 393–394
  plural forms, 384
  possessive forms, 387

R

Radio program titles, 375
Radiology reports, 223
  transcription of, 302, 306, (illus.), 310
    (illus.)
RAM, 116
Random-access memory. *See* RAM
Randomized controlled trials, 88
Range of numbers. *See* Inclusive numbers
Ratios, 329, 358, 425
RBRVS. *See* Resource-based relative value
  scale
RCTs. *See* Randomized controlled trials
Read only memory. *See* ROM
Readiness, as patient service indicator,
  180
Receipt processing, accounts receivable,
  272
Reception area design, 125–127 (illus.)
Receptionist, 145–146
  environment of, 186–187
Record keeping, 36–37
Record storage, 249
Recruiting methods, 153–156
  physicians, 153–154
  support staff, 154–156
Reducing costs, gatekeeper concept and,
  83
Reduplication compounds, 391–392
Reference list. *See* Bibliographies
Reference material
  CD-ROMs and, 120
  for medical transcription, 292
Reference number, in books, 427
References (bibliographic), 427–429
  documentation of articles in, 428–429
  documentation of books in, 428
  documentation of newspapers in, 429

documentation of periodicals in, 428–429
  numbered, 427
  parenthetical, 427
References (employment), 435–436 (illus.)
  checking, 159–161
  contacting, 436
  written, 160
Referral letter, 314–315 (illus.)
Referrals, 28
Refusal of treatment, 27–28
Regional variations in medical care quality, 46
Registered medical assistant, 144
Registered nurse, 143
Rehabilitation Act of 1973, 170
Reimbursement, 266
  internal control of, 278–279
  third-party payers and quality of care, 46
Relative Values for Physicians, 259–260
Religious groups, 372–373, 424
Religious terms, 372–373
Religious titles, filing, 242
Remuneration, 15
Repair, of files, 245
Report cards, 67–68
Reports system, computerized, 254
Representative, 409
Requests, polite, 351
Required reports, 37
Research needs, health record retention and, 248
Resolved, 361
Resource-based relative value scale, 206, 234–235, 261
Respect, for patient, 6–7
Respondeat superior, 41
Responsibility to attend patient, 25
Responsiveness, as patient service indicator, 180
Rest periods, 173
Restrictive appositive, 333
Restrictive clauses and phrases, 332
Restroom design, 139, 140
Résumé, 432–434
  format, 433–434 (illus.)
Retention schedules, for health records, 248–249
Retirement plans, 284–286
  401(k), 286
  combined profit sharing and money purchase pension plans, 285–286

Keogh plan, 286
  money purchase pension plan, 285
  profit sharing plan, 285
  salary reduction simplified employee pension plan, 285
  simplified employee pension plan, 285
Retrospective review, 84–85
Reverend, Rev., 409
  filing, 242
Review of systems, 217
RMA. *See* Registered medical assistant
RN. *See* Registered nurse
Roll film, 250
ROM, 117
Roman numerals, 413–414
  in outlines, 414, 423
  in proper names, 413
Round numbers, 412–413
  in monetary amounts, 423
Rulers' names, 413
Run chart, 62–63 (illus.)

S

Sacred works, 373
Saint, St., 407, 408
  filing, 242
Salary, discussion of at job interview, 444
Salary reduction simplified employee pension plan, 285
Salary vs. wages, overtime and, 172
Salutation of letter, 329, 339, 361
Sample script for irate callers, 192–195
SARSEP. *See* Salary reduction simplified employee pension plan, 285
Schedule, for collection, 267
Scheduled appointments, 207
Schedules of controlled substances, 449–451
Scheduling appointments, 206–210
  appointment book, 207–208
  guidelines, 208–209
  reminders, 209–210
  scheduling, 206–207
Science, 20
Scientific terms, 373–374, 409, 414
Scope of practice, 30
Screening process, in job search, 438–439
Scripted responses, telephone, 189
Seasons, capitalization of, 374
Second, 2nd, 2d, 413
  filing, 242

Second job interview, 443
Secretary, personal, 147
Security, of health information, 237–239
Security passwords, computer, 101–102
Self- compounds, 398
Semicolon, 356–358
   and comma compared, 357–358
   and conjunctions, 356–357
   and period compared, 356
   between clauses, 334, 356–357
   in a series, 357–358
   with conjunctive adverbs, 357
   with dash, 341–342
   with phrases, 356
   with quotation marks, 355, 358
   with *so* and *yet*, 357
   within parentheses, 349, 358
Senator, 409
   filing, 242
Senior, Sr., 338, 408, 409
   filing, 242
Sentence fragments, 347, 359
Sentences
   beginnings of, 359–361, 411
   interrogative, 351
   parallelism in, 331
   within sentences, 336–337, 353, 358
SEP. *See* Simplified employee pension
   plan
Serial comma, 335
Serial numbers, 415
Series
   interrogative, 351
   numbered, 348, 351
   of main clauses, 335
   of numbers, 412
   of percentages, 424
   of questions, 351
   punctuation of, 329, 338, 351, 358
Server, 112
   location, 113
Service charges, 276
Sexually transmitted diseases
   confidentiality and, 11
   consent to release health information
     and, 27
   prevention of, 448
Shapes, indicated by letters, 377–378
Shareware, 115
Shelf guides, 244
Sign language interpreters, 145
Signature forms, 119
Signs in capital letters, 379

Simplified employee pension plan, 285
Single quotation marks, 355–356
Sister, filing, 242
Slander, defined, 43
Slash, 358–359
   in dates, 359, 418
   in poetry, 354–355, 359
   in ratios, 358, 425
   spacing of, 358
   with abbreviations, 359, 401
Small capitals, with dates, 379, 419
So, as conjunction, 357
SOAP, 214, 302
   in follow-up notes, 294, 297 (illus.)
Soaping, 214
Social Security numbers, as filing method,
   241
Social Security withholding. *See* FICA
Society, ethical obligations of health care
   professionals to, 19–20
Software, computer. *See* Computer soft-
   ware
Solidus. *See* Slash
Sorting files, 245–246
Sounds, representations of, 352, 378
Source-oriented health record, 212–213
Spacecraft names, 376
Specialized managed care models, 79–82
Specialty technicians, 144
Species names, 373
Speech. *See* Dialogue
Spreadsheets, 254
Sr. See Senior, Sr.
St. See Saint, St.
Staff lounge design, 140
Staff managed care models, 73–74
Staff ownership models, 95
Staff relations, respect among physicians
   and staff members, 195–196
Staffing, telephone, 187–189
Staff-model health maintenance organiza-
   tion, 453
Standard of care, 38
State disability insurance, 281
State employment agencies, 440
State Medicaid regulations, 80–81
State names, 338, 348, 406
State regulations
   confidentiality of health information,
     226
   health record and, 203
   health record disposition, 251
   health record retention, 247

Medicaid, 80–81
 of drugs, 32
State taxes, 280
 unemployment tax, 281
Stationery, 119
Statutory and regulatory requirements,
 for health records retention, 247
STD. *See* Sexually transmitted diseases
Stimulants, 449–451
Stock-market quotations, 427
Stop payment, 275
Storage, of files, 243–244
Storage and retrieval, of health informa-
 tion, 237
Storage space design, 140
Story titles, 375
Straight numerical filing method, 240
Street names. *See* Addresses, street
Stress, reducing at job interview, 444
Stroke, prevention of, 448
Structure of care, 48–49
Style manuals, 465
Subject headings, 361
Subordinate clauses and phrases, 331–332
Subspecies names, 373
Substance abuse
 confidentiality and, 11, 37
 consent to release health information
 and, 27
 managed care and, 81–82
Subtitle, 329
Suffixes, 397, 398, 399
 with abbreviations, 401
 with hyphen, 346
 with numbers, 398, 401
Suits, responding to, 40
Sun, 374
Supplementary clauses and phrases,
 340–341, 347–348
Supplies, filing, 244–245
Support services, computer, 101
Support staff. *See also* Business personnel;
 Clinical personnel; Personnel policies
 interviewing for employment, 158–159
 recruiting, 154–156
Supreme being, references to, 372
Surge protection, computer, 108
Surgical pathology reports, transcription
 of, 302–305 (illus.)
Surveillance systems, 449
Suspension of structure, 344
Suspension points. *See* Ellipsis points

Symbols
 plural forms of, 384
 units of measurement, 426
 with inclusive numbers, 417
System security, health information and,
 239

T

Task list, written, 41–42
Taxes, 280–281
 federal and state unemployment, 281
 FICA, 280–281
 state and federal, 280
 state disability insurance, 281
Team development, TQM and, 57–58
Team TQM tools, 58–59
Telecommuter, telephone staffing and,
 187, 189
Telephone, 184–195
 collection calls, 268–271
 equipment, 186
 evaluating service, 195
 importance to medical office, 184–186
 quality assurance and, 190
 resolving complaints, 190–195
 responding to newspaper ad, 439–440
 staffing and training, 187–189
Telephone environment, 186–187
Telephone etiquette, 189–190
 patient service and, 179–181
Telephone lines, number of, 186
Telephone numbers, CD-ROMs and, 120
Telephone performance, evaluating, 195
Telephone procedures handbook,
 189–190
Telephone professional, job description,
 188 (illus.)
Telephone quality assurance question-
 naires, 190
Telephone surveys of patient satisfaction,
 182
Telephone-call handling procedures, 189
Television program titles, 375
Temporary compound, 388
Temporary employment agency, recruit-
 ing support staff and, 156
Terminal digit filing method, 240–241
Terminals, computer, 114
Terminating employees, 165–169
 employer rights, 167–168
 final steps, 169
 reduction in force, 165
 WARN act and, 165–167

Termination of physician-patient relationship, 16, 25–26
Testing, at job interview, 443
That, replaced by comma, 337
The Chicago Manual of Style, 428, 465
Third, 3rd, 3d, 413
Third-party payers. *See also* Insurance billing
 as users of health information, 205
 capitation and, 35–36
 coding, billing, and collection, 36
 contracts, 34–35
 health record and, 203–204
 prior approvals and, 35
 relations with, 34–36
Third-party requests for information, 11
Thousand, 411
Three aspects of quality, 50 (illus.)
Tickler system
 collection calls and, 270
 for license renewal, 29
Time management, scheduling appointments and, 209
Time of day, 329, 409, 425–426
Time off in lieu of pay, 173
Time periods, 374
Time records, overtime and, 172
Time zones, 409
Title VII of the Civil Rights Act of 1964, 170
Titles of persons
 corporate, 371
 courtesy, 409–410
 governmental, 371–372
 honorific, 409–410
 professional, 371, 409–410
 punctuation of, 338
Titles of works, 375–376
 art, 375
 articles, 375–376, 428
 books, 375, 428
 musical compositions, 376
 parts of books, 376
 periodicals, 375
 poetry, 375
To do no harm, 13–14
Tobacco, health promotion and, 447
Topographical terms, 363–364
Total Quality Management. *See* TQM
TQM, 46, 51–53
 compared to QA, 52
 continuous quality improvement and, 54

 integrating with QA, 65–68
 medical office case study, 63–65
 multiple projects and, 65
TQM cycle, 54–55 (illus.)
TQM in the medical office, 53–65
 case study, 63–65
 first phase, 54–60
 fourth phase, 62–63
 second phase, 60
 third phase, 60–62
TQM tools for problem identification and performance measurement, 56–59
Trademarks, 376
Training
 for new employees, 162
 telephone etiquette, 187–189
Transcription. *See* Medical transcription
Translations, with parentheses, 347
Transportation, 376
Treaties, 367
Treatment
 refusal of, 27
 uniform agreement on, 46–47
Treatment plans, 214
Triage nurse. *See* Phone nurse
Trustworthiness, as patient service indicator, 181

U

Ultrasound reports, transcription of, 302, 307–309 (illus.)
Underlining, 379
Undue advantage, 15
Unfinished sentences, 343–345
Uniform agreement, on medical treatment, 46–47
Unintentional injuries, health protection and, 448
Unit (number) combinations. *See* Inclusive numbers
Unit modifiers, 392
United States, U.S., 407
Units of measurement. *See* Measurement, units of
UNIX, 111–112
Unpaid wages, 173–174
UR. *See* Utilization review
Urgi-centers, 207
Urology procedure room design, 136
U.S. Food and Drug Administration, 31
U.S. Public Health Service, 446
U.S. Supreme Court, capitalization, 365

USP standards, 322–323
Uterine ultrasound report, 309 (illus.)
Utilization management, 82
Utilization review, 51, 84–85, 453

V

v. (*versus*), 368, 407
Vacation pay, 173
Vacations, pay for foregoing, 173
Values, of health care team, 18
Varieties (botany), 373
Vehicle names, 376
Venipuncture area design, 139
Verbal release of information, 230 (illus.)
Verbs
    in compound words, 390–391, 396–397
    inflection, 346
    with apostrophe, 326
    with hyphen, 346
versus, vs., 368, 407
Vertical drawer files, 243
Vessel names, 376
Veterans Administration, 446
Vice- compounds, 398
Violent and abusive behavior, health pro-
    motion and, 447
Virgule. *See* Slash
Vocabulary standards, health care,
    321–324
vol., vols., 427
vs., versus, 368, 407

W

Wage and benefit statement, 165, 166
    (illus.)
Wages, 172–174
    in lieu of benefits, 176
    penalties for unpaid, 173–174
    raises, 164–165
Wages vs. salary, overtime and, 172
Waiting room design, 125, 127 (illus.)
Waiving right to confidentiality, 11
Want ads, recruiting support staff and,
    154–156
WARN Act, 165–167

Wars, names of, 367
Watson, James D., 20
Wave scheduling, 209
Whereas, capitalization of, 361
Whole numbers, 411
Willingness, as patient service indicator,
    179
Word division, hyphen and, 346
Word processing, 254
Word processing computer software, 119
WordPerfect, 254
Words referred to as words, 352
    plural forms of, 384–385
Words, frequently confused and misused,
    318–321, 486–491
Work habits, computer-related, 107–111
Work organizer, 289
Worker Readjustment and Retraining No-
    tification Act. *See* WARN Act
Workers' compensation, 282
Workforce, reducing, 165
Working relationship
    benefits of, 174–176
    federal regulations governing, 169–171
    motivation, 162, 164–165
    orientation, 161–162
    overtime policies, 171–172
    terminating, 165–169
    training, 162
    wage and hour requirements, 172–174
Workstation, medical transcriptionist,
    289–290
Writing checks, 275
Written authorization, to release health in-
    formation, 227, 229 (illus.)
Written task list, 41–42

XYZ

X-ray and health care equipment permits,
    31
X-ray department design, 139–140
X-ray reports. *See* Radiology reports
X-ray technician, 144
Year numbers, 326, 418–420
Yet, as conjunction, 357
Zero, 423
Zoological terms, 373